Demon Possession in Anglo-Saxon England

Medieval Institute Publications is a program of
The Medieval Institute, College of Arts and Sciences

WESTERN MICHIGAN UNIVERSITY

Demon Possession in Anglo-Saxon England

Peter Dendle

MEDIEVAL INSTITUTE PUBLICATIONS
Western Michigan University
Kalamazoo

This book is printed on acid-free paper.

Library of Congress Cataloging-in-Publication Data

Dendle, Peter, 1968-
Demon possession in Anglo-Saxon England / Peter Dendle.
p. cm.
Includes bibliographical references and index.
ISBN 978-1-58044-169-8 (clothbound : alk. paper)
1. English literature--Old English, ca. 450-1100--History and criticism. 2. Demoniac possession in literature. 3. Deviant behavior in literature. 4. Psychology, Pathological, in literature. 5. Exorcism in literature. 6. Christian hagiography--History. 7. Devotional literature, English--History. 8. Medical literature--England--History--To 1500. 9. Civilization, Anglo-Saxon, in literature. I. Title.
PR179.D48D43 2012
829'.09353--dc23

2012032060

Manufactured in the United States of America

C 5 4 3 2 1

Contents

For my mother,
Catherine Dendle

Acknowledgments

I AM GREATLY INDEBTED to Kirsten C. Uszkalo for her continuous support of this project, and for her dynamic insights into the processes of demon possession. Also I would like to thank Richard Raiswell for his detailed comments on the work, and for our ongoing discussions (in many forms) of premodern cultural constructions of the demonic. Karen L. Jolly and Brian Dendle read the complete work in manuscript and provided many helpful suggestions; I have relied abundantly on their comments. The positions adopted in this book, however, have not been universally shared by those who have read it and discussed the ideas with me.

I am thankful to Dr. Renuka Prasad of the Neurosurgery Division, University of Kentucky College of Medicine, for welcoming me as part of his team and for teaching me a great deal. My experiences in his lab contributed to many of the directions this study has taken. For additional professional consultation, manuscript reading, and discussion, I owe thanks to Todd Feinberg, Mary Lou Reaver, Amy Baxter, Louis Calderon, and many other participants at conference presentations and in email correspondence whom I cannot possibly list in full.

For invaluable research support for this and many other endeavors, I wish to thank Alica White, Lalana Powell, Margaret (Peggy) Angelovich, Carol Maholtz, Thomas Reinsfelder, and Johanna Ezell. Nick Pastura, Jason Silverstein, and Leidi Shaw were very diligent as research assistants. Lisa Selser helped considerably with citation and formatting, which she performed meticulously.

This project evolved in response to presentations given for the following organizations and institutions, to whose organizers and participants I am indebted: American Historical Association; International Society of Anglo-Saxonists; the University of Tennessee; the University of Nottingham; the Institute for the Arts and Humanities, University Park, The Pennsylvania State University; the Azerbaijan Association of Medical Historians; the Southeastern Medieval Association; the Medieval Academy of America; and the Plymouth State College Medieval Forum.

I am grateful to the National Endowment for the Humanities for a summer stipend and to the Institute for the Arts and Humanities at Penn State for a resident fellowship in support of this project. The Commonwealth College (now University College), the Office for the Vice President of Commonwealth Campuses, the Mont Alto campus, and other divisions within The Pennsylvania State University have been very generous in facilitating my work. In particular I wish to thank Michael Doncheski, Francis Achampong, Shirley Ketrow-Crawford, David Gnage, Sandra Gleason, Richard Kopley, Laura Knoppers, Sue Reighard, and Kevin A. Boon.

Abbreviations

ACW	*Ancient Christian Writers*
ANF	*The Ante-Nicene Fathers*
ASE	*Anglo-Saxon England*
ASPR	*The Anglo-Saxon Poetic Records*
CCCC	Cambridge, Corpus Christi College
CCCM	Corpus Christianorum, Continuatio Mediaevalis
CCSL	Corpus Christianorum, Series Latina
CSEL	Corpus Scriptorum Ecclesiasticorum Latinorum
DOE	*Dictionary of Old English*
DSM-IV	*Diagnostic and Statistical Manual of Mental Disorders*, fourth edition
DSM-V	*Diagnostic and Statistical Manual of Mental Disorders*, fifth edition
EETS	Early English Text Society
EETS o.s.	EETS original series
EETS s.s.	EETS supplementary series
HBS	Henry Bradshaw Society
HE	Bede, *Historia ecclesiastica* (ed. Colgrave and Mynors)
JEGP	*Journal of English and Germanic Philology*
MGH	Monumenta Germaniae Historica
MGH, AA	Monumenta Germaniae Historica, Auctores Antiquissimi
MGH, SRM	Monumenta Germaniae Historica, Scriptorum rerum Merovingicarum
NM	*Neuphilologische Mitteilungen*
NPNF	*A Select Library of Nicene and Post-Nicene Fathers*
OE	Old English
PGM	Papyri Graecae Magicae
PL	Patrologia Latina
SC	*Sources Chrétiennes*
WHO	World Health Organization

Biblical quotations in English are from *The New Revised Standard Version* (ed. Metzger and Murphy); references to the Latin Vulgate are from *Biblia Sacra* (ed. Webert). Unless otherwise indicated, all translations are mine.

Preface

THE PRESENT WORK GREW out of an earlier study that examined the devil as a character in Old English narrative literature. That study found that the devil's narrative appearances are contrived and malleable, suiting context as required by internal literary logic rather than adhering to any consistent underlying theological conception of his nature or activities. The devil is usually introduced as a causal agent only ad hoc, to serve as a literary symbol or a rhetorical expression of moral judgment. In Old English literature the demonic is cast in a small range of character molds, from the wormy and contemptible hagiographic demon (such as the one who confesses his sins at length in *Juliana*) to the epic devil whose defeat marks several of the broad turning points of salvation history (such as the devil of *Genesis B* or *Christ and Satan*).[1]

Alongside these, lurking in less prepossessing texts such as Bald's *Leechbook* and the *Lacnunga Book*, are what we might call the "medical demons": those demonic agencies perhaps implicit in the "elves" and "devil's temptations" mentioned in the medical books, and certainly presupposed in the raving, flailing demoniacs brought to saints' tombs. These demons are blamed for contorted bodies, frozen limbs, and uncontrollable outbursts. They germinate illness in humans and livestock alike. These demons did not fit neatly into my earlier study and seemed to offer a glimpse—outside of the self-contained world of monastic letters—into the day-to-day lives of ordinary Anglo-Saxons. The demons of the medical texts hint at a facet of medieval demonology entirely different from the clean, stylized devil of *Genesis B* or *Christ and Satan*. Here are pain, ulcers, and madness, and here the focus is on offering immediate help rather than on quoting learned patristic commentary or gaining advantage in episcopal rivalries. In their role as disease agents—in the twisted, broken people at healing shrines and saints' tombs, in self-destructive and antisocial behavior, and in the blasphemies that shocked parents, neighbors, and pastors—the "medical" demons provide the points of tangible contact between everyday people and the demonic. It is in this role that demons form the subject of the present inquiry.

There are grand debate scenes between saints and demons in many surviving Old English works, both poetry and prose. An audience accustomed to seeing demoniacs and witnessing exorcisms would experience Cynwulf's *Juliana* or Ælfric's *Life of St. Martin* differently than audiences who have only read about such things in books. Were possessions and exorcisms as commonplace as the domestic chores described in Ælfric's *Colloquy*, or were they rather as exotic as some of the foreign customs encountered in the Old English *Orosius* or the *Wonders of the East*? Are we justified in reading scenes of demon-saint conflict as mirroring reality in some way, or are they purely literary constructs?

In writing this book I have come to believe that there is only very little connection between these scenes and anything happening with any frequency outside the monastery in Anglo-Saxon society. If this is true, then scenes of demon-saint conflict in Anglo-Saxon literature should be interpreted not as responding to lived, authentic occurrences in society but as operating within the fairly closed world of ecclesiastical letters. The quasi-exorcism scene in *Juliana*, in this case, tells us more about Cynewulf's literary precedents than about adversarial dialogues that might have taken place during an Anglo-Saxon exorcism. These scenes, of course, have been generally read as literature rather than realistic description to begin with, and—I will be the first to admit—it has thus taken me a number of years to discover what everyone else has probably known all along. And yet, I think the current study (if its conclusions are accepted) challenges in several important respects our tacit assumptions concerning Anglo-Saxon church and society. This study has reinforced for me the competing aims of diverse literary genres to which we must necessarily turn as our only possible evidence. Factoring out the inherent predispositions of these genres, we find that there is scant evidence left from which to reconstruct the nature or frequency of possession and exorcism in Anglo-Saxon England. Furthermore, the glimpses into select psychiatric and neurological conditions that may have existed in Anglo-Saxon England may help provide a more vivid and contoured understanding of some of the more severe problems that a handful of Anglo-Saxons must have certainly experienced, and how that society was, on those occasions, potentially equipped to respond to them.

Social scientists sometimes find it useful to distinguish between emic and etic approaches to the study of a given culture. Emic models look to a society's own conceptual categories and seek to make sense of a worldview in terms that would make sense to members of that community. These approaches are useful in helping to make a belief or practice which might initially seem alien more comprehensible, more "rational," to the observer. Etic models, on the other hand, remain external to the culture: these strive for objectivity by drawing from comparative parallels and by deploying the latest knowledge (e.g., conceptual categories, theories, and data) available within a given discipline. Etic approaches derive, necessarily, from the observer's conceptual categories, rather than from those of the culture under study.[2]

The current study, in attempting to negotiate a relationship with the past which allows us to visualize what may or may not have been happening, relies necessarily on an etic approach. I am interested in trying to "see" what Anglo-Saxon possession may have looked like, from the point of view of a twenty-first century observer.

What Paul Lloyd has written regarding linguistic reconstruction of Latin in early medieval Europe is equally applicable to the history of medicine: "We can never truly understand how those people thought and felt; the weight of subsequent history bears too heavily upon our minds, since, after all, we cannot help knowing how it all turned out."[3] A broken bone was not a different physiological event for an Anglo-Saxon than it is for a modern English person, however different the individual experience or contemporary cultural interpretation of it. We understand that the right tibia of a middle-aged Anglo-Saxon buried in Hampnett, Gloucester, had been broken during life and subsequently fused together again with the fibula, whatever categories the man himself may have had to interpret the injury.[4] The brain is also capable of being "broken" in certain recognizable ways that sometimes transcend cultural boundaries. At the same time, such an approach brings into sharper focus the limitations of our current constructs. I have tried to avoid some of the more obvious pitfalls of a teleological or "Whig" history of medicine, but the reader will not find in this book an extensive methodological defense of using modern constructs to interpret England's medical past, any more than archaeologists defend the use of meters in describing a medieval site, or any more than literary theorists deploy modern categories such as "masculinity," "hegemony," or "meta-text" in understanding medieval texts.

The reader should know from the outset that I have built this study on a premise that the vast commonality of human experience far surpasses local variations in cultural expression. While many paradigms of social structure, natural world, and spirit world are incompatible and even untranslatable from one culture to another, in my experience the thousand little things in the course of a day that make us laugh, frown, squeal, and scowl are readily understandable. In all but a few curious cases, intonation and body language regarding basic affective states are instantly understood among humans, among higher animals, and even between humans and higher animals. This is principally a book about demons of the body. This study has led me, in certain respects, to the complicated dynamics inherent in a society governed by competing discourses of illness, spirituality, power, and community, and I have had the impression of briefly glimpsing into corners of the personal lives and pains of people dead for thirteen hundred years. Whether or not I am mistaken in this impression, this study attempts to take a fresh look at primary documentary records—the august heroic literature, the disarmingly intimate and personal saints' lives, the puzzling medical literature, and the magisterial liturgy—and to guess somewhat at the phenomenon variously cast by these refracting lenses.

NOTES

1. On the distinction between the "hagiographic" and the "epic" demon, the two major character types for the devil in Old English literature, see Abbetmeyer, *Old English Poetical Motives*; Dendle, *Satan*, pp. 40–41.

2. See Headland, Pike, and Harris, *Emics and Etics*.

3. Lloyd, "On the Names of Languages," p. 15.

4. Burn Ground site (Hampnett, Gloucestershire), grave 9 (Grimes, *Excavations*, vol. 1, pp. 123–24, 128).

Introduction

THIS PROJECT COLLECTS the known documentary evidence that records demon possession in Anglo-Saxon England, and reinterprets its significance in light of modern views of possession. By "demon possession" I mean the array of observable behaviors (falling to the ground, thrashing about, lashing out violently, shouting abusively, raving) in which the subject's personality has, in the eyes of the community, been supplanted by a sentient agent intending harm. Then as now, demon possession was at the nexus of a number of conflicting cultural dimensions—individual and society, religion and medicine, custom and taboo. While post-Enlightenment advances in psychiatry and medicine have rendered the demon possession paradigm virtually obsolete in contemporary medical discourse, the endurance of possession beliefs and behaviors attests to the ongoing utility of the construct as a component of even twenty-first century society. The challenge of a book such as this one is to contextualize and interpret this fascinating set of behaviors (a subset of broader demonic beliefs and broader possession beliefs alike) of a thousand-year-old culture largely opaque to us, without placing undue faith in either medieval or modern attempts to interpret this complicated matrix of behaviors rooted in pain and separation.

Demon possession, introduced along with exorcism by Christian missionaries, may have provided the Anglo-Saxons with a behavioral and theoretical paradigm for the expression of certain biological, psychological, and even sociopolitical dysfunctions. An epileptic was provided an explanation of what was happening to him; a woman torn by rape and war-related loss, perhaps fractured to the deepest sense of self, had a means of enduring; the political or religious dissident incapable of openly admitting frustrations subconsciously found a means of venting them. Demon possession can perform a much wider range of roles than these, but dysfunction is central to the construct, then as now: possession states or behavioral anomalies that do not cause suffering and discord are not generally attributed to demonic agency. There is no satisfactory way to tell what sorts of dysfunctions and what sorts of "demons" the pagan Anglo-Saxons had prior to conversion, but the

Christian model which had long taken root by the time of our principal documentary records—and which flourished later in the great healing shrines and hospitals of Anglo-Norman England—grew and adapted to a society under continuous change and instability.

The "demonic" is a potent and layered concept, one which at a certain level is inextricable from broader representations of evil. Grendel, heathens, and monsters such as those found in *Wonders of the East*, for instance, are all rhetorically assimilated with demons in many respects. In Anglo-Saxon liturgical books, adjurations against lightning appear alongside exorcisms for the possessed. The current study, however, is exclusively concerned with demons in so far as they are believed to enter the body, insinuate the limbs and organs, and supplant the mind and personality. For Christianized Anglo-Saxons, these demons are one and the same with the angels who rebelled against God and were expelled from heaven in a time before the creation of humanity (or else who are descended from those apostate angels). They are sentient, powerful, and malicious, intent on foiling God's plan for humanity by assailing humans whenever possible in body and mind. Demons appear in Anglo-Saxon literature most often as the gods of heathen nations or as abstract psychological instigators of sin and vice, but there remains a small handful of texts in which demons are portrayed as taking over the bodies and minds of Anglo-Saxons themselves.

It is possible that demon possession was as widespread an occurrence in the Anglo-Saxon countryside as it seems to have been in first century Palestine or in Gregory of Tours's Gaul. A methodical survey of the evidence, however, points away from the assumption tacitly held in Anglo-Saxon studies that demon possession was a thriving phenomenon in Anglo-Saxon England. Most of this evidence comes from seventh- and eighth-century Northumbria and Anglia; virtually all references to particular cases of possession have dropped out of the documentary record by the eleventh century. Of course, the occasional epileptic or psychotic may have been perceived as a demoniac (or "energumen"): such a person could be perceived as having a medical condition, an indwelling spirit, or both, depending on local custom, surrounding circumstances, and the subjective assessment of available priests and healers. These cases may have been quite rare, though, and when hagiographers wrote of demoniacs crowding around saints' tombs or besieging a saint with supplication, the writers may have been drawing from literary models rather than from personal experience. I explore this provisional hypothesis as a possible corrective for currently held beliefs about demon possession in Anglo-Saxon society, but beyond this, given that a few cases certainly would have existed and would have been considered the work of demons, my hope is also to paint a portrait of what some cases of demon possession may have actually looked like in the early Middle Ages based on the current state of medical and psychiatric thinking. At the very least, this study (as with so many studies of early medieval society) should serve as a sobering reminder of the paucity and limitations of the sources at our disposal.

Certain oversimplified generalizations often circulated about medieval demon possession do not withstand close scrutiny. Demon possession is not just an early misunderstanding of mental illness, though mental illness was sometimes interpreted as possession.[1] A wide range of aberrant behaviors, from muscle control disorders to political and theological heterodoxy, were periodically regarded as the work of demons (sometimes described as indwelling, sometimes not)—and this despite the fact that medieval thinkers also acknowledged the existence of nondemonic muscle control and mental disorders. No one condition or behavior unequivocally incurred the label "possession." Occasionally a writer may seem to equate demon possession with madness, such as Gregory of Tours's equation of *a daemonio correptus* with *insano furore* or Bede's claim that King Eadbald of Kent "crebra mentis uaesania et spiritus inmundi inuasione premebatur" (was overwhelmed by frequent mental insanity and possession by an unclean spirit).[2] Such appositional formulations may find inspiration in biblical equations such as the Jewish accusation against Jesus in John 10:20, "daemonium habet et insanit" (he has a demon and is out of his mind), but the overlapping of madness and demon possession is well attested throughout the ancient world. The wording is ambiguous as often as not, and a statement listing madness and possession in parallel might be taken either as apposition or disjunction. When Ælfric of Eynsham states that Christ returned the *deofulseocum* ⁊ *wodum* (the possessed and the mad) to their right minds, for instance, does he visualize two separate classes of people, or is this rhetorical apposition?[3]

More often than not, possession was considered distinct from insanity throughout the medieval era, though it is rarely clear precisely how any given author envisions this distinction.[4] In one passage Augustine uses a seemingly supernatural symptom—clairvoyance—as a means of deciding whether a given person's illness is simply physiological or whether an indwelling demon is implicated as well:

> Erat autem iste febriens et tamquam in phrenesi ista dicebat. Et forte reuera phreneticus erat, sed propter ista daemonium pati putabatur. . . . Nec tamen eidem saltem presbytero illa cessit mentis alienatio siue daemonium, nisi cum sanus esset a febribus, sicut phrenetici sanari solent, nec aliquando postea tale aliquid passus est.[5]
>
> [There was a certain man with a fever who spoke as if in a frenzy. And maybe he was in fact a *phrenetic*, but because of this (his apparent clairvoyance) people believed that he suffered from demons. . . . Nor did this derangement or evil spirit abate for the priest until the man had gotten over the fevers—just as *phrenetics* often get well. He never suffered any such thing after that.]

Here Augustine is puzzling over the evidence. Apparently, additional symptoms must be considered (clairvoyance) to decide that the man has a demon; fever and gibbering are themselves insufficient. However, though distinct, they are still linked: the exorcism of the demon continues to remain ineffective so long as the fever persists. Similarly, meditating on King Alfred's symptoms, Asser records in the *Life of Alfred* that some attributed the king's illness to the evil eye, some to the devil, some to a fever, and some to the piles.[6] These candidates are presented as disparate diagnoses. The fact that neither the spiritual nor the medical model ever fully displaced the other over such a large course of time suggests that both paradigms—the spiritual and the physiological—were performing necessary functions in the Middle Ages.

Gregory the Great writes in his *Dialogues* that he once invited a certain priest named Amantius, known for his healing powers, to visit a hospital in Rome. There Amantius was able to cure a mentally disturbed patient—who suffered so much that he would howl wildly and loudly at night—by praying and laying on hands. Gregory notes that this patient suffered from a "seized mind" (*mente captus*), adding, "quem medicina graeco uocabulo freneticum appellat" (which in medicine is called a *phrenetic*, to use the Greek term).[7] At no point in his account is there a mention of demonic possession or diabolic influence; as far as we can tell from his description, this for him is nothing more than a medical phenomenon. Gregory certainly believes in possession: his *Dialogues* are otherwise filled with demons driven out by saints.[8] Aberrant behavior—in fact, *any* belief or action a given author considers objectionable—could easily be attributed to demons. Demonic agency was as often a metaphorical or moral assertion as an empirical diagnosis. This interpretive freedom does not imply that madness and possession were one, however: writers were simply free to make autonomous interpretations concerning (what they considered) the empirical facts of a given case.

Additionally, there is a delicate relationship between sin and illness throughout the Middle Ages, an association which at times finds expression in passages implying that all illness was at some root level attributed to prior guilt or sin.[9] When the "illness" in question is demon possession, the question is even more complicated. Deuteronomy states that the Lord will visit the unrighteous with all manner of illness, disaster, and madness, and implies a one-to-one correspondence between health and righteousness (28:28). On the other hand, Job's sufferings are expressly visited on him despite his steadfast righteousness.

In the absence of a consistently elaborated demonology of the early Middle Ages, the individual passages from various sources that serve as our primary evidence only yield impartial and seemingly contradictory information. For instance, the anonymous author of the Merovingian *Life of Rusticula*, in describing an encounter between St. Rusticula (or Rusticola) and a band of possessed men, presumes that all demonic possession implies prior sin of some sort:

> Inquirenti vero Christi ancillae, quo casu vel neglegentia spiritus maligni in hominibus introissent, confitebatur unusquisque per singular, unus, quia poculum aquae absque signaculo hausisset, alius, quia per gulam, alius, quia per periurium, alius per furtum, alius per homicidium, vel reliquis malis.[10]
>
> [After the handmaid of Christ inquired from what lapse or neglect the evil spirits had entered into them, the men each confessed individually: one, because he had drawn a cup of water without the sign (of the cross); another, because of his gluttony; another for oath breaking; another for theft; and the next because of murder or from other evil deeds.]

The saintly woman seems to know a priori that the demoniacs have transgressed in some way by the very fact that they suffer from a demon. Gregory of Tours, upon mentioning a girl whose hand is stiffened, adds that he does not know what her sin was: and so here he too seems to presuppose that all physical infirmity is the result of guilt.[11] Elsewhere, however, Gregory writes that St. Martin appears to a man who is at a loss to understand the guilt behind the sudden pain and paralysis of his hands, and Martin answers that not all illness implies sin. Here, Gregory explains, "neque ille peccaverat neque parentes eius" (neither the man had sinned, nor his parents).[12] Gregory is quoting John 9:2, in which Jesus specifically rebukes his disciples for believing that all illness is guilt: "Jesus answered, 'Neither this man nor his parents sinned; he was born blind so that God's works might be revealed in him.'" Individual authors thus had free reign, in any set of circumstances, to presume prior guilt as a causal mechanism in demon possession.[13] This was generally not the case, however.

In the New Testament demons are primarily medical nuisances while the devil is more of a moral metaphor. That is, the guiltless may be stricken in the usual course of things with a demon as easily as with an illness, but allowing the devil into one's heart implies complicity and a perversion of the will.[14] This distinction between demons and the devil is largely lost by the Middle Ages. By this time demonic agency is malleable and interchangeable in its expression. The potential issue of implicit prior guilt, though, endured and often required extra commentary. If partisan writers occasionally accused opponents of sin and pointed to physical infirmity as proof, pastors and holy men also had to reassure devoted parishioners that their infirmities did not necessarily imply divine reproof. A man named Hildmær in Bede's *Life of Cuthbert*, for instance, is ashamed to tell people that his wife is possessed, for fear that they will think she has sinned in some way. Cuthbert strives to assure the man that possession does not imply fault:

> Neque enim tali tormento soli subiciuntur mali, sed occulto Dei iudicio aliquotiens etiam innocentes in hoc saeculo non tantum corpore sed et mente captiuantur a diabolo.[15]

> [It is not only the evil who are subjected to such anguish, but—through the hidden decree of God—now and again even the innocent of this world are taken by the devil, not just in body but also in mind.]

Ælfric still emphasizes this aspect of the story when he retells it two centuries later.[16] In an analysis of some three thousand miraculous cures at medieval English shrines, Ronald Finucane finds that "sin is nearly as rare [as demons] as a *stated* cause of illness . . . most people did not regard sin as an important cause of illness."[17] Jerome Kroll and Bernard Bachrach likewise found that of 464 instances of early medieval illness examined, only 89 (19 percent) attributed the illness to sin. Of these, almost all could be explained by the particular author's political, religious, or moral quarrel with the person in question: "disease as divine punishment was selectively invoked only when the medieval author wished to castigate an enemy or immoral person."[18] In another study specifically examining the association of mental illness and sin, the connection was even weaker: only 9 out of 57 instances of mental illness (16 percent) implicated sin as the causal factor (and in all nine, once again, a "strong propaganda motive" was evident).[19] The connections are significantly stronger between possession and sin (one in three cases of possession were linked with sin in this study), but still relied primarily on the ad hoc, personal judgment of the author.[20]

Anglo-Saxons would have learned from their local priests that they were all sinners in an abstract sense (e.g., original sin). The philosophical implications of guilt and illness, however, were probably of more interest to theologians than to most rural pastors or Anglo-Saxon lower orders, who were not likely to treat their sick friends, family, and neighbors—from infants to the elderly—uniformly as having committed particular crimes or trespasses. The care and empathy for the ill evinced in the sources reflect an attitude in which illness is simply part of the human condition. The few relevant items in laws and penitentials point toward a society just as concerned for preserving the well-being of the mentally ill as for punishing the effects of their violence.[21] Generalizations implying that in the Middle Ages sin was not considered distinct from illness, then, belie the complexity of the evidence. In fact, such claims are part of a broader tendency toward painting medieval societies as irrational and alien. Sin and illness were of course loosely linked, on many occasions, but no more than they still are today in both professional medicine (e.g., the implicit moral judgments when doctors warn about smoking, diet, and exercise) and popular discourse (e.g., calling people "insane" when their behavior is disliked or poorly understood).

When we speak of "demon possession" today, we have in mind a much more restrictive phenomenon than the myriad activities potentially attributable to demonic agency in the early Middle Ages. Nonetheless, that restrictive set of behaviors—that specific type of demonic causality—enjoys an unbroken line of descent from the Middle Ages to the present, surviving even such radical religious paradigm shifts as the Protestant Reformation and secular modernism, and such scientific ones as Freudian psychoanalysis and molecular biology. This study will devote substantial attention to currently recognized medical and psychiatric conditions that may be relevant to medieval possession. This is not meant to imply reductively that demon possession is nothing more than misunderstood psychiatric disturbance, nor that the complicated social processes embodied in the dynamics of possession can be exhaustively reduced to chemical imbalances. It is only a single facet of possession that this book explores: the supplanting of an individual's personality with another being, a being that behaves wildly and violently and that (if it speaks at all) expressly adopts the persona of a mythological fallen angel. Behavioral disorders (many of which are rooted in physiological dysfunction) certainly constituted an important part of demon possession, though, and reviewing what we currently know about the body and mind in distress can help us form a more vivid and informed picture of what was going on in a number of cases. It is these neurological conditions, furthermore, that provided the models from which possession behaviors more broadly take their cue. It is because epileptics fall to the ground and foam at the mouth, for instance, that those functionally possessed (i.e., those who adopt possession behavior unconsciously, following conventional, culturally sanctioned patterns) often fall to the ground and foam at the mouth.[22]

Reconstructing Medieval Madness

Societies define insanity against their own constructs of normal behavior, which are only translatable to a limited degree across diverse cultures and ages. Earlier generations of psychiatry textbooks recognized a number of conditions such as hysteria and conversion disorders which have been found largely bankrupt as diagnostic concepts. Some of these changes reflect fixed behaviors that have simply been reclassified: homosexuality in its basic mechanisms, for instance, presumably did not change much through the twentieth century, even though the medical community stopped classifying it as a pathology in 1974. Helen Ullrich provides an interesting case study in which two competing descriptions of dysfunctional behavior seem little more than a case of semantics. Two generations of women in a Southern Indian family exhibited a common core of symptoms indicative of severe depression, but the individuals described their afflictions differently: "For the older woman, ghost possession provided an explanation for difficulty functioning in an expected role [of traditional wife]. . . . The younger woman considers herself depressed and attributes her depression to the cognitive dissonance between her expectations for the marriage and the marriage itself."[23] Both women exhibited decreased interest, weight loss, insomnia, fatigue, and a general inability to fulfill the duties of a traditional Indian wife.[24] A reattribution of causality, resulting from a shift in worldviews between two generations at the cusp of modernity, distinguishes perhaps artificially what otherwise struck the outside clinical observer as a similar cluster of symptoms. Differentiation becomes crucial, however, in prescribing a course of therapy. These two women live in such different perceptual worlds that it is not at all clear that one course of therapy—either exorcism or antidepressants—would be equally meaningful or effective for both women.

A number of conditions recognized differently today than in earlier schools of medicine reflect actual changes in physiological response. For instance, some conditions which once existed have disappeared or radically altered their profile. Middle- and upper-class white women do not faint anymore, as they often did in the nineteenth century (perhaps for cultural—even sartorial—reasons, as much as organic ones).[25] Some medical categories are transparently ideological rather than empirical, such as the infamous nineteenth-century diagnosis "drapetomania": a condition particular to African-American slaves, which makes them want to run away. Conversion disorders (in which, for instance, a perfectly healthy limb does not function, or a person witnessing some horrible event goes blind, without any apparent physiological basis) are rife in early psychiatric sources but are now rare, though it is unclear why. It is entirely possible that early medieval demon possession reflected psychological or physiological disturbances which are no longer available for study, however much the symptoms and surrounding circumstances of those cases available for observation in the modern world may resemble them.[26]

On the other hand, there is good reason to believe that the behavior patterns associated with demon possession in the modern world are cultural cognates of their medieval counterparts. Although "demon possession" is proposed for inclusion in the *Diagnostic and Statistical Manual* (DSM), diagnosis and treatment usually occurs entirely in a religious rather than a psychiatric context.[27] Demon possession in this sense is a perceptual construct employed by the members of the group in which it occurs, usually a congregation or ministry. "Deliverance ministries," as they are called, are currently on the rise in both developed and developing nations. The private and highly secretive exorcisms of the contemporary Catholic Church no longer preserve the public dimension of medieval exorcism, but the sensational dramas enacted before many Protestant congregations do recapture the public dynamic so important in early medieval sources.[28] The symptomology of early medieval possession is sufficiently detailed in the documents to allow at least provisional comparison with modern profiles of exorcism behavior, and it is clear that both continuity and evolution are present. Michael Cuneo, documenter of contemporary American exorcism activity, reports witnessing subjects (in addition to assuming alternate personae) vomiting, "flailing and slithering . . . shrieking and moaning . . . grimacing and growling," and was apparently the only person at a certain event who did *not* perceive the subject to have levitated off the ground: "But you must have seen the body rising," he quotes another attendant as telling him afterwards. "The rest of us saw it. It clearly rose, maybe three feet off the chair. How could you not have seen it?"[29] These phenomena are in keeping with the ancient traditions of Christian possession; early medieval demoniacs also vomit, howl, groan, and levitate.[30] Furthermore, many of the complicating factors implicated in modern possession—profiteering, malingering, and the influence of example—are also well attested in medieval sources, reminding us that the phenomenon cannot be reduced to any single psychological, cultural, economic, or theological explanation. Possession is a fluid, adaptive model that is simultaneously available to fill a variety of purposes in an individual, a community, or an age.

Of course, not all possession states are pathological. Speaking in tongues, for instance, is a contemporary trance state communally sanctioned (valorized, even, in many congregations) and so not considered in need of treatment. A case can be made that possession and exorcism form an equally theatrical rite, not "pathological" at all when enacted within the tacitly understood, prescribed boundaries of a given community. In labeling early medieval demon possession as a disorder, however, we are not arbitrarily pathologizing a cultural practice from a modern secular bias. It is the medieval sources themselves that indicate this series of behaviors is an illness: demon possession is invariably described as causing pronounced distress in the subject, disrupting social relationships, and inhibiting the individual's economic and emotional contributions to the community.[31] The subject's distress distinguishes demonic possession from ecstatic communion or mystical revelation, forms of religious expression increasingly common and culturally sanctioned in the later Middle Ages.[32] In the later Middle Ages a wider range of personal, mystical experiences became common, and by the end of this period theologians had great difficulty in trying to sort out demonic impulses and visions from divine ones.[33] That is not yet a problem for our period, however: divine or ecstatic visions (including dream visions and near-death experiences) uniformly bring a sense of peace, and these are clearly distinct from the sort of demon possession that requires exorcism, medical attention, or both.

The Literary Contexts of Demon Possession

Unexplained behavior and apparent rifts in an individual's sense of identity, if severe or destructive in expression, were often attributed in the Middle Ages to an indwelling demon. At other times, the attribution of demonic possession comes across rather as a figurative shorthand for simple displeasure: for example, when a group of Jews in early sixth-century Syria (as related shortly afterwards, in a letter by Bishop Simeon of Beth Arsham in 524 CE) complain of Mahya of Najran's vehement Christian polemic by ambitiously asserting, "This woman is the very Satan of the Christians: there is not a single devil that does not live in her."[34] This is invective, not diagnosis. There was, accordingly, awareness of the subjective nature of positing demon possession in a given case. When the drunken treasurer Eberulf accosts Gregory of Tours and a priest with reviling accusations and insults, Gregory tells us that "we observed that he was driven by a demon, as I would say."[35] Here there is no proof of spirit possession other than the perceived inappropriateness of the offender's tirade itself; the added phrase "as I would say" (ut ita dicam) reminds us of the provisional nature of such a claim, or of the potentially complicated relationship (in this case) between drunkenness and demonic instigation.

Any impulse to evil action was often imputed to the devil; in the medieval mindset, such a psychological impulse is often hard to distinguish from the potential presence of an indwelling demon. Felix's *Life of Guthlac* provides an instructive instance of diabolic instigation as (ostensibly) distinct from demon possession. Guthlac's disciple Beccel plans to kill his mentor, once the devil sews the idea in his heart: "Cuius praecordia malignus spiritus ingressus, pestiferis vanae gloriae fastibus illum inflare coepit" (the evil spirit, having entered his heart, began to inflate him with the pernicious conceits of vainglory).[36] Guthlac presciently discovers the plot and confronts the would-be assassin:

> O mi Beccel, ut quid hebido sub pectore antiquum hostem occultas? Quare amari veneni mortiferas limphas non vomis? Scio enim te a maligno spiritu deceptum; quapropter flagitiosas meditationes quas tibi generis humani hostilis criminator inseruit, ab illis convertendo, confitere.[37]
>
> [Oh, my Beccel—why do you hide the ancient enemy in your dull breast? Why do you not vomit up the deadly fluids of bitter venom? You see, I know you have been deceived by an evil spirit: therefore, confess the disgraceful thoughts the hostile accuser of humankind has inserted in you, by turning away from them.]

In this instance, it is clear that Beccel's own will is what has been swayed and that Beccel himself (as opposed to an indwelling demon) is still in control. Thus it is Beccel, not the demon, whom Guthlac addresses, and there is no demon to rail, complain, and be messily expelled. The distinction is possible, then, even if it is not systematically maintained nor applicable to all cases.

With these caveats in mind about the potentially unsystematic nature of references to possession in the early Middle Ages, we can distinguish four broad deployments of the demon idiom in medieval Christian thought and letters: (1) Demons are closely associated with human vices, either as their causes or else as embodiments of them. In this role, demons are employed in sermon literature, for instance, to offer concrete images for rhetorical effect. (2) Demons are treated as sentient entities with individual histories, characters, and pursuits. In this capacity, demons are often believed to inhabit specific locations (such as the air, a house, a forest, a mountain, or a desert). They can be encountered in material form, and thus present the danger of physical harm to travelers, not unlike other wild beasts. (3) Demons are well-recognized characters in the broader Christian narrative of salvation history, and their influence can be traced throughout the unfolding of human affairs. In this capacity, demons provided writers with a powerful explanatory model for a wide range of historical and theological topics. For instance, the undeniable power and glory of ancient kingdoms—which Anglo-Saxons well knew to be greater than their own civilization—can be explained as a treacherous farce once it is understood that it was in fact demons inhabiting the idols and perilously duping these heathens into worshipping false gods. (4) Demons are believed to be capable of entering into and taking control of bodies; in this role, they are associated especially with a select range of what we might consider neurological, muscle control, and psychiatric disorders. Thus they help members of the community understand and cope with an otherwise frightening series of dysfunctions that challenge core notions of identity. This fourth role is the subject of the present book.

Medieval sources themselves do not acknowledge these distinctions. There is no early medieval treatise on demonology, laying out a consistent series of principles by which these various functions can be reconciled.[38] It is difficult for the modern—especially the secular modern—observer to understand how at one moment a demon might be believed to represent a vice (such as drinking or fornicating) with almost metaphorical breadth, and at the next moment to be lurking behind a tree. There are cases in which multiple demons inhabit a single person, and even the occasional case in which a single demon inhabits two or more people simultaneously.[39] Sometimes the demons are equated with (collectively identified as) Satan, the devil himself; at other times they are portrayed as his subordinate angels. The list of ambiguities and outright inconsistencies could continue at great length. In fact, I argued in *Satan Unbound* that this resistance to clear definition and conceptual demarcation is essential to the place of the demonic in early medieval literature and thought. Thus, before narrowing the current study to the last of the four roles outlined, it may be helpful to spell out in further detail the nature of all four, to reiterate the multivalent nature of early medieval demons, and to provide more complete context for the focused study of the medical demons.

Demons as Metaphors for Vice

By the patristic era demons in the Christian tradition had become closely associated with the stirring passions of the human soul that threaten to distract the individual from spiritual advancement. In many cases, demons and vices are identified so completely that there is little indication that the demon is a separate, conscious being. The term "demon" becomes virtually a poetic shorthand for sin: thus, a Blickling homily notes that those who reject God's will are "like heathens" (on hæþenra onlicnesse), and that "many devils dwell in him" (manig deofol on him eardaþ). This implies not that the unrighteous are all possessed but that they are infested with sins.[40] The *Old English Martyrology*, likewise, explains that when Mary Magdalene had seven demons, it simply means that she succumbed to all the major sins: "seo wæs ærest synnecge, ond heo wæs mid seofon deoflum full, þæt wæs mid eallum uncystum" (she was at first a sinner, and she was filled with seven demons—that is, with all vices).[41]

The term spirit (*spiritus*) can refer either to a sentient being or, more abstractly, to any "motive, gift, inspiration." When Gregory the Great says that Constantius of Aquino has the "spirit of prophecy," he is not stating that the former bishop is possessed by a sentient being, whether desirable or not; he simply means that Constantius is gifted with this characteristic, that it is predicable of him.[42] By the same token, to be possessed by a "spirit of drunkenness" usually means no more than that the subject drinks too much. Such idioms remain deliberately ambiguous, at the intersection between didacticism and diagnosis.

The abstract identification of demons with human passions or with sudden, uncharacteristic impulses is evident in the Old Testament and in the Qumran scrolls.[43] The "spirit of confusion" (Isaiah 19:14) and the "spirit of whoredom" (Hosea 4:12) in the Bible, and the "demons of falsehood" in Qumran, probably have more figurative than literal sense.[44] The reference to a "spirit of the community" is unequivocally a figure of speech.[45] The Testaments of the Twelve Patriarchs, a pseudepigraphal work drawing from both Christian and Jewish tradition, enumerates seven spirits of error: the spirits of sight, hearing, smell, speech, and taste, together with those of sex and (interestingly enough) of "life."[46] This creative period in formative Christianity reveals the wide appeal of the demonic (and spiritual agencies in general) as a multivalent conceptual tool in forging communal ideals, as expressed in religious narratives.

Medieval thinkers were experienced at interpreting texts polysemously. The famous exegetical model of the "four senses of Scripture" helped to guide conceptual categories and rhetorical patterns throughout the Middle Ages, though we should not overestimate that categorization as either exhaustive or uniformly employed. A scriptural passage, according to this model, can be simultaneously read literally (historically), typologically (analogically, specifically with reference to Old Testament prefigurations of New Testament ideas), tropologically (morally), and anagogically (eschatologically).[47] Aldhelm expounds this fourfold model in *De virginitate*, for instance.[48] The second (typology) is sometimes referred to as allegory, though in fact typology here refers primarily to a specific form of allegorical signification (the Old Testament prefiguring of New Testament people and events), and all three of the nonliteral approaches can be roughly thought of as "allegorical." This model was a sophisticated theological justification among the educated elite for the interpretive flexibility already being exercised at local pulpits: in practice, priests and homilists could draw freely from scriptural phrases and images—regarding both the divine and the demonic—to make connections in crafting their sermons and devotional works. Thus preachers kept alive throughout the Middle Ages the peripheral tradition that passions are demons, though probably more for the powerful finesses of rhetoric it allowed than from any commitment to a systematic demonology. The rhetoric represents an attractive pastoral tool, empowering the individual to direct internal energies and to reflect upon personal motives. There is something satisfying in battling one's own weaknesses as though they are foes: "apparuit ei corporaliter spiritus fornicationis, et dixit ei: tu me vicisti, Sara" (The spirit of fornication appeared to her corporeally, and said to her: "You have conquered me, Sarah").[49] Such clear-cut identifications only appear sporadically and ad hoc, however, with little development from the beginning of the Middle Ages to the end. A strict allegorical view of demons as reified passions was and still is ill at ease in the mainstream Christian tradition.

More commonly, demons are not equated with vices but are held to be their direct or indirect cause. This can be envisioned variously: classical Greek and Hellenistic thinkers often posited a "daemon" or guardian spirit accompanying each individual, sometimes elaborated as two distinct spirits—a good and an evil one.[50] Preserving similar lore, the Old English *Solomon and Saturn II* ends with a meditation on the two spirits accompanying each individual, one urging the individual to good and the other to evil:

Đonne hine ymbegangað gastas twegen;
oðer bið golde glædra, oðer bið grundum sweartra....
oðer him læreð ðæt he lufan healde
metodes miltse, and his mæga ræd;
oðer hine tyhteð and on tæso læreð ...[51]

[Therefore two spirits surround him: one is brighter than gold, the other is darker than the abyss... One teaches him to keep to the advice of kin and to his love for the mercy of God; the other provokes him and draws him toward ruin ...]

The poetic trope also appears in *Guthlac A*:

hine twegen ymb
weardas wacedon, þa gewin drugon,
engel dryhtnes ond se atela gast.[52]

[Two guardians watched over him, sustaining battle: an angel of the Lord and the evil spirit.]

Ælfric writes, "ælcum geleaffullum menn is engel to hyrde geset þe hine wið deofles syrewungum gescylt" (to each faithful person an angel is set as a guardian who shields him against the devil's traps).[53] Alternately, an important tradition traceable at least to the ancient Near East posits only two spirits directing all of humankind, one of truth and one of perversity.[54] Yet another early paradigm, which became widespread through its prevalence in the early Christian writings on the desert fathers, depicts each demon as having a particular vice or sphere of influence.[55] Evagrius Ponticus in his *Antirrheticus* (or Talking Back) speaks of eight demons, one for each deadly sin.[56] Rufinus of Aquileia's *History of the Monks in Egypt* implies a one-to-one correspondence of demons to passions, though remaining careful not to eliminate either factor from the equation:

> esse quosdam daemones, qui certis quibusque vitiis obsequantur quique, cum affectus animae passibiliter et vitiose viderint moveri, convertunt eos ad omne facinus malum. Si quis ergo est, qui vult daemonibus dominari, prius vitiis suis et passionibus dominetur. Quodcumque enim vitium propriae passionis abieceris huius vitii daemonem poteris etiam de obsessis corporibus effugare.[57]
>
> [(There are) demons who incline toward certain vices, and when they perceive the soul to be turning vulnerably and wickedly, they push them wholly to that wicked sin. So whoever wishes to have control over the demons must first control his own vices and passions. Whatever vice and corresponding passion you cast off, you will thus be able to drive the demon of that vice from the bodies of the possessed.]

In a passage not appearing in the Greek original, Rufinus's version of the *History of the Monks* further clarifies that the vices prepare room in the sinner's heart for the devil: "Si ergo sint vitia in corda nostro, cum venerit princeps eorum diabolus, quasi proprio auctori dant locum et introducunt eum velut ad possessionem suam" (so if there are vices in our heart, when their leader the devil comes, they will make room as though he were their own author, and they will welcome him as though to his own property).[58] Well into the Christian era, a wealth of models were available to writers for visualizing the relationship between the human psyche, sin, and demons.

Demons were of course believed to be real—often tangible. For most early medieval thinkers, the logical distinction between demon as metaphor or abstract principle and demon as independent, sentient entity was not a productive one. They preferred to keep the boundaries blurred. This results in such hybrid conceptual potpourris as we find in Boniface's letter to Æthelbald, for instance. Boniface describes the possession of King Ceolred of Mercia, who apparently suffered a breakdown of some sort: the fit comes on suddenly (*subito*) while at the dinner table, and the king is overcome with a madness (*insaniam mentis*) that leaves him, according to Boniface, "conversing with devils" (*cum diabolis sermocinans*) and refusing Christian rites until his dying day.[59] From this description, Boniface passes to King Osred, whose unconscionable romantic liberties with cloistered nuns are said to be caused by a "spirit of wantonness" (*spiritus luxoriae*). Boniface implies immediately afterwards that in both of these cases the perpetrator succumbed to the "darts of the ancient enemy" (*iacula antiqui hostis*).[60] If Boniface wished this explanatory agent to be understood literally as an indwelling spirit, he did not stress the point; in this passage he is more obviously concerned with the king's alleged moral trespasses than his mental health. It seems that the "spirit" is shorthand for the immoral impulses leading to the king's transgressions: thus the demon who strikes Ceolred physiologically only appears subsequently, as a punishment rather than a cause.[61]

The monk of Wenlock famously granted a vision of hell describes a fascinating scene in which his own vices appear to him as demons and threaten to block his entry into heaven. Boniface relates the story in a letter of 716 to Abbess Eadburga of Thanet:

> Et se ipsum audisse omnia flagitiorum suorum propria peccamina, quae fecit a iuventute sua et ad confitendum aut neglexit aut oblivioni tradidit vel ad peccatum pertinere omnino nesciebat, ipsius propria voce contra illum clamitasse et eum dirissimæ accussasse et specialiter unumquodque vitium quasi ex sua persona in medium se obtulisse dicendo quoddam: "Ego sum cupiditas tua."[62]
>
> [And he heard all his own wicked sins, which he had committed from his youth and had neglected or forgotten to confess or which he did not even know were sinful. Each declaimed against him with its own voice and accused him harshly, and each of the vices individually—as though in person—introduced itself, saying, "I am your lust."]

Ten more vices come forward thus ("I am your vanity," etc.), and then the entire passage concludes with an open-ended "and so forth thus" (*et cetera his similia*) that implies a still greater litany of sins. No one in the Middle Ages would have taken such scenes as this one as literal, historical descriptions of the soul's conflict with passions; the distancing marker "as if in person" (*quasi ex sua persona*) flags this scene as an elegant simile.[63]

Old English use of the genitive often reflects such a figural conceptualization of "spirits." The Old English *Life of Margaret* mentions a "spirit of truth" (*sopfæstnesse gast*, translating *spiritu ueritatis*).[64] Wærferð's translation of Gregory's *Dialogues* refers to a "spirit of pride" (*oferhigde gaste*, rendering *superbiae spiritu*).[65] The OE *Rule of Benedict* notes that God relieved a certain cenobite of the "spirit of arrogance" (*upahefednesse gast*, for Benedict's *spiritum elationis*).[66] Translations from the Bible often preserve the idioms of the Latin Vulgate: thus the *spiritus irae* (spirit of anger) of Psalm 17:16 becomes *gastys yrrys*; the *spiritum infirmitatis* (spirit of illness) of Luke 13:11 becomes *untrumnesse gast*.[67] The spirit of fornication who presents himself to St. Anthony is called by his Latin name in the

Old English Martyrology (Spiritus Fornicationis—this is presented as his proper name), with the Anglo-Saxon translator or redactor adding the explanation, "þæt is dernes geligeres gast" (that is, the spirit of deceitful fornication).[68]

The instances cited thus far have all been translations from Latin source texts, but the trend is also evident in original vernacular passages. The "demon of love" (*amoris dæmonem*) referred to in Jerome's *Life of Hilarion* is expanded, in the *Old English Martyrology*, more descriptively: "ðæt deofol ðe hyne lærde ða unclænan lufan" (the devil that taught him sinful love).[69] The genitive case is thus potentially capable of creating new "spirits" in Old English no less than in Latin. In the *Old English Vision of St. Paul* the "spirits of sin" appear as reified entities:

> And se ængel hine ða gelædde, Paulum, on nyowelnessa ðær hylware wæron, and he him ðær æteowode on hwilce stowe arleasra sawla gelædde beoð ðanne hi of ðæm lichaman ut gegangeð; and Paulus ðær geseah ondryslic weald ðara mænaga gasta, ðe manna hyrtan beswicað: þæt is tælnessa gast, and forhealdnyssa gast, and hathyrtnyssa gast, and leasunga gast, and ofermodignyssa gast, and eaðbylhnyssa gast . . . yrra gast,[70] and æwergednyssa gast, and ðas wæron buton ælcere mildheortnesse.[71]
>
> [And the angel then led Paul into the depths, where there were hell denizens, and there he showed him all over the place wicked souls being brought once they had departed the body. And there Paul saw the terrible power of the many spirits that seduce the hearts of humankind: that is, the spirit of slander, and the spirit of unchastity, and the spirit of anger, and the spirit of lying, and the spirit of pride, and the spirit of irascibility . . . (and) the spirit of ire, and the spirit of wickedness, and they were without any mercy.]

Antonette di Paolo Healey, editor of the Old English *Vision*, observes that the Old English translator envisions the role of these various spirits differently than the Latin source texts: "OE has confused the spirits who dwell beneath the firmament, whose duty it is to challenge the soul on its way to heaven, with the merciless angels, whose duty it is to lead out the evil soul at the moment of death. The text conflates the two groups which the Latin keeps distinct."[72] Such creative fluidity may signal that these demons are to be taken as literary figures or metaphors. For the authors in question, however, interpretive categories such as literal and metaphorical were not exclusive. Thus, a secular modern reader might be tempted to ask whether Boniface's moral indictment of King Osred mentioned above (that he was afflicted by the *spiritus luxoriae*, "spirit of wantonness") implies that Osred harbored a vice initially implanted there by a demon, or whether it implies that the demon actually possessed him. For most medieval thinkers, the question posed in this way would represent a misunderstanding of the underlying nature of the demonic. The demonic and a demon could become interchangeable: for instance, a demon might implant a vice in someone and then become, by degrees, increasingly manifest in that person as an independent, indwelling personality.[73] An exorcist, therefore, could cast out a vice or even a physiological disease using the same methods that he would in casting out a demon. For our present purposes, however, it will be necessary to cull out those instances of possession that clearly signify a prominent behavioral disorder from those which appear to be figures of speech or which are more naturally read as moral censure. The much wider pool of accusations and idioms, although independently interesting, are more justly treated in a history of early medieval rhetoric than in one of early medieval organic dysfunction.

Demons as Wild Beasts

The natural world, in medieval imaginative literature, is populated by all manner of monsters. The Anglo-Saxon saints Cuthbert and Guthlac—like Anthony before them—had to tame unforgiving lands inhabited by wild animals and demons in order to stake out a quiet place for meditation and prayer. The *Voyage of Brendan* tells of strange and perilous monsters at the far corners of the earth, as do popular traditions of exotic travel stories as represented in the *Wonders of the East* and the *Letter of Alexander to Aristotle*. The *Beowulf* poet is fascinated by the monsters he weaves into his narrative, pausing on occasion to consider their ancestry and their place in God's cosmos. Since wild animals can be portrayed as demonic, and since demons often assume the shape of animals, it is not always easy to distinguish between them. Not all monsters were necessarily "demons," but certainly any monster—just as any animal, storm, psychological impulse, or indeed any inconvenient obstacle—could potentially be interpreted as demonic in the medieval mindset, in so far as it poses danger or appears to frustrate the efforts of humankind.[74]

No culture (and certainly not ours today) is without a menagerie of folkloric creatures lurking in the wastes, just beyond the perimeter of well-explored paths. Such creatures (the study of which is currently hiding behind the more scientific-sounding term "cryptozoology") serve important sociological functions, such as the construction of explored vs. unexplored boundaries and the articulation of primordial fears of darkness and the unknown.[75] In the early Christian stories of the desert fathers, demons scuttle about the wilderness alongside lions and crocodiles, wolves and basilisks. In this capacity demons are largely amoral: they are simply trials to be suffered on the path for salvation—together with thirst and storms—and often perform narrative functions for which an animal, a thief, or even an inopportunely situated rock could be substituted just as easily. The devil in Gregory's *Dialogues* is largely a prankster: he throws rocks, sits on a stone that some monks are trying to move, and pushes a wall over onto an innocent monk.[76] Augustine writes of a man in his vicinity whose house and livestock had been plagued by attacks from evil spirits until he hung up a clod of the sacred earth from Jerusalem in his bedroom.[77] Gregory of Nyssa's *Life of Gregory the Wonder Worker* speaks of a "demon of the bath" who assailed those trying to use the bath after dark, as does the Merovingian *Life of Caesarius of Arles*.[78] The royal physician mentioned in the *Life of Caesarius of Arles* is pelted with stones in his own house by the demons also inhabiting it.[79] In Adomnan's *Life of Columba*, demons occupy a well and an empty milk pail.[80] In the *Annals of Fulda* for the year 858, an evil spirit throws stones and bangs on the walls to annoy the inhabitants of a certain house.[81] The Anglo-Saxon St. Dunstan comes close to having his head struck by a large rock, apparently thrown by the devil.[82]

The distinguishing feature of this second class of demons is their obstinate physicality. They present saints with problems of passage (traversing a river or settling in a certain location), which can then be interpreted, subsequently, as problems of spiritual advancement. In *Guthlac A*, when Guthlac settles in the remote fenlands, the demons and monsters that assail him are not easy to read as his own evil passions or his human potential to turn away from God: he has already confronted the devil and overcome him prior to these encounters.[83] In fact, these demon assaults form type scenes, of a sort also familiar from the *Life of Cuthbert* and the *Life of Gall*, for instance. They can be traced to the remarkable series of ordeals that St. Anthony suffers in the *Life of Anthony*. A thirteenth-century artistic rendition (figure 1, roundel 7 from BL Harley Roll Y.6) shows a host of demons besieging the saint and carrying him into the air.[84] Similarly, a common psalter drawing shows the subject of Vulgate Psalm 37 afflicted by tiny, winged "enemies" (Vulgate *inimici*).[85] In such encounters the demons are described as external threats, never successful in their attempts to tempt the saint or to turn his or her will. In modern parlance the term *obsession* has (tenuously and intermittently) come to be used to distinguish external assaults of this sort, in which the personality is never displaced, from *possession*, in which the individual adopts a different persona.[86] Indwelling demons, such as those that Guthlac casts out from Ecga in figure 2, afflict secondary characters, never the saint. Though highly dramatic, scenes of external temptation—the scenes of *temptatio* or *obsessio*—fall outside the scope of our study, both because the subject does not lose control of his or her personality, and because such obsession was not by itself considered a pathology in the Middle Ages. As Simon Kemp argues, "perhaps the most interesting feature of medieval obsession is that those suffering from it do not usually seem to have been regarded as insane or mad at all."[87] To be tested in such a way was a sign of divine attention; to undergo the trials successfully was a sign of sanctity, not insanity.

Just as a demon could take physical form as a monster or animal, so too could it physically occupy a location. The Catholic liturgy preserves to this day the ancient idea that demons can inhabit a landscape as well as the human heart: this is technically known as "infestation," the Christian version of a *genius loci* (spirit of the place).[88] Springs, houses, wells, crossroads, trees, and other features of the natural terrain were rife with spirits of various sorts in the Greco-Roman world, as well as in the Semitic traditions of the ancient Near East, and these traditions remained vibrant throughout the Latin Middle Ages. Audrey L. Meaney has recently argued that these spaces remained venerated—if not quite worshipped—in the consciousness of rural Anglo-Saxons throughout the Anglo-Saxon period, much to the dismay of church reformers.[89] Gregory the Great records Bishop Datius of Milan first exorcizing a long-abandoned house of the devil before Datius can occupy it. According to Braulio of Saragossa, a demon inhabiting the house of a certain senator slips animal bones and manure in his food, steals clothes and puts them on the roof, and terrorizes the occupants with other such pranks.[90] Infestation presumes that a building or place (itself amoral) can host demons regardless of the moral state of its human inhabitants. This is a form of misfortune, along with illness and possession, that can befall an individual, a household, or a community.

In his *Life of Willibrord*, Alcuin writes of a particularly persistent case of infestation on the continent that does not respond to repeated attempts at exorcism:

> Contigit cuidam patri familias et domui suae dira demoniacae inlusionis temptatio, ita ut apertae malignus in eius domu spiritus ex horrore et maleficiis habitare agnoscebatur. Nam subito cibos vel vestimenta vel alia domui necessaria rapere solebat et in ignem mittere, immo parvulum inter amplexus parentum pausantem, illis dormientibus, tulit et in ignem proiecit; sed vagitu infantis parentes suscitati, vix parvulum de incendio eruerunt. Et multa atrocia eadem familia a nefando spiritu perpessa est.[91]
>
> [It happened that there was an attack of dreadful, demoniacal illusion to a certain father and his household; it was readily apparent from the horrible and wicked things that an evil spirit inhabited his house. It was in the habit of suddenly grabbing food or clothes or other household items and would then throw them into the fire. It even took a very small child from the embrace of the sleeping parents and threw it into the fire—but woken by the child's crying, the parents picked it back out of the fire. And the family endured many frightful things from this abominable spirit.]

After the house spontaneously bursts into flames, a new house is built on the same spot and consecrated with holy water. This new one is free of demons. Even the furniture, presciently removed from the house shortly before the fire broke out, must be independently doused with holy water before it can be introduced again to the new house.

A family's relationship with its own domestic space can sometimes be a tense and ambivalent one, leading even in the modern world to popular belief in hauntings and poltergeists. Perhaps one's own home is too familiar a place, too small a world in which to lead one's entire life. Painful memories linger; inconveniences fester in the mind and become exaggerated over time. Bedbugs, spiders, and other vermin populated the medieval household, some potentially quite noxious. Moving into a new space, likewise, can gestate a different range of potential anxieties, especially when moving to a new community. Medieval inhabitants responded to such tensions as these in several ways, including hanging herbs or amulets around the house and having the house sprinkled with holy water (known as "aspersion" or "aspergation").[92] We have little evidence to tell us why or under what circumstances this would be done for private homes.[93] Aspergation is among the most common of the occasional rites appearing in Anglo-Saxon liturgical manuscripts, however. The consecration of a church required asperging, and rites are also extant for monastic cells.[94] Such practices presumably served, among other things, to develop a sense of personal and communal control over the household and living space, which—no less than the natural world outside—was capable of presenting medieval families with a host of dangers, both real and imagined.

Humankind will probably always indulge in the archetypal belief in monsters: David Quammen has eloquently articulated why it is not frivolous but psychologically healthy for us as a species to live in proximity with perceived harmful predators more powerful than ourselves.[95] The critical inclination (practiced by medieval and modern commentators alike) to "save" such stories from the appearance of superstition—for instance, by reading them allegorically as spiritual struggles within the human soul—can inadvertently deny an important dimension of the human relationship with the natural world, if the belief in literal monsters is too categorically denied.

Demons as Characters in the Broader Mythological Narrative

In societies with prominent traditions of possession, the possessing entities can be conceived in a number of ways. Two of the most common forms the possessing agent tends to take are the dead (ancestors or ghosts, common in Africa and the Near East), and demons (common in India, China, and Christian Europe).[96] While belief in the restless dead is arguably compatible with orthodox Christianity,[97] on the whole early missionaries considered it a remnant of pagan beliefs and endeavored to replace native models of ghostly revenants with the Christian narrative of fallen angels.[98] Thus there is very little evidence for ghosts or ancestors as possessing spirits in early medieval Europe. The recent work of Éva Pócs, on the other hand, has helped demonstrate that popular belief in ghosts as possessing spirits (in her study, in small Hungarian villages) can exist alongside more ecclesiastically sanctioned models of demon possession, without arousing great attention, for very long periods.[99] We should keep in perspective that for the early Middle Ages we only have church writings at our disposal, but there was probably a much wider spectrum of beliefs and activities that escaped documentation.

The only consistently available model for possessing agents in early medieval Europe that appears in our extant records, then, was possession by demons—the invisible, sentient beings familiar from scripture and apocryphal texts, as expounded through centuries of theological commentary and assimilation with popular beliefs. Demons are not always equated strictly with the fallen angels expelled from heaven, but the belief that demons were fallen angels or that they were somehow descended from them was thoroughly entrenched by the Anglo-Saxon period.[100] Having been exiled from their former abode in the heavens, the demons now inhabit pagan idols, sow discord, and deceive humans with delusions and lies, either in a futile attempt to spite the Creator or else from engrained malice.

Sometimes we can occasionally "meet" these demons directly, through the mouths of suffering demoniacs during the wrenching confession scenes in histories and hagiography. At least, this is the story the demoniacs—each in the persona of a possessing demon—tell the exorcist regarding who they are and what crimes they have committed. Certainly, many of the dialogues between demon and exorcist that appear in the sources were never actually spoken by anyone: they are literary constructs or reconstructions, devised by pious authors, following a long tradition of saint versus demon literary models.[101] To what extent the actual populace assimilated and then repeated the erudite confessions that demons elaborate in hagiographic models—to what extent they "stuck to the script"—can justly be doubted. However, if on the whole people had internalized the gist of the demonic role at the thresholds of salvation history, and within the fundamental momentum and trajectory of a Christian exorcism, they would be equipped with the essential tools for participating in dramatic altercation with the exorcist. They would have available to them a basic repertoire of things to say and stances to adopt. Alongside the possible expression of individual preoccupations or anxieties, in these harangues and laments the "demons" could also remember their primordial trespass and the ensuing exile from heaven, confess to a wide range of cosmic evils, and hint darkly that they know what awaits them after the Second Coming.

On the continent, Einhard writes of a woman from Baldradesstat who is possessed by an evil spirit and who engages the priest in a lengthy dialogue during the exorcism. The demon, "in caelo se fuisse et inde propter superbiam deiectum esse, confessus est" (confessed that he had been in heaven, and that he was cast down from there because of his pride).[102] When the priest finally asks where the demon will go once expelled from the demoniac, it answers through the woman, "'Ego,' ait, 'in viam pessimam perrecturus et longinquas desertasque regiones petiturus sum'" ("I," he said, "am to proceed along the worst path, and seek out remote and deserted regions").[103] Before Einhard's time the demons in Gregory of Tours's Gaul likewise adopted the personae of cosmic antagonists. At the death of Disciola (in Gregory's *History of the Franks*), an energumen tearing at his hair laments before all of those assembled:

> "Heu, heu, heu nobis, qui tale damno perpessi sumus! Vel licuisset prius causas inquirere, et sic de potestate nostra fuisset ablata haec anima." Inquirentibus vero his qui aderant, quod esset hoc verbum, quod loquebatur, respondit: "Ecce anima puellae Michahel angelus suscepit, et ipsi eam ad caelos evexit. Princeps vero noster, quem vos diabolum nominatis, nihil in ea participatur."[104]
>
> ["Oh no! Oh no for us, that we suffer such a loss! Before we were permitted to look into the case, this soul has been stolen from our power." Then, being asked by those present what it was he was talking about, he responded: "Behold! The angel Michael has received that young woman's soul, and taken it up to heaven. Our prince—known to you all as the Devil—cannot have any part of her."]

In actively assuming their alternate personae, demoniacs thus appeal to the Christian narrative of fallen angels in framing their putative identities. All the relationships that logically ensue from that are preserved: Satan is the master, God the enemy, the demoniac's body a convenient (if temporary) abode, and the intervention of the saint an unforeseen circumstance—a travesty, even.

However, there are very few extant descriptions of possessions that take place in Anglo-Saxon England, and none provide such a detailed "confession" on the part of the demon as the abundant continental sources. Indeed, no putative Anglo-Saxon demoniac speaks a single word that has been recorded in direct dialogue. For Anglo-Saxon analogues to the protracted interrogation scene, we must turn instead to a distinct but related genre, the demon vs. saint dialogue in hagiography. In these scenes, an external demon—not one inhabiting a human—engages the saint in a debate. Perhaps the most memorable such scene is that in Cynewulf's *Juliana*. The virgin martyr, tortured by the pagan prefect and thrown into a dungeon, gains the upper hand when a demon comes in attempting to trick her. She seizes the demon, and demands that he relate at length his current mission, his past crimes, and his methods. He grudgingly says that his father, *hellwarena cyning* (king of hell's dwellers), sent him on the present mission, and that he and his fellow demons have committed countless crimes among humans:

> Þus ic wraðra fela
> mid minum broþrum bealwa gefremede,
> sweartra synna, þe ic asecgan ne mæg,
> rume areccan, ne gerim witan,
> heardra heteþonca.[105]
>
> [Thus, with my brothers, I have perpetrated many malicious evils—

dark sins, cruel and malign designs—which I cannot express or explain in detail; I don't even know how many.]

He says that he and his compatriots instigated Herod to decapitate John the Baptist, Simon Magus to accuse the apostles of sorcery, Nero to execute Peter and Paul, Pilate to execute Christ, and on and on. His identity as a fallen angel is clear from Juliana's rebuttal:

Þu wið Criste geo
wærleas wunne ⁊ gewin tuge,
hogdes wiþ halgum; þe wearð helle seað
niþer gedolfen, þær þu nydbysig
fore oferhygdum eard gesohtes.[106]

[Faithless, you contended with Christ, once, and brought about enmity, plotting against God; for you the pit of hell was dug below, and there, harrowed and distressed, you found a home, because of your pride.]

The demon repeatedly laments that he is in torment as the result of her interrogation, and that further torments await him once he is forced to return to hell having failed his mission. Similar moments occur in the poetic *Guthlac A* and *Andreas*, and in prose passions such as the *Lives of Margaret*. These scenes provide fascinating insights into the battle between good and evil as Anglo-Saxon authors, compilers, and translators envisioned it, but the events remain conspicuously divorced from the human realm. The interrogation scene in *Juliana*, for instance, takes place in a dungeon, in the dark, with no human spectators. The demonic in these texts remains external; these are not exorcisms.

Pagans, heretics, and apostates are all, a priori, under the influence of the devil and his minions. In medieval Christianity, following Paul (1 Corinthians 10:20), the gods of the pagans were considered to be demons. For early apologists such as Justin Martyr, Athenagoras, Origen, and Tertullian, the demons inhabited idols and demanded sacrifices, to glut their sensory appetites: "they engross themselves in the blood from the sacrifices and lick all around them."[107] In *De falsis diis*, Ælfric spells out the Christian apologetic tradition that the demons pose as heathen gods, inhabiting idols and demanding sacrifices.[108] It is in this role—their posture as false pagan gods—that we most frequently encounter demons in early Anglo-Saxon authors such as Bede and Boniface.[109] The majority of Bede's references to demons are not to indwelling spirits but to false gods. In the *Historia ecclesiastica*, demons are primarily beings who inhabit pagan idols and lead people astray. The demons foment apostasy and resistance to conversion. In his exposition of Matthew 4:24 (Vulgate reading: "obtulerunt ei . . . qui daemonia habebant et lunaticos et paralyticos . . . et curavit eos" [they brought to him demoniacs, lunatics, and paralytics, and he cured them]), he explains:

> Tunc quoque curati sunt daemoniaci, id est, gentiles ad fidem conversi idola relinquebant, nec non lunatici et paralytici sanati sunt, id est, instabiles et per varios errores nutantes confortabantur.[110]
>
> [Then the "demoniacs" were cured—that is, the pagans, having converted to the faith, relinquished their idols; and furthermore, the "lunatics" and "paralytics" were healed—that is, the inconstant and people teetering among various errors were strengthened.]

Bede is less interested in demons as a medical phenomenon than he is in their metaphorical potential in the narration of broad sweeps of conversion history according to his ideological program. Similarly, Alcuin employs possession as a trope of evil and the desire for vengeance, rather than as diagnosis. In the *Life of Willibrord*, the devotee of a pagan cult strikes the saint with a sword for destroying the local shrine. In response the man "demoniaco spiritu arreptus est" (is seized by a demonic spirit) and dies three days later *infeliciter* (unhappily).[111] Throughout the period of Anglo-Saxon letters, the demonic is very much an abstract "other" against which correct religious alignment can be established.

Demons as Mental, Behavioral, and Neurological Disorders

Each of the prior three semantic deployments of the demonic are important and each probably warrants a book to itself. The current study focuses exclusively on the fourth, however: the demons of the body and mind. Since early in the history of civilization itself, extreme personality shifts and muscle control disorders such as epilepsy have often been attributed to independent, sentient spirits. Figures 3 and 4 for instance, show early medieval visual depictions of possession as muscle control disorders. In figure 3, a bas-relief of a water vessel which Paciaudi identifies as an early medieval baptismal font from Perugia, Italy, four priests (or exorcists) are confronted with a convulsing energumen.[112] This iconography demonstrates the early association of catechumens (those undergoing Christian instruction and preparing for baptism) with energumens (those somehow under the devil's power).[113] The scene provides an invaluable depiction of early medieval demon possession, visualized here as unnatural contortion of limbs and the head. In figure 4, the eleventh-century Ottonian Aachen Gospel Book, Christ expels the demon from the "epileptic boy" (Matthew 17:14–21, Mark 9:14–29, Luke 9:37–43). J.-M. Charcot and Paul Richer believe this to be the oldest depiction of a possessed person (at least in a manuscript illustration) that incorporates realistic elements of seizure—elements that the Renaissance masters would later paint with haunting sublimity.[114] For visualizations of demoniacs and possession we must turn to such continental examples, because there are no visual depictions of demoniacs, possession, or exorcism from Anglo-Saxon England.

Sudden behavioral anomalies are thus described as the work of hostile, invasive spirits; this provides an explanatory framework and suggests specific courses of therapy. On this account even a spooked horse or rabid dog could be considered "possessed," and, indeed, animal possession is well-attested in the early Middle Ages. A horse in the *Earliest Life of Gregory the Great* is possessed by demons, and the devil prompts another to *insolitam ferocitatem* (unusual ferocity) in Hucbald of St. Amand's *Life of Rictrude*.[115] Also, particularly vexatious ailments, such as blindness, lameness, paralysis, and contortions of the back or limbs, over a long period of time can be attributed to a demon. The demonic as invasive pathogen or indwelling spirit can become a highly visceral, biological series of metaphors, with the demons inhering in organs, limbs, sinews, and ligaments, and being expelled as vomit, excreta, pus, and blood. There is a very real sense, then, in which demons *are* the body—they represent matter and especially the unpleasant aspects of human physiology, or of the body in distress or decay.

Naomi Janowitz writes that exorcism, as it was forged in late antiquity and bequeathed to the Christian Middle Ages, "was based on a deep-seated suspicion of the body."[116] Accounts of demon expulsion in the early Middle Ages—as with many accounts of miraculous healing—often focus on specific parts of the body, emphasize fluids and tissues, and present the whole business as messy. In having demons cast out, demoniacs vomit forth *sanguinem fetidum* (fetid blood), *purulentum nescio* (I don't know what kind of pus), and *purulentum nescio . . . cum sanguine* (I don't know what kind of pus, and blood).[117] In the *Life of Rusticula*, a man jumps from a window, rushes up to the saint, and tries to eat her hand; when she makes the sign of the cross over him, he vomits forth blood in the shape of a man.[118] In Jonas's *Life of Columban*, the devil comes out of a man "cum viscerum motione ac vomitu multo" (through a motion of his bowels, and with great vomiting), leaving a great *fetorem* (stench).[119] Gregory of Tours writes of a demon entering into a man's thumbnail, and when holy oil is applied, the skin breaks, emitting both blood and the demon.[120] In Venantius Fortunatus's *Life of Radegund*, a woman named Leubila has her back cured by the saint, a cure which is made manifest to all when "in scapula crepante cute et verme foras exeunte" (there was a rustling under the skin of her shoulder and a worm came out).[121] In the same work the devil leaves the wife of a carpenter through her ear, and in yet another chapter, St. Radegund orders a possessed woman to lie on the pavement and then stands on her neck, thus causing the devil to be flushed out *fluxu ventris* (in a flow from her innards).[122] One demon who threatens to leave through a woman's eyes departs instead, at Saint Genovefa's bidding, through her bowels, *foeda relinquens* (leaving behind some filth).[123] In Augustine's *City of God*, a demon departing from a young man names the various body parts it intends to maim on the way out, but then only winds up ripping the eye out of the socket, such that it dangles by a single vein.[124] In Palladius's *Lausiac History*, there is a possessed boy who eats his own excrement and drinks his own urine, and another who—when subjected to exorcism—swells up like a wineskin and then returns to normal after emitting water through all of his "sense organs."[125] Germanus of Auxerre, in treating a demon-possessed eunuch brought to him (the boy apparently suffers falling seizures every month, at the new moon), finds that the demon "miserandi iuuenis medullas et interiora penetrauerat ut quasi uas proprium certis temporibus possideret" (had entered the marrow and the innermost parts of the miserable young man such that, at certain times, it was as if it controlled him as its own body).[126] The idiom of demon possession provided a conceptual model for expressing dysfunctions of the body and its processes, especially the more visceral and unpleasant ones.

Monks read about the distant temptations of the desert saints by demons, and of the oft-repeated dialogues between the martyrs and the devil. The demons of the body, however, were different. This is something that could be experienced firsthand by the farmers, fishers, spinners, and herders, and the mothers, fathers, sons, and daughters who came to their town healers or to the local clergy with suffering and hope.

Theoretical Models of Demon Possession

Possession medieval or modern is, at the broadest level, a relationship—at first between the sufferer and the immediate family, subsequently between the sufferer and the healer (priest, physician, etc.). This relationship is fundamentally adversarial, either because the community cannot tolerate the behavioral aberrations of an individual, or because (in the case of functional possession) the energumen him- or herself desires at some level to resist behavioral strictures. Simply criminalizing and punishing a potentially subversive or violent demoniac would be an easy, understandable mode of containing the problem, but in fact most traditional societies (including those of early medieval Europe) evince a wide range of responses. The perception of the individual as not being him- or herself anymore—that instead an indwelling spirit has taken over—largely absolves the individual and community of any immediate guilt, and allows for a formal ritual in which the subject can be reintegrated with the community after a process of heated venting, debate, and reconciliation.[127] What Anthony of Egypt says of a young man possessed by a demon—a man who physically attacked Anthony—generally holds for the treatment of the possessed throughout the Middle Ages: "Nolite alienam culpam juveni misero ascribere: furor iste obsidentis est, non obsessi" (Do not attribute the guilt of another to the pitiable young man: this fury comes from the possessor, not the possessed).[128]

While the primary caregivers (the family) respond to demoniacs in a variety of ways, motivated by any combination of emotions including empathy, anxiety, confusion, fear, and love, the priest or physician's essential task is to appear in control. The patient's own belief in the skills of the exorcist and in the efficacy of the rite contributes materially to the patient's regaining of personal control. For minor psychic or emotional disturbances, an exorcism may quickly restore mental health for an appreciable period. Fits or seizures of short duration, which subside on their own anyway, would appear as though responding to whatever popular rites and prayers (sometimes referred to as "charms"), herbal medicine, or exorcism therapy were immediately applied.[129] For more serious conditions, such as severe psychosis, and for primarily organic conditions, such as epilepsy, exorcism will at the very least provide the community with a narrative of what is happening, and thus allay broader social anxieties and maintain social order. Thus even failed exorcisms serve the important role of validating the energumen's behavior, allowing public expressions of pain and humiliation, and reassuring the community that no behavior—however erratic in appearance—is unprecedented or unmanageable.

In modern academic discussions, theoretical models of demon possession—which is still widely observable in churches, ministries, and other religious gatherings, as well as in isolated cases brought privately to the attention of a local priest or pastor—approach the phenomenon from two directions. On the one hand are biological and psychological models, which see the individual as principal locus. On the other are social and anthropological models ("functionalist" models), which see the community as principal locus. The first situate the phenomenon in an individual's brain chemistry, medical profile, or personal experience, while the latter read possession as a social behavior grounded in the human relationships within a community. Both approaches can potentially contribute to an understanding of possession in the early Middle Ages, with the understanding that in applying conclusions retrospectively, we move from the realm of observable phenomena to exclusively written documents.

For Freud, "'possessions' correspond to our neuroses . . . the demons are our depraved and rejected desires—our repressed instincts." He continues, "We reject only the projection of these psychic entities to the outside world, which the Middle Ages accepted. We hold they originate in the inner life of the patients, where they abide."[130] Pierre Janet likewise theorizes that the devil "is frequently embodied in human regrets, desires, and vices."[131] Such schools of thought as instinct theory and object-relations theory refined and developed these early models during the course of the twentieth century.[132] According to object-relations theory, for instance, the infant early on develops notions of good or bad objects, as perceived in the satisfaction or frustration of desires. The mother is inevitably viewed as both a provider and a depriver, since not all desires can be fully satisfied. As the infant progresses through childhood, the release of aggressive impulses is socially permissible to a certain extent, or else becomes channeled into socially acceptable behaviors. As a young adult or adult, however, a subject with particularly deep-rooted frustration or anger projects these emotions onto an external object—thus they are cast as a ghost or demon.[133] Such entities can even be projected within the subject's own body (sometimes called "introjects"): pregnant mothers commonly perceive their own babies to be foreign objects invading their bodies, for instance, and similar feelings of intrusion are well documented in transplant organ recipients and cancer patients.[134] Such individual-centered approaches guided clinical thinking on possession throughout the better part of the twentieth century.

In recent decades, socio-anthropological approaches have supplemented such models with the awareness that an individual only develops in the midst of intricate social networks.[135] According to this newer model, behavioral dysfunction or "illness" is a social construct operating within a matrix of cultural symbols given meaning by the community at large: "possession always implies a kind of theatrical interaction between actors and audience who share a repertory of cultural meanings and behavior."[136] Possession, for instance, might reinforce the power structures of community, priest, and God: "Exorcisms orchestrate a highly disciplined, hieratic message of authority and subordination, which they both enact and explain."[137] Conversely, the rite has been read as giving voice to the underrepresented in some societies; thus J. H. Chajes notes that women can sometimes "'use' the idiom of possession as an 'oblique aggression strategy' to overcome the limitations inherent in their position in society."[138] The drama of possession enacted at shrines and in churches allowed people the opportunity to articulate frustrations and vent emotions which would otherwise be unacceptable.

Gregory of Tours relates an interesting confrontation between King Theudebert and Bishop Nicetius of Trier, which becomes an opportunity for a certain man to rail against the king and express popular support for the bishop. The king tries to attend mass with several members of his retinue who have been excommunicated, and refuses to send them away when asked to do so. The bishop, in turn, refuses to say mass so long as they stay. The cause is championed unexpectedly by a local citizen, who breaks the stalemate:

> Subito exclamat unus de populo, arreptus a daemone puer iuvenis, coepitque voce valida inter supplicia torturae suae et sancti virtutes et regis crimina confiteri. Dicebatque episcopum castum, regem adulterum; hunc timore Christi humilem, illum, gloria regni superbum; istum sacerdotio inpollutum a Deo in posterum praeferendum, hunc ab auctore sceleris sui velociter elidendum.[139]
>
> [Suddenly one from among the people there—a young man seized by a demon—cried out and began to proclaim loudly, through the pains of his writhing, the virtues of the saint and the crimes of the king. And he declared that the bishop was chaste, the king adulterous; that the first was humble in his fear of Christ, the other proud in his royal magnificence; that this one would be found by God in the next life to be pure in his priestly duties, while that one would be summarily crushed by the author of his wickedness.]

This is not the sort of thing subjects tell their monarchs under common circumstances. After a half-hearted attempt to have the demoniac thrown out of church, however, the king acquiesces and instead sends out his own excommunicated followers. Immediately afterwards, as though willing to meet the king half way, Nicetius orders the unruly demoniac removed as well (although, due to his superhuman strength, it proves impossible to remove him without expelling the demon first). Here, the shocking spectacle may have defused a volatile and highly public showdown between the king and the bishop by introducing a common enemy (the demon) and by diluting the tense moment through a neutral distraction. Gregory specifies that relations are somewhat smoother between Theudebert and Nicetius following this episode. Peter Brown reads this scene as an instance of saint as mediator: the saint in late antiquity often served to reconcile the stalemate of power among village populaces and representatives of external, institutional authority. Public possession and exorcism as it evolved in the medieval church may often have performed the same role.[140] Elsewhere, Gregory writes of demoniacs "spewing forth abuses" against St. Julian: this provides a literary foil for the hagiographer's protagonist, but it may also reveal glimpses of mixed popular opinion concerning figures of standing.[141] Such functionalist approaches have brought us forward a great deal in understanding how possession can manifest itself in different cultural contexts, and how it can respond to important social anxieties.

Thus, while some researchers on possession stress physiological causes and others stress social causes, in most cases both can play a role. Few of the extant accounts from Anglo-Saxon England, however, give us much to go on in reconstructing power balances or social dynamics within a given case's family or community. Some of the most prominent aspects of possession as an expression of resistance against restrictive authority—for instance, the graphic sexual demonstrations or expostulations of possessed women in the Early Modern period—are virtually absent from early medieval sources.[142] Furthermore, when taken to the extreme, sociological models can make demoniacs into heroes, of sorts—pioneers of self-expression and empowerment in societies staunchly averse to disruptive behavior. While such a characterization may be applicable to Merovingian Gaul (to some extent) and the later Middle Ages (more certainly), the few sources from Anglo-Saxon England do not encourage such a valorizing assessment. Ours is a humbler story to tell. The Anglo-Saxon sources show us not victims of society but of their own bodies and brains. Thus I focus exclusively on possession rooted in organic, physiological processes (in so far as they can be reasonably inferred from the available descriptions), since they have more universality and thus serve more confidently as a bridge between our disorders and those of the early Middle Ages. It is only a single piece that I hope to illuminate of a much broader and more complicated puzzle.

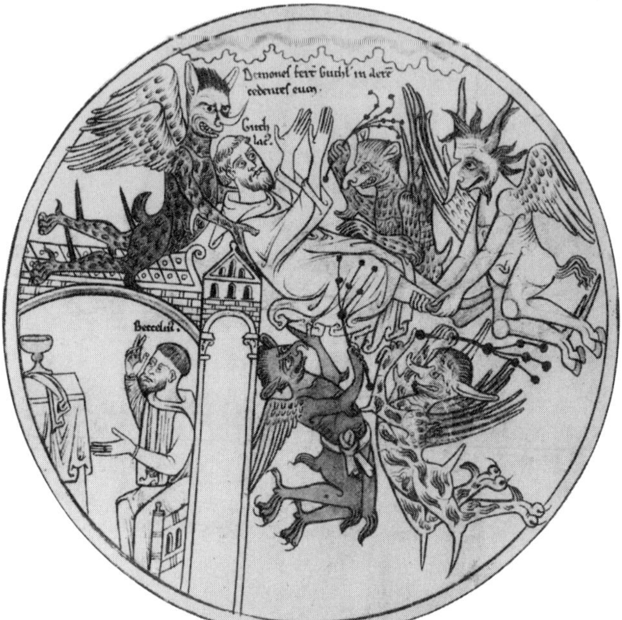

Figure 1. Roundel 7. British Library MS Harley Roll Y.6. (Photo: © The British Library Board.)

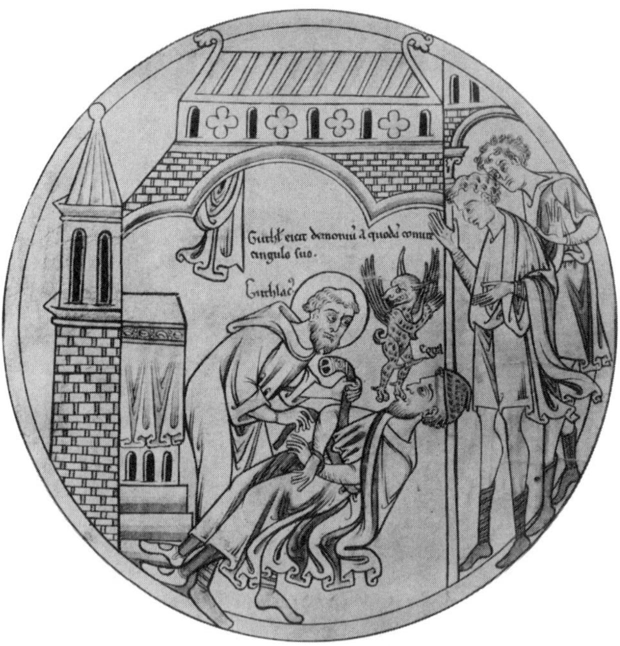

Figure 2. Roundel 10. British Library MS Harley Roll Y.6. (Photo: © The British Library Board.)

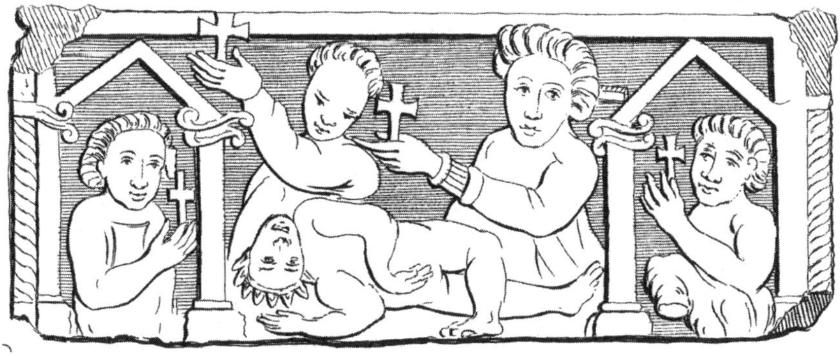

Figure 3. Bas-relief of an early medieval baptismal font from Perugia, Italy. (Photo: Reproduced from Paciaudi, *De Christianorum Balneis*, p. 212; Courtesy Pitts Theology Library, Emory University, Atlanta, GA.)

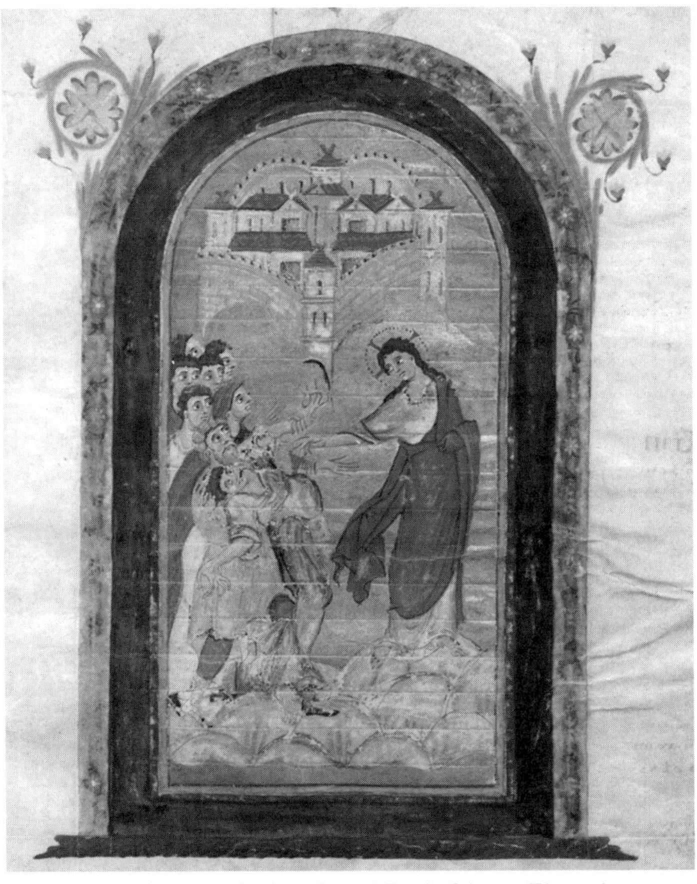

Figure 4. The Ottonian Aachen Gospel Book, fol. 88v. Eleventh century. (Photo: Ann Münchow; © Domkapitel Aachen.)

NOTES

1. See Kemp, "Ravished"; Kroll, "A Reappraisal."

2. Gregory of Tours, *Historiae* 8.34 (Krusch, *Historiarum*, p. 403); Bede, *Historia ecclesiastica* 2.5 (*HE*, p. 150).

3. Ælfric, *De initio creaturae* (Clemoes, *Catholic Homilies*, pp. 187–88). See also Ling, *Significance*, pp. 13–14, for discussion of apposition vs. distinction in passages relating to possession and illness.

4. Boureau, *Satan*, pp. 124–32.

5. Augustine, *De Genesi ad litteram imperfectus liber* 17 (Zycha, *Sancti Aurelii*, pp. 403–4).

6. *Vita Ælfredi* 74: "Multi namque furore [MS favore] et fascinatione circumstantis populi hoc factum esse autumabant; alii diaboli quadam invidia, qui semper bonis invidus existat; alii inusitato quodam genere febris; alii ficum existimabant, quod genus infestissimi doloris etiam ab infantia habuit" (Stevenson, *Asser's Life*, p. 55; "Many people asserted that this was brought about through the malice and evil incantation of those people around him; others thought it was from the envy of the devil, who always comes forth envious of the good; others, from an unknown kind of fever; and others judged it to be the piles, because he had had this kind of most troublesome pain from infancy"). On this passage, see Kershaw, "Illness"; Pratt, "Illnesses." Scholarly consensus maintains the traditional ascription of the *Life of Alfred* to a ninth-century contemporary of Alfred named Asser, though some prefer a tenth-century date with Byrhtferth of Ramsey as putative author (thus Smyth, *The Medieval Life*; Hart, *Learning*, vol. 2, bk. 1, p. 91).

7. Gregory the Great, *Dialogi* 3.35; *Dialogues*, vol. 2, p. 406. For discussion see McCready, *Signs*, pp. 230–32.

8. E.g., Gregory the Great, *Dialogi* 1.4, 1.10, 2.16, 2.30, et al.; *Dialogues*, vol. 2, pp. 44, 98, 186, 220. For general discussion see Petersen, *Dialogues*, pp. 51–52, 133–34.

9. Penelope Doob claims that illness is essentially a moral question in the Middle Ages (*Nebuchadnezzar's Children*, pp. 1–2), quoting Hrabanus Maurus to the effect that sickness implies guilt. She offers that this applies especially for possession: "Possession usually signifies wickedness" (16). Mirko D. Grmek concurs: "Despite the vigorous criticism of scholarly physicians or rationalist philosophers, most of the common folk—and indeed probably the majority of those working in the healing arts—refused to abandon the archaic belief that disease was the result of moral stains or the breaking of a taboo" (Grmek, "Concept," p. 257). Likewise Henderson, "Exorcism," p. 129; Rampolla, "A Mirror," p. 103.

10. *Vita Rusticulae* 13 (Krusch, *Passiones* [MGH, SRM 4], pp. 346–47).

11. Gregory of Tours, *Liber in gloria confessorum* 28 ("nescio quo exsistente peccato"; Krusch, *Miracula et opera*, p. 315). On sin and illness in Gregory, see Van Dam, *Saints*, pp. 87–89, 94.

12. Gregory of Tours, *Liber de virtutibus S. Martini* 2.40 (Krusch, *Historiarum*, p. 173).

13. See Janowitz, *Magic*, p. 35.

14. Thus, for instance, demons are routinely cast out alongside fevers and other infirmities in the New Testament (e.g., Matthew 17:14–18, Mark 1:32–34, Luke 4:40–41, Acts 5:16), while the devil is a moral agent who inclines souls to evil (e.g., Judas in John 13:21–27 and Ananias in Acts 5:1–3). See Kelly, "Devil," p. 195; Langton, *Satan*, p. 32; Yates, "Jesus," p. 43.

15. Bede, *Vita Cuthberti* 15 (Colgrave, *Two Lives*, p. 206).

16. Ælfric, *Depositio Sancti Cuthberti* (*Catholic Homilies* 2.10; Godden, *Second Series Text*, p. 85).

17. Finucane, *Miracles*, p. 72.

18. Kroll and Bachrach, "Sin and the Etiology," p. 411. In a somewhat different context, Valerie Flint makes a similar observation: "Demons come in and out, as it were, as counters, depending partly upon the writer, partly upon the audience to be addressed, partly upon the political and psychological circumstances within which the pastor believes he operates" (*Rise*, pp. 150–51).

19. Kroll and Bachrach, "Sin and Mental Illness," p. 511.

20. Kroll and Bachrach, "Sin and Mental Illness," p. 512.

21. Additions to Ecgbert's Penitential, item 29: "si homo quis animo suo vel mente sua exciderit, et ei aliquem occidere evenerit, solvant pro homine propinqui ejus, et eum contra simile quid servent" (Thorpe, *Ancient Laws*, p. 237; "if a man has lost control of his soul or his mind, and he should happen to kill a person, his relatives may pay satisfaction, and they may protect him against similar [charges]"). A provision in the *Laws of Henry I* which, as Nigel Walker and Basil Clarke believe probably reflects pre-Conquest custom, urges the criminally insane to be "compassionately" (*misericorditer*) left in the charge of their own family: "Insanos et eiusmodi maleficos debent parentes sui misericorditer custodire" (*Leges Henrici I*, 78.7 [Liebermann, *Die Gesetze*, vol. 1, p. 595]; "the insane and similar sorts of enchanters should be compassionately cared for by their parents"). See Walker, *Crime*, pp. 15–18; Clarke, *Mental Disorder*, p. 60.

22. Thus Oesterreich, *Possession*, p. 136. The modeling of possession behavior on more severe, demonstrably physiological disorders is intriguing. A new "spirit" appearing in 1976 in the French colony of Mayotte (an island off of Mozambique) adopted epileptic behavior as a model: "Only individuals possessed by this kind of spirit frothed at the mouth, and they did so only when actively manifesting the spirit . . . the frothing stopped as soon as certain substances were applied, such as a white sheet, said to be appreciated by this kind of spirit. People acknowledged the severity of the entry into trance, and the spirit did not become popular. They also acknowledged the similarity to epilepsy, but they pointed out that the spirit only mimicked the latter . . . epilepsy was only signifier but not signified" (Lambek, "From Disease," p. 42). Those with organic physiological disorders must, in fact, *learn* to interpret their own conditions as demonic: "Although it is generally believed that suggestible individuals develop the symptoms of possession as a result of a culturally influenced process, the chronically psychotic patients in our series presumably became persuaded that they were possessed secondarily to experiencing these symptoms of their underlying psychotic disorder" (Goff, Brotman, and Kindlon, "The Delusion," p. 570).

23. Ullrich, "Cultural Shaping," p. 649.

24. Ullrich, "Cultural Shaping," p. 649. For "bride sickness" manifesting itself as possession, see also Obeyesekere, "The Idiom," pp. 104–5; Colleen Ward, "Possession," p. 132.

25. Alarcón, Foulks, and Vakkur, *Personality Disorders*, p. 202.

26. Henderson, "Exorcism," p. 131.

27. Until recently, demon possession fell under "Dissociative Disorders Not Otherwise Specified" in the DSM-IV as "possession trance." The diagnostic guidelines caution, "The proposed disorder should not be considered in individuals who enter trance and possession states voluntarily and without distress in the context of cultural and religious practices that are broadly accepted by the person's cultural group" (DSM-IV, pp. 727–728). For recent findings and current status of the category, see First and Tasman, *DSM-IV-TR*, pp. 1043–46.

28. On contemporary exorcism, see Cuneo, *American Exoricsm*; and for a more global view, Goodman, *How about Demons?* (esp. pp. 52–63 for Pentecostalism in an international context).

29. Cuneo, *American Exorcism*, pp. 276, 275.

30. Vomiting: Sulpicius Severus, *Dialogi* 1.22 (Halm, *Sulpicii Severi*, p. 175). Shrieking and moaning (*ululare, ingemiscere*): Jerome, *Vita Hilarionis*, chap. 22; PL 23: col. 39A. Levitating: Palladius, *Lausiac History* 22, p. 64; Sulpicius Severus, *Dialogi* 3.6 (Halm, *Sulpicii Severi*, p. 204). For some important differences in the ongoing evolution of Christian healing in context from the New Testament to the present, see Porterfield, *Healing*.

31. Alarcón, Foulks, and Vakkur, *Personality Disorders*, p. 153.

32. See Kroll and Bachrach, "Medieval Visions."

33. Caciola, "Breath"; Caciola, *Discerning Spirits*; Newman, "Possessed by the Spirit."

34. Brock and Harvey, *Holy Women*, p. 110.

35. Gregory of Tours, *Historiae* 7.22: "vidissimus eum, ut ita dicam, agi a daemone" (Krusch, *Historiarum*, p. 341).

36. Felix, *Vita Guthlaci* 35 (Colgrave, *Felix's Life*, p. 112).

37. Felix, *Vita Guthlaci* 35 (Colgrave, *Felix's Life*, p. 112).

38. For expository discussions of demonology in late antiquity and the early Middle Ages, one must turn to sources such as Tatian's *Oratio ad Graecos* and Apuleius of Madaurus's *De deo Socratis* (for an early Christian and pagan view of demons, respectively, both from the second century); Athanasius, *Vita Antonii*, chaps. 15–20; Cassian, *Collationes*, bk. 7 (esp. 7.9–32) and bk. 8; Evagrius of Ponticus, *Praktikos*; Augustine, *De divinatione daemonum* and *De civitate Dei*, bks. 8–10; Isidore, *Etymologiarum libri XX*, esp. 8.11. For basic orientation (including both expository and non-expository backgrounds), see Walzel, "Sources"; but the most comprehensive and accessible overview is Jeffrey Burton Russell's four-volume study of the devil (for early Christianity, see *Satan*; for the Middle Ages proper, see *Lucifer*). In *Satan the Heretic*, Alain Boureau investigates the legal and theological causes of the birth of systematic (Scholastic) demonology in the late thirteenth and early fourteenth century.

39. Man possessed by legion (*legio*) of demons: *Miracula S. Austrebertæ* 19 (*Acta Sanctorum*, February 10, p. 425); Gregory of Tours, *De virtutibus Martini* 1.38 (Krusch, *Miracula et opera*, p. 156). One demon inhabiting two people: Braulio of Saragossa, *Vita Aemiliani* 15 (PL 80: col. 708A).

40. *Dominica Tertia in Quadragesima* (Morris, *Blickling Homilies*, p. 49).

41. *OE Martyrology*, July 22 (Kotzor, *Martyrologium*, vol. 2, p. 156).

42. *Spiritum prophetiae*; Gregory the Great, *Dialogi* 3.8 (*Dialogues*, vol. 2, pp. 285–86). Several chapters later (3.14), however, when an attendant is said to have a "spirit of pride" (*superbiae spiritu*), this may well imply an indwelling being because that spirit is exorcized (Gregory the Great, *Dialogues*, vol. 2, p. 304). Bede suggests that Queen Æthelthryth may have had the *prophetiae spiritum* (*HE* 4.19, p. 392).

43. Ferguson, *Demonology*, pp. 118–19.

44. Qumran Text 11 in Eisenman and Wise, *Dead Sea Scrolls*, p. 67.

45. Qumran Text 49 in Eisenman and Wise, *Dead Sea Scrolls*, p. 273.

46. *Testaments of the Twelve Patriarchs*, *ANF* 8, p. 9.

47. See Henri de Lubac's *Exégèse médiévale* (1959), available now in English (*Medieval Exegesis*). For the application of the fourfold model to Anglo-Saxon England, especially with reference to Bede's exegesis, see Gatch, *Loyalties*, pp. 83–94.

48. Aldhelm, *De virginitate*, chap. 4 (Gwara, *Aldhelmi Malmesbiriensis*, 2:59).

49. *Verba Seniorum* 5.11 (PL 73: col. 876B).

50. Flint, "Demonisation," pp. 284–85.

51. *Solomon and Saturn II*, lines 477–83 (Menner, *Poetical Dialogues*, p. 103).

52. *Guthlac A*, lines 114–16 (*ASPR* 3, p. 53).

53. Ælfric, *Dedicatio Ecclesiae S. Michahelis Archangeli* (Clemoes, *Catholic Homilies*, p. 473). See Richard F. Johnson, *Saint Michael*, p. 71.

54. See, for instance, the Qumran *Manual of Discipline* for a particularly bald statement of the principle (Dupont-Sommer, *Essene Writings*, p. 78 ff.). The tradition stems ultimately from the dualistic religions spreading from the East, most notably early Iranian Zoroastrianism.

55. This informs the *Shepherd of Hermas*, for instance, and the fourth-century writings of Evagrius Ponticus. In the *Praktikos* Evagrius catalogs an army of specialized demons, including the demons of impurity, vanity, *acedia* (spiritual sloth), pride, despair, and blasphemy (John Bamberger, *Evagrius*, chaps. 8, 12, 14, 19, 23, 25, 27, 28, 31, 33, 51). *Shepherd of Hermas*, chaps. 27, 100 (Joly, *Hermas*, pp. 146, 340). See also Jeffrey Burton Russell, *Satan*, p. 138 (for Origen) and pp. 182–84 (for Evagrius). In his *Collationes* (7.17), Cassian follows Evagrius: "unicuique uitio certos spiritus incubare" (Petschenig, *Iohannis Cassiani*, p. 195; "certain spirits nurture each individual vice").

56. O'Laughlin, "Evagrius Ponticus," p. 248. For the role of the demonic in Evagrius, see also O'Laughlin, "Bible."

57. Rufinus of Aquileia, *Historia Monachorum* XIII.3–4, pp. 333–34.

58. Rufinus of Aquileia, *Historia Monachorum* I.3.9, p. 257.

59. Boniface, Letter 73 (Tangl, *Die Briefe*, p. 153).

60. Boniface, Letter 73 (Tangl, *Die Briefe*, p. 153).

61. In this passage Boniface censures Ceolred for his sins (*peccantem*; Tangl, *Die Briefe*, p. 153), implying that the evil spirit's attack is just.

62. Boniface, Letter 10 (Tangl, *Die Briefe*, p. 9).

63. For a similar literary allegorization of demons as vices, see Ælfric's *Dominica v in Quadragesima*: "swa manegum leahtrum swa he gehyrsumað, swa manega deofla him beoð to hlafordum gesette" (*Catholic Homilies* 2.13; Godden, *Second Series Text*, p. 129; "as many sins as he gives in to, that many devils are set as masters over him"). This is an original passage by Ælfric, not appearing in the sources (Godden, *Introduction*, pp. 468–69).

64. Old English: Tiberius A.iii, chap. 19 (Clayton and Magennis, *Old English Lives*, p. 132); Latin: p. 214.

65. Hecht, *Dialoge*, p. 200; Gregory the Great, *Dialogues*, vol. 2, p. 304. The "spirit of prophecy" (*witegunge gast* in CCCC 322 or *witedomes gast* in Oxford, Bodleian Library, MS Hatton 76; Hecht, *Dialoge*, p. 130) appears frequently in the work also.

66. Chap. 38 (Schröer, *Die Angelsächsischen Prosabearbeitungen*, p. 62; Fry, *The Rule*, p. 236).

67. Wildhagen, *Cambridger Psalter*, p. 33; Liuzza, *Old English Version*, p. 131.

68. *OE Martyrology*, January 17 (Kotzor, *Martyrologium*, 2:18).

69. Jerome, *Vita Hilarionis* 24 (PL 23: col. 38c); *OE Martyrology*, October 21 (Kotzor, *Martyrologium*, 2:237).

70. The manuscript is too faded to make out the letters immediately following "eaðbylhnyssa gast."

71. Healey, *Old English Vision*, pp. 65–67. Since, as Wright points out, the work is apparently referred to by both Aldhelm and Ælfric, it evidently enjoyed popularity throughout the Anglo-Saxon period (*Irish Tradition*, p. 108).

72. Healey, *Old English Vision*, p. 78.

73. For a meditation of this problem in relation to Aldred, a tenth-century Anglo-Saxon glossator, see Boyd, *Marginalia*, pp. 17–19.

74. For basic orientation on monsters in Anglo-Saxon England and in the Middle Ages, see Bildhauer and Mills, "Introduction"; Mittman, *Maps*; Orchard, *Pride*; Verner,

Epistemology. Helpful essays also appear in Jones and Sprunger, *Marvels*, and Olsen and Houwen, *Monsters*. There is a basic awareness throughout the Middle Ages that demons constitute, in an important sense, an order distinct from animals—that they are "spiritual" beings. Demons do not appear in bestiaries, for instance. Jeffrey Burton Russell comments, "Still, monsters are not properly demons but are at least one step removed from them" (*Lucifer*, p. 79). See also, however, Francis Carmody, who traces the increasingly prominent place of the devil as the motivating spirit behind animal evil in the bestiaries ("Le diable").

75. For the significance of monsters in the construction of the relationship between humans and nature, see Gilmore, *Monsters*; Dendle, "Cryptozoology"; and Mittman and Dendle, *Ashgate Research Companion*.

76. Gregory the Great, *Dialogi* 2.1 (throws rock, *Dialogues*, vol. 2, p. 132), 2.9 (sits on stone, *Dialogues*, vol. 2, p. 170), 2.11 (pushes wall over, *Dialogues*, vol. 2, p. 172).

77. Augustine, *De civitate Dei* 22.8 (Dombart and Kalb, *Sancti Aurelii*, 2:572).

78. Gregory of Nyssa, *Life and Wonders* 92, p. 81; *Vita Caesarii ab eius familiaribus scripta* 2.22 (Morin, *Sancti Caesarii Episcopi Arelatensis*, p. 334). In Gregory of Nyssa's account, the demon only attacks those who come to the baths after dark. See Bonner, "Demons," for analogues and discussion.

79. *Vita Caesarii ab eius familiaribus scripta* 1.41 (Morin, *Sancti Caesarii Episcopi Arelatensis*, p. 313).

80. Adomnan, *Vita Columbae* 2.11 (Anderson and Anderson, *Adomnan's Life*, pp. 348–50), 2.16 (p. 360).

81. Pertzii, *Annales Fuldenses*, p. 52.

82. *Vita Dunstani auctore B* 18 (Stubbs, *Memorials*, pp. 28–29).

83. Thus *Guthlac A*, lines 151–53: "þæt lond gode fægre gefroþode, siþþan feond oferwon Cristes cempa" ("that he might protect the fair land of God, once the soldier of Christ overcame the enemy").

84. A refreshing exception to this type scene appears in the metrical *Vita Iudoci* (probably from tenth-century Winchester), in which the saint—upon discovering that his chosen location for a hermitage is beset with evil spirits—asks his patron Duke Haymo if he can go find another place instead (*Vita Iudoci*, lines 228–30; Lapidge, "A Metrical *Vita*," p. 284).

85. These figures (and their close counterparts in the Utrecht Psalter and the Eadwine Psalter) have been often interpreted as early depictions of elves, but Jolly demonstrates that they derive from Christian conceptualizations of spiritual foes rather than native ones ("Elves in the Psalms?").

86. Oesterreich, *Possession*, p. 77 ff. Rodewyk traces the origin of the terminological distinction to the eighteenth century (*Possessed by Satan*, p. 179; see pp. 178–85 for full discussion).

87. Kemp, "Ravished of a Fiend," p. 71. For a reading of early saints' lives that distinguishes the psychological deployment of demons from the merely sensational, see Kurtz, "From St. Antony," pp. 103–46. Kurtz argues that Felix's *Life of Guthlac* is the only early saint's life to recapture the psychological realism so deftly used in the *Life of Anthony*, while other early sources show more interest in "zoology" than in "spirituality" (130–31).

88. The term "infestation" is early: it appears for instance in the sixth-century *Vita Caesarii* (*diabolica infestatione*, Morin, *Sancti Caesarii Episcopi Arelatensis*, p. 313). There are still provisions for infestation in the 1999 revisions to the *Rituale Romanum*, though the infestation rite is now relegated to an appendix (appendix 1: "Supplicatio et exorcismus qui adhiberi potest in peculiaribus adiunctis ecclesiæ," in *De exorcismis* 71–77). I am grateful to

Fr. Andrew Cucchiari for relating to me his personal experiences with administering the rite of infestation, and for helping me interpret the spirit of the newly revised exorcism rites (June 29, 2001). For an analysis of the revised rites in their historical and theological context, see Van Slyke, "Ancestry."

89. Meaney, "And we forbeodað," pp. 486–93; also Blair, *Church*, p. 226.

90. Braulio of Saragossa, *Vita Aemiliani*, p. 17 (PL 80: cols. 708–9).

91. Alcuin, *Vita Willibrordi*, chap. 22 (Krusch and Levison, *Passiones*, p. 133).

92. The *Leechbook* bk. 3 (item 58) recommends hanging *rudniolin* ("water pepper"?) over the door to guard against *feondes costunge* ("temptation [or affliction] by the enemy"; Cockayne, *Leechdoms*, vol. 2, p. 342).

93. See Penitential of Theodore, chap. 146: "Ex aqua benedicta domus aspergendae sunt" (Finsterwalder, *Die Canones*, p. 250: "houses are to be cleansed by holy water"). Keefer suggests that the bridal chamber would probably be blessed before newlyweds employed it ("Manuals," p. 107). Note that many liturgical rites for asperging a "house" (e.g., Benedictio aquae spargendae in domo) refer to a "house of God" (*domo Dei*): that is, they are for the consecration of a church and not necessarily for a private habitation (see Willis, *Essays*, pp. 153–56, 164).

94. See Keefer "Manuals," p. 107.

95. Quammen, *Monster*, p. 431 (speaking specifically of natural predators, but equally applicable, I believe without violence to his context and intentions, to imaginary monsters as well).

96. Goodman, *Demons*, pp. 95–98.

97. E.g., the witch of Endor passage (1 Samuel 28:7–25).

98. Schmitt, *Ghosts*, pp. 6, 29; and see also Finucane, *Appearances*, pp. 29–48. For select medieval ghost accounts in translation, see Joynes, *Medieval Ghost Stories*.

99. Pócs, "Possession Phenomena," esp. pp. 89, 94–99, 111. For ghosts as possessing agents in the later Middle Ages, see Boureau, *Satan*, pp. 132–35.

100. On the relationship between fallen angels and demons, see Genesis 6:22 ff., 1 Enoch 15:8, 2 Enoch 18:3–5, Jubilees 5:2. See Bernard Bamberger, *Fallen Angels*, pp. 20–35, 74–81; Nash, *The Other Satan*, pp. 1–43; Jeffrey Burton Russell, *Devil*, pp. 191–97 and *Satan* (*passim*).

101. See Lohr, *Patristic Demonology*, pp. 43–57.

102. Einhard, *Translatio et miracula sanctorum Marcellini et Petri* 4.16 (Waitz, *Translatio*, p. 263). See also Augustine *De civitate Dei* 8.26 (Dombart and Kalb, *Sancti Aurelii*, 1:366).

103. Einhard, *Translatio et miracula sanctorum Marcellini et Petri* 4.16 (Waitz, *Translatio*, p. 263). See Matthew 12:43 and Luke 11:24 for an expelled demon forced to seek out "waterless" (*inaquosa*) regions.

104. Gregory of Tours, *Historiarum Libri X*, 6.29 (Krusch, *Historiarum*, p. 296). On the Archangel Michael as psychopomp, see Richard F. Johnson, *Saint Michael*, pp. 71–86.

105. Cynewulf, *Juliana*, lines 322 (*hellwarena cyning*), 311–515 (Woolf, *Juliana*, p. 35).

106. Cynewulf, *Juliana*, lines 420–24 (Woolf, *Juliana*, p. 40).

107. Athenagoras, *Plea* 26 (Schoedel, *Athenagoras*, p. 65). For more references, see Dendle, "*Solomon and Saturn*," pp. 392–94.

108. Pope, *Homilies*, vol. 2, pp. 667–712. See also David Johnson, "Euhemerisation."

109. See, for instance, Bede, *HE* 1.7, 1.21, 1.30, 2.4, 2.5, 2.10, 2.15, et al.; Willibald, *Vita Bonifatii* 6 (Levison, *Vitae Sancti Bonifatii*, p. 27); Boniface, Letters 21, 57 (Tangl, *Die Briefe*, pp. 35–36, 102–5).

110. Bede, *In Matthaei evangelium expositio* 1.4 (PL 92: col. 23D).

111. Alcuin, *Vita Willibrordi* 14 (Krusch and Levison, *Passiones*, p. 128).

112. Paciaudi, *De sacris Christianorum balneis*, pp. 136 ff., 143 ff. Dating of the vessel ranges from the fourth or fifth century (Lacroix, *Military and Religious Life*, p. 212) to the seventh (Paciaudi).

113. This evidently represents a symbolic conflation of catechumen and energumen, since no one in the midst of such throes would be suitable for the actual rite of baptism. For this reason, Smith and Cheetham postulate that it may not have been a baptismal font at all but a vessel perhaps for holy water in the atrium of a church (*Dictionary*, pp. 652–53).

114. Charcot and Richer, *Les démoniaques*, p. 8.

115. Colgrave, *Earliest Life*, chap. 22, p. 112; Hucbald of St. Amand, *Vita Rictrudis* 2.22 (*Acta Sanctorum*, May 12, p. 85).

116. Janowitz, *Magic*, p. 37.

117. *Sanguinem fetidum*: Gregory of Tours, *De virtutibus Martini* 2.37 (Krusch, *Miracula et opera*, p. 172); *purulentum nescio*: Gregory of Tours, *De virtutibus Martini* 2.34 (Krusch, *Miracula et opera*, p. 172); *purulentum nescio . . . cum sanguine*: Gregory of Tours, *De virtutibus Martini* 2.20 (Krusch, *Miracula et opera*, p. 166) and also *Vitae Patrum* 8.11 (Krusch, *Miracula et opera*, p. 250).

118. *Vita Rusticulae* 16: "quasi effigiem hominis sanguine plenam evomuit" (Krusch, *Passiones* [MGM, SRM 4], p. 346; "he vomited forth blood in the full likeness of a man").

119. Jonas of Bobbio, *Vita Columbani* 49 (PL 87: col. 1039A).

120. Gregory of Tours, *Liber in gloria confessorum* 9 (Krusch, *Miracula et opera*, p. 304).

121. Venantius Fortunatus, *Vita Radegundis* 1.28 (Krusch, *Fredegarii*, p. 373). Radegund crushes the worm under her foot.

122. Ear: *Vita Radegundis* 1.33 (Krusch, *Fredegarii*, pp. 374–75); pavement: *Vita Radegundis* 1.30 (Krusch, *Passiones*, pp. 374–75). Gregory of Tours likewise speaks of a man expelling a demon *per fluxum ventris* (*Liber in gloria confessorum* 9 [Krusch, *Miracula et opera*, p. 304]). *Fluxum ventris* may be envisioned variously as wind or liquid matter, expelled through the bowels. There is an interesting meditation on the expulsion of demons through the bowels in the *Liber Eliensis* (see Fairweather, *Liber Eliensis*, pp. 247–48).

123. *Vita Genovefae*, chap. 9, p. 142.

124. Augustine, *De civitate Dei* 22.8 (Dombart and Kalb, *Sancti Aurelii*, 2:573).

125. Macarius of Egypt: "saepe sua comedebat excrementa, et lotium bibebat" ("often he would eat his own excrement, and drink his own urine," *Historia Lausiaca*, chap. 19; PL 73: col. 1111C); Macarius of Alexandria: "per omnes sensus aquam emisit" ("he emitted water through all his senses," *Historia Lausiaca*, chap. 20; PL 73: col. 1117D).

126. Constantius of Lyon, *Vie de Saint Germain* 39, pp. 194–96.

127. Asch, "Depression," p. 152; Brown, *Cult*, p. 111.

128. Evagrius, *Vita Antonii* 36 (PL 73: col. 152D–153A). Venantius Fortunatus writes of a girl who suffers from long-term paralysis "undeservedly" (*non merito*; Krusch, *Venanti*, p. 10), and the *Sayings of the Desert Fathers* advises the reader to "hate sickness but not the sick person" (Benedicta Ward, *Sayings*, p. 233).

129. Murdoch, "Charms," pp. 64–67; see also Murdoch, "*Peri Hieres Nousou*," p. 147. Scholarly language is leaning away from use of the word "charms," which often carries presuppositions unwarranted in early medieval context (e.g., "magical" as opposed to devotional, superstitious as opposed to religious, supernatural as opposed to natural, heterodox as opposed to orthodox). Karen Jolly has pioneered this recalibration of terminology with regard to Anglo-Saxon texts (and of the associated shift in underlying critical approaches

to this material) in favor of terms such as "remedies," "popular rites," and "formulas," as, for example, in *Popular Religion*.

130. Sigmund Freud, "Eine Teufelsneurose im Siebzehnten Jahrhundert" ("A Case of Devil-Neurosis in the Seventeenth Century"), pp. 317–18: "Die Besessenheiten entsprechen unseren Neurosen . . . Die Dämonen sind uns böse verworfene Wünsche, Abkömmlinge abgewiesener, verdrängter Triebregungen. Wir lehnen bloß die Projektion in die äußere Welt ab, welche das Mittelaler mit diesen seelischen Wesen vornahm; wir lassen sie im Innenleben der Kranken, wo sie hausen, entstanden sein."

131. Janet, "Un cas," p. 56: "Le diable incarnait souvent les remords, les désirs et les vices des hommes." See also pp. 41–57.

132. See Graeme Taylor, "Demoniacal Possession," pp. 53–60.

133. Asch, "Depression," pp. 158–62; Henderson, "Exorcism," pp. 132–33.

134. Asch, "Depression," p. 159.

135. Thus, for instance, Lewis, "Spirit Possession"; Marsella, "Culture," p. 374. For application to early medieval saints and exorcism, see Brown, "Rise and Function," pp. 88–89.

136. Garrett, *Spirit Possession*, p. 7; see also Van Dam, *Saints*, pp. 84–85. For an overview of general anthropological approaches to possession behavior in social context, see Crapanzano and Garrison, *Case Studies*; Ferracuti, Sacco, and Lazzari, "Dissociative Trance Disorder"; Leavitt "Trance," p. 55; Colleen Ward, "Possession," pp. 128–30.

137. Caciola, *Discerning Spirits*, p. 267. Brown explains, "The dialogue between the possessed and the community, therefore, tends to have the stylised, articulated quality of an operetta. Possession and its working through is a way in which a small community can both admit and control disruptive experiences by playing them out" ("Rise and Function," p. 88). Elsewhere he argues that the drama serves important social functions: "To a late-Roman man the drama of exorcism was the one demonstration of the power of God that carried unanswerable authority" (*Cult*, p. 107).

138. Chajes, "Jewish Exorcism," p. 389. See also Lewis, "Spirit Possession"; Colleen Ward "Possession," p. 130, for women and possession.

139. Gregory of Tours, *Liber Vitae Patrum* 17.2 (Krusch, *Miracula et opera*, p. 279).

140. Brown, "Rise and Function," pp. 86–87. Van Dam concurs: "the ritual of healing therefore involved a process of reconciliation on several intersecting levels as disrupted communities and shattered selves were mended" (*Saints*, p. 93).

141. Gregory of Tours, *Liber de passione et virtutibus sancti Iuliani martyris* 30: "Inergumini vero cum advenerint, plerumque evoment in sanctum Dei convitia" (Krusch, *Miracula et opera*, p. 126; "When energumens came to him, they usually spewed forth abuses at the man of God").

142. See, for instance, Elliott, *Fallen Bodies*; Karlsen, *Devil*; Mary Keller, *Hammer*; Roper, *Oedipus*; Stephens, *Demon Lovers*; Zika, *Exorcising Our Demons*. By the end of the Middle Ages, with the growth of witchcraft beliefs, possession becomes inextricably linked with witchcraft: the indwelling spirit is believed to have been summoned deliberately by another member of the community. Thus, in Early Modern England the guilt that had been largely deflected to the spirit realm for many centuries is directed toward humans instead (see Raiswell and Dendle, "Demon Possession").

Chapter 1

Backgrounds to Anglo-Saxon Exorcism

Evil spirits haunt even the first extant literary records, and the primordial fears they embody—illness, death, darkness, and misfortune in general—may reach back to the earliest epochs of humankind's carving of the world into words. We will probably never know what the striking and sometimes monstrous figures appearing in the cave paintings of the Paleolithic represent, but in the inceptive literary records of the ancient Near East, evil spirits are already presupposed in sophisticated, highly elaborate demonologies. Many of these constructs survived in the scholarly textual traditions as well as in popular belief systems, changing and adapting continuously to new circumstances. The Anglo-Saxons were distant inheritors of both biblical and non-biblical vestiges of ancient Near Eastern scientific and religious beliefs, from the unlucky ("Egyptian") days and astrological materials so amply recorded in Anglo-Saxon prognostic manuscripts, to many of the rhetorical patterns appearing in the medical books and the liturgy.[1]

Demon possession, of course, extends well beyond the West, constituting an important dimension of ancient and medieval belief systems in, for instance, Indian, Chinese, and Arabic traditions as well.[2] It is not my intention here to provide a world overview, nor to trace routes of influence exhaustively, nor to provide a complete list of medieval demonological motifs derived from disparate ancient cultures. Select examples should suffice to suggest the overall picture. Independent routes of transmission through the Germanic and the Greco-Roman traditions came together in the conceptualizations of disease and forms of exorcism presupposed in Anglo-Saxon medicine, liturgy, and popular rites.[3] These conceptualizations find their distant roots in the underlying disease constructs of early Indo-European and Semitic cultures. Scholars have long puzzled over some of the striking parallels between widely disparate traditions, such as the rhetorical similarities between the second Merseburg Charm from medieval Germany and a recipe from the Sanskrit *Atharva Veda*.[4] I will indicate a number of parallels with some early traditions to provide a sense of the great diversity of potential beliefs that could persist for long periods of time, and to provide greater context for the Anglo-Saxon conceptualization of demons.

My main purpose in this chapter, however, is to set the stage for the emergence and development of exorcism within the early Christian tradition, to show that demon possession is not a uniform and universal phenomenon, and is not something that existed in stable, undifferentiated form—or even something that existed at all—in all the regions through which Christianity spread. Formative Christianity developed a particular series of behaviors and responses in concert with the peoples and traditions that adopted the religion as it spread. This is important because, as with so many elements of early medieval Roman Christianity, it is possible that outlying cultures such as the Anglo-Saxons and the Irish did not come fully under the sway of these behavior patterns. The educated churchmen of Anglo-Saxon England wrote about possession and exorcism much as they found it described in their source texts, but it is an entirely separate question whether possession "took" locally in the Anglo-Saxon population in the way that it did in a number of other Christianized cultures.

The Ancient Near East

Sumer has the earliest known literary tradition, preserved in abundant detail thanks to the resilient clay tablets that served as the writing medium, the dry conditions of the desert environment, and the laborious scholarly efforts of the Babylonians and Assyrians who studied that tradition for many centuries. Already the incantation and exorcism tablets of Sumer (starting ca. 2500 BCE) reveal a pervasive fascination with evil spirits, elaborated in a kaleidoscope of demons, beasts, and witches whose precise meanings and relationships are probably lost beyond adequate reconstruction. Misfortunes from a variety of causes are woven together in the incantation tablets, forming a seamless rank of the ills besieging humankind: disease, blight, bankruptcy, unrequited love, insomnia, and natural menaces such as serpents and scorpions. There are occasions in which medicine (physical remedy) seems to have been conceptually distinct from exorcism (spiritual remedy), though either or both could apparently be brought to bear on a given case.[5]

Some references in Mesopotamian incantations, which have significant narrative content, imply that a special class of priests conducted the rituals described therein. This class of priests apparently became more specialized over time: a shift in person of the speaker (from third person to first person) in the incantations suggests that what was originally spoken by the sufferers themselves was eventually assumed by the exorcist.[6] Whether or not there were originally secular, independent exorcists who could ply their magic or apotropaic skills, by the period of Standard Babylonian literature (the first millennium BCE), the exorcist (or *āšipu*) is associated primarily with the temple.[7] This well respected class of initiates—the keepers of occult knowledge—was principally entrusted with preservation of the king, the royal family, and wealthy clients.[8] A "*gudu* priest of Ningirim" is described as "releasing illness," and Ningirim is the deity invoked most often in the early Sumerian incantations.[9] She was apparently considered a goddess of magic and healing. The incantations invoke the aid of divine help, and so they blend effective magic and prayer; indeed, if divine help can be counted on in response to a direct appeal, the distinction between magic and prayer becomes illusory. Some passages imply that ritual gestures accompany the incantations—the laying on of hands or the sprinkling of water, for instance[10]—but entire rites from beginning to end cannot usually be reconstructed.[11] Curses are as common as cures in many early traditions; they too remained popular throughout the eastern Mediterranean well into the Christian era.

Many spirits in these texts are morally ambivalent. In pre-Sargonic Sumer we are first introduced to the notorious *udug-hul*, or "evil udug," though temple inscriptions also refer to *udug-sig*, or "good udug."[12] Gods as well as spirits can appear in these texts as harmful beings. Some incantations imply that the patient has transgressed in some way, but the majority treat illness as simple misfortune. Illness, as Hector Avalos notes, is often seen as divinely sanctioned, but this does not mean it represents divine reproof: the gods of Mesopotamia were creatures of whim.[13]

Incantations can be either therapeutic (curative) or apotropaic (preventive). Notions of binding and release are central to the conceptualization of illness presumed in these texts, with patients constricted or "tied" by their misfortunes, and priests and deities "releasing" them.[14] This metaphor survived into the European Middle Ages through a number of narrative and liturgical channels, and was still available to Ælfric of Eynsham, for instance.[15] A scene in his "Passio Bartholomei," from the first series of *Catholic Homilies*, has a possessed girl bound with fetters brought to the apostle. He orders her unbound, proclaiming to the reluctant attendants, "Ic hæbbe gebunden þone feond þe hi drehte, ⁊ ge gyt hi ondrædað? Gað to ⁊ unbindað hi" (I have bound the enemy that tormented her, and you still fear her? Go to her and unbind her).[16] Anglo-Saxons justified St. Peter's primacy as the first pontiff of Rome, and (through apostolic succession) as the establisher of the Catholic Church's primacy among all churches, by citing specifically his power to "bind" and to "loose."[17] An Anglo-Saxon ritual formula for joint pain reads, "Diabolus lignauit, angelus curauit" (The devil has bound, an angel has cured).[18] So thorough is the rhetoric of binding used to describe disease, in fact, that scholars are uncertain whether the first of the two tenth-century Old High German Merseburg Charms is meant to free a prisoner or to cure someone of a disease.[19] This insistence on who can bind whom as the operative trope for relative power draws from an ancient, well-established tradition traceable to the earliest texts of the ancient Near East. Bede seems to refer to popular beliefs of the seventh century regarding a written amulet employed to prevent physical restraint. A man who cannot be bound—chains fall off of him as soon as they are fastened—is believed by contemporaries to possibly have protective "loosing letters" (*litteras solutorias*) somewhere on him, "like those related in fables" (*de qualibus fabulae ferunt*).[20]

Groups of seven appear as a common motif in Mesopotamian healing incantations, usually as seven assailing demons or seven succoring deities. Of course, the number seven has long enjoyed symbolic status in Hebrew and other traditions, but seven can also abstractly represent "totality" or "unlimited number" in Sumerian, just as it would later for St. Augustine.[21] Thus it is possible this number is simply meant to represent demonic powers in the abstract or to imply that the full categorical range of demonic assaults is involved (as opposed to a single demon associated with a specific sin or infirmity). The New Testament refers to a demon that has been driven out of a person returning to that person with seven others (the strong man parable); elsewhere Mary Magdalene is said to have had seven demons driven from her.[22] Seven demons accompany the devil into Andreas's cell in the Vercelli Book poem *Andreas*—or else, on another reading, there are seven demons total (six plus the devil).[23] By the Middle Ages these passages were often interpreted allegorically, the demons being readily associated with the deadly sins. Thus Ælfric identifies the demon and his seven companions from the strong man parable as greed, fornication, avarice, ire, sloth, sadness, vanity, and pride.[24] Groups of seven demons form a tidy opposition to groups of seven archangels (Rev. 8:2).[25]

A common principle of Mesopotamian exorcism is the transfer of evil to a neutral carrier (usually a goat or a pig), a practice later recalled in the Gerasene demoniac episode in the Gospels. For instance, in one text preserved in Akkadian, the "evil eye" is transferred to a black, virgin ewe, which is then slaughtered, flayed, stuffed with some unidentifiable plant, and submerged in a river.[26] As a preliminary, the ewe is lifted up to each of the four corners within the afflicted man's house (to "absorb the evil," according to the editor).[27] Evil is viewed as an active force or substance—like the poison, or *attori*, of Anglo-Saxon medicine—rather than an imbalance of humors as in classical Hippocratic and Galenic medicine. This conceptualization of illness or misfortune as a reified entity is ubiquitous in these incantations, and so exorcism (driving out or expelling) is the central means of curing.[28] The rhetorical means of driving this "stuff" of evil from an infected person or house is to fragment and dissipate it, conceptually—to reduce it to its essential elements, each one of which is "isolated, and without strength."[29] Thus early exorcisms often consist of lengthy lists: lists of the demons implicated and their various activities, lists of body parts affected or societal misfortunes, and lists of things the demon will no longer be able to do once the rite is completed.[30] These catalogs of demonic natures, activities, strengths, and weaknesses are the precursors to medieval Christian exorcisms, through the implication that the exorcist has power over the demon primarily by having detailed, categorical knowledge of it. Numerous Latin prayers such as the Celtic Christian "Lorica of Gildas" and the "Alia super energumino baptizato" (item 2479 in the Leofric Missal) enumerate all the body parts to be protected by the power of prayer.[31] Old English vernacular texts also employ lists against demons, as in the litany of crimes extracted from the devil in *Juliana*, or the letters of the Pater Noster assaulting demons in orderly sequence in the poetic *Solomon and Saturn I*.[32] Remedies written in the margins of CCCC 41 by an Anglo-Saxon scribe imply that certain demons have dominion over certain parts of the body or certain provinces of illness, and the remedies call on angels to combat the demons specifically: Raphael is asked to help "shut out" (*exclude*) a certain Fondorahel from the ears, and Dormiel to help shut out the evil angel (*angelum malum*) Lanielem from the stomach.[33]

A general poison or "venom" appears as the disease agent in many tablets from the ancient Near East, similar in many ways to the "venom" charms of early Germanic and Anglo-Saxon demonology. One variant invokes the image of natural poisons ("on the man a wounding snake, a wounding scorpion, a wounding rabid dog has spat its venom"), while another attributes the poison to mythical entities named *ushumgal* and *shegbar*.[34] The almost metaphorical nature of these "venoms" reaches the surface in an Old Babylonian incantation which states that evil spirits are "the venom of the bile of the gods," and in a cylinder text that claims, "when my heart is angry . . . it produces venom for me."[35] Nine "poisons" referred to as *attre* and *onflyge* are the enigmatic villains of the Old English "Nine Herbs Charm."[36] A recipe against "flying poison" (*fleogendum atre*) is mixed with remedies for snake bites in the *Leechbook*.[37]

The worm (or serpent), another disease agent common in early medieval medicine, also abounds in the demonology of ancient Mesopotamia.[38] Bonser collects the various *wyrmas* from the medical texts of Anglo-Saxon England, including *ana-wyrm* (translation uncertain), *deaw-wyrm* ("dew worm"), *flæsc-wyrm* ("flesh worm"), *hond-wyrm* ("hand worm"), *rengc-wyrm* ("round worm" or "ring worm," translating the Latin *uermes circa umbilicum*), *smea-wyrm* ("penetrating worm" or "subtle worm"), and *þeor-wyrm* (translation uncertain).[39] The worms are said to "grow on" or "grow in" a person (*on men weaxe*), to "trouble" him "inside" (*innan eglað*), and to "eat his flesh" (*flæsc etað*).[40] The worm evidently embraced a broad spectrum, from actual worm parasites to airborne contagious diseases. Worm charms are also attested in Old High German and Old Low German (Old Saxon), contemporary with the Anglo-Saxon period. An Old Saxon charm of the tenth century exorcizes the worm, commanding it and its subordinates to depart in an elaborate chain of egress:

> Gang ut, nesso, mit nigun nessiklinon,
> ut fana themo marge an that ben, fan themo bene an that flesg,
> ut fan themo flesgke an thia hud, ut fan thera hud an thesa strala.[41]

> [Go out, worm, with nine lesser worms, out from the marrow into the bone, out from the bone into the flesh, out from the flesh into the skin, out from the skin into this arrow.]

At this point in the ritual, Stephen Glosecki surmises, an arrow held by the practitioner has become sympathetically identified with the worm or disease, and may perhaps be thrown or shot away as a symbol of casting away the disease.[42] It is difficult to reconstruct exactly what a healing ceremony might have actually looked like, either for the northern Europeans or for their Near Eastern forebears, but the continuity of rhetorical patterns in the extant rites suggests a continuity of underlying conceptions of illness.

In the ancient world, healing and harming magic often went hand in hand. For over a thousand years—stretching from around the fifth century BCE to around the seventh century CE—Palestine, Egypt, and large parts of the Greek-speaking world preserved in the magical papyri of Egypt and the ubiquitous curse scrolls and tablets many aspects of ancient Near Eastern magic and demonology. A variety of gods and powers are invoked in these records, and just as many demons and alleged witches are warded off. Alongside prayers and spells meant to protect from gods or spirits are prayers and spells to send the same spirits against an enemy. Lead tablets came to replace clay ones, and though their use was increasingly private, rather than public and ceremonial, the continuity of tone and content is evident.[43] This tradition was strong in imperial Roman Britain also: sizeable caches of lead and pewter curse tablets have been unearthed in Bath and Uley, Gloucestershire.[44] Some five hundred curse tablets are extant in Latin, mostly from the second century CE onward.[45] John Gager argues that the Christian loricae of the early Middle Ages, such as that found in the *Lacnunga*, were indebted to the curse tablet tradition.[46]

There are no curse tablets, however, from Anglo-Saxon England. Lester Little discusses some poetic echoes of cursing in the *Battle of Maldon*, but the curses of the Latin charter tradition are more obvious analogues.[47] Following continental exemplars, hundreds of extant charters include curse provisions for those who alter or repeal the charter's dictates. Appearing in both Latin and Old English, these curses often threaten the wrath of God and eternal damnation, as part of a spiritual economy whose practical currency is property rights.[48] Popular cursing also surely continued to exist in some form; some of the formulas offer protection against what might be cursing, such as "wiþ ælcre yfelre leodrunan" ("against every evil sorcery" or "sorcerer").[49] The vast bulk of surviving curses, though, are bookish boilerplate from the monasteries, and are more the provenance of the literate clergy than of uneducated seers and wonder workers. In this sense, the overall profile of Anglo-Saxon curses represents a notable departure from the curse traditions of Roman Britain. The spectrum of magic and demonology documented in Anglo-Saxon England evinces some fundamental differences from the late Roman world, perhaps reinforcing the need for caution when extending late Roman patterns of possession to the Anglo-Saxons.

Late Roman patterns of possession, in fact, may have been largely alien to the ancient Near East, even though so many other rhetorical and conceptual tropes emerge from that cultural milieu. Since virtually all of the various ills and afflictions of the Mesopotamian magico-medical records are attributed to "demons" of various sorts, demonic assault in early Mesopotamia and Egypt did not necessarily mean possession as we think of it, involving a radical change in the patient's personality. Doubtless those possessed had insanities, and doubtless many considered these the work of demons, but insanities or personality disorders are not markedly differentiated as a distinct type of demon or a specific kind of ailment. Marten Stol objects to the use of the word "exorcist" at all in describing these ancient Near Eastern texts (he prefers "conjurer"): "So far as I am aware there is no Babylonian evidence for possession at all."[50]

Perhaps the earliest story that does possibly indicate possession as we think of it comes from a stele at Karnak, Egypt (probably fourth century BCE). Rameses II's sister-in-law Bentresh is stricken with a demon: a sickness has invaded her body or limbs, and she is said to be "in the condition of one possessed of a spirit."[51] Upon arrival of the god Khonsu (one of whose epithets is Smiter of Evil Spirits), sent by Rameses, Bentresh is immediately cured.[52] We know that this case is one of personality displacement rather than a muscle disorder or generic physical ailment, since an alien spirit speaks through Bentresh's voice:

> Then said this spirit which was in her before Khonsu-the-Plan-Maker-in-Thebes: "Thou comest in peace, thou great god . . . I am thy servant. I will go to the place whence I came. . . ." Then the spirit departed in peace to the place he desired, by command of Khonsu.[53]

The indwelling spirit and the exorcizing deity are reconciled, and a feast day is celebrated to commemorate the arrival of Khonsu in Bekhten. Though admittedly confusing, the wording suggests that Bentresh's condition (1) is considered an illness (rather than a positive trance state), (2) involves a dysfunction in her limbs, and (3) involves an alien presence within her—all of which resemble demon possession. The amicable settlement reached between this spirit and the god who cures her, however, implies a social understanding of possession far different from the adversarial dramas of later forms of exorcism.[54] In contrast with this reconciliatory exchange, the antagonistic and uncompromising dialogue between energumen and exorcist would become one of the more consistent hallmarks of exorcism in the Western tradition.

The Early Jewish Tradition

The question of whether or not demonic possession had already appeared in the Old Testament must inevitably turn to the only unequivocal analogue there, the intriguing attacks that plague Saul in 1 Samuel.[55] Saul is said to be tormented by an "evil spirit," referring to a series of sporadic fits of frenzy,[56] and he becomes violent, once throwing a spear at David.[57] David is usually able to soothe him and return him to his normal state by playing the lyre: "the evil spirit [*rah-ruwach*] would depart from him."[58] Saul has been cited as suffering from manic depression, bipolar disorder, and nonspecific psychotic states, to name but a few.[59] In any event, no other mental disturbance in the Old Testament—such as Nebuchadnezzar's period of living in the wilderness as an animal, eating grass and growing his hair and nails (Dan. 4:28–33)—is explicitly demonized. Medieval commentary traditions would, of course, retrospectively read the activity of demons into many scriptural episodes.

In the first century CE Josephus clearly thought there was possession in the Old Testament period: in his *Antiquities* he repeats the common belief that Solomon bequeathed to posterity the knowledge of driving out demons.[60] Probably this tells us more about Josephus's time than about Solomon's, however (in retelling the story of King Saul's madness, for instance, Josephus recasts the king as being inhabited by plural *daimonia*—reminiscent of New Testament demonology—rather than the Old Testament's single "spirit").[61] Josephus believed that demons were disembodied souls (of the dead, for instance) that could enter victims' bodies and kill them. These spirits could easily be driven out through the root of the "baaras" plant.[62] Jewish apocryphal and pseudepigraphal writings contain rich and colorful descriptions of demons, but these are often abstract, symbolic visions of cosmic forces, set against mythological backdrops.[63] The writings are not much help in gathering information about mundane occurrences, such as human illness and possessing demons. Explicit references to possession only appear in later, and very likely Christianized, redactions (e.g., Testament of Solomon and Testaments of the Twelve Patriarchs).

Frederick Cryer surmises that exorcistic and apotropaic magic must have been common in Syria-Palestine throughout the formative period of the Old Testament, despite the reluctance of the Old Testament to address it.[64] The archaeological evidence of incantation bowls from the last few centuries BCE and the first few centuries CE reveals a different dimension of Jewish popular belief than that preserved in the orthodox textual tradition. According to Rebecca Lesses, "The incantation bowls thus preserve a glimpse into a particular area of Jewish culture not ruled by the rabbis: spells and rituals that ordinary people employed to rid themselves of demons and the ills they caused."[65] For instance, she traces in detail how the early Jewish apotropaic texts metaphorically employ the terminology of divorce to drive away the unwanted spirit or *lilith*.[66] Erica Hunter notes that Jewish, pagan, Gnostic, and Christian material culture reflects notable overlap and integration among these various communities, and in fact it is sometimes difficult to decide to which tradition a given bowl is to be ascribed.[67] Jewish popular rites of the early Middle Ages—such as that for a "man who has had a stroke and half of him is dried up, either by an [evil] spirit or by witchcraft," and one to "drive off an evil spirit so it will not come to a woman when she is in childbirth and so it will not kill her child"—are strongly reminiscent of Babylonian magico-medicine.[68]

Acts 19:11–16 speaks of itinerant Jewish exorcists in Ephesus contemporary with Paul's life, although in that episode the seven sons of the Jewish high priest Sceva are unsuccessful in their exorcism attempts. Just as Josephus believed that demon possession was part of Old Testament Hebrew culture, so also he cites contemporary demoniacs in the time of Vespasian (69–79 CE), and recounts an instance which he claims to have personally witnessed:

> I have seen a certain Eleazar, a countryman of mine, in the presence of Vespasian, his sons, tribunes and a number of other soldiers, free men possessed by demons, and this was the manner of the cure: he put to the nose of the possessed man a ring which had under its seal one of the roots prescribed by Solomon, and then, as the man smelled it, drew out the demon through his nostrils, and, when the man at once fell down, adjured the demon never to come back into him, speaking Solomon's name and reciting the incantations which he had composed.[69]

The efficacy of the exorcism is demonstrated by means of a vessel of water placed a little way from the demoniac, which is overturned at the demon's departure. Somewhat later, in the Rabbinical commentary tradition, Rabbi Simeon ben Jochai (mid-second century CE) mentions a demon who enters the daughter of the current emperor. The rabbi calls the demon by name and commands it, "Ben Temalion, get out! Ben Temalion, get out!"[70] The Rabbinic traditions also refer to a certain Chanina ben Dosa (first century CE?) as an exorcist, but none of the extant stories about him relate the sort of exorcism (casting demons out of a person) familiar from the New Testament.[71] The traditions of the Mishnah generally have more to say about demons inhabiting physical locations or being made to perform errands than about demons entering bodies and displacing personalities. The *dybbuk* of more recent Jewish tradition is an evil spirit who enters the body and displaces the person's identity, but the word does not appear before the sixteenth century.[72] Jewish belief in spirit possession evidently blossomed in the sixteenth century, accompanying the general European explosion of witchcraft and demoniac phenomena also occurring at that time.[73] As in the ancient Near East and throughout the Hellenistic Mediterranean world, references to "demons" and "exorcism" in early Judaism were so broad as to encompass most diseases and misfortunes, and so it is hard to sift out when references to "demons" may have designated indwelling demons that take over the mind.

The tantalizing references in the Dead Sea Scrolls, for instance, of the first century CE, generally sound more allegorical than descriptive of actual behavioral phenomena.[74] The Scrolls are formal, stylized texts steeped in the metaphorical language of light and darkness. Demons are not necessarily distinguished from illness or from moral corruption as a whole. The Dead Sea Scrolls certainly contain passages that envision demons entering the body; in the Genesis Apocryphon, Pharaoh asks Abraham to heal him:

> "And now pray for me and my house that this evil spirit may be expelled from it." So I prayed [for him] . . . and I laid my hands on his [head]; and the scourge departed from him and the evil [spirit] was expelled [from him], and he lived.[75]

Douglas Penney and Michael Wise draw attention to a (somewhat fragmentary) incantation amidst a series of proverbs, detailing more specifically what sorts of spirits can enter the body:

> . . . Beel]zebub, you/to you [. . .
> . . .] the midwife, the punishment of childbearers, an evil visitant, a de[mon . . .
> . . . I adjure you all who en]ter into the body, the male Wasting-demon and the female Wasting-demon
> . . . I adjure you by the name of YHWH, "[He who re]moves iniquity and transgression," O Fever and Chills and Chest Pain
> . . . [and forbidden to disturb by night in dreams or by da]y in sleep, the male Shrine-spirit and the female Shrine-spirit . . . [76]

Given the background of ancient Near Eastern demonology in general, it is hard to be sure that these references are to indwelling demons who alter personality and behavior. In this context, all diseases and misfortunes (such as fever and chills or chest pain) could be reified as demons that descend upon a person or enter into him, without implying displacement of identity. Nonetheless, recent commentators such as Sorensen and Penney and Wise argue for the existence of possession and exorcism among the Qumran community.[77] Penney and Wise argue that the more the Dead Sea Scrolls are made accessible (especially since 1991, with the release of a facsimile edition), the clearer it is becoming to what extent early Jewish sects could turn to popular magic, rather than Mosaic law, for their conceptualizations of the demonic.[78]

The literate rabbinic tradition on the whole, however, shied away from what it considered magic and popular superstition, and in fact some early Jewish writers were manifestly skeptical of popular belief in possession. The *Pĕsikta dĕ-Rab Kahăna* (fifth century CE) records Rabbi Johanan ben Zakkai—a rough contemporary of Josephus—as engaging a gentile in a discussion on impurity, and citing demon possession as an off-hand analogy. The non-Jewish interlocutor accuses the Jews of witchcraft and superstition because they claim to remove "impurity" through the sprinkling of ashes. The rabbi rebuts the gentile interlocutor thus:

> Rabban Johanan asked the heathen: "Has the spirit of madness ever possessed you?"
>
> He replied, "No."
>
> "Have you ever seen a man whom the spirit of madness has possessed?"
>
> The heathen replied: "Yes."
>
> "And what do you do for such a man?"
>
> "Roots are brought, the smoke of their burning is made to rise about him, and water is sprinkled upon him until the spirit of madness flees."
>
> Rabban Johanan then said: "Do not your ears hear what your mouth is saying? It is the same with a man who is defiled by contact with a corpse—he, too, is possessed by a spirit, the spirit of uncleanness."[79]

The rabbi correctly presumes that spirit possession and exorcism will be a scene familiar to the gentile, but this does not mean that the rabbi himself subscribes to those beliefs. As soon as the interlocutor leaves, in fact, the rabbi's disciples ask him why he gave the gentile such an unsatisfactory answer, and ask for a straight response now that the outsider is gone. He answers that it was simply an analogy: the corpse itself does not have the power to defile, any more than the ash and water mixture has intrinsic power to cleanse. If the rabbi here means to combat the charge of superstition, which is clearly the context, then the obvious implication is that the "uncleanness" of the corpse is no more an entity or force than the "demon" within the mad person. Both are convenient symbolic codes, and the "demons" of madness are thereby demythologized.[80]

These sources—gathered from different genres, centuries, and geographic provenance, and many of them hard to date—leave only an imperfect sense of the prominence of possession in early Jewish societies from the Old Testament period through the early Middle Ages. Many commentators presume that possession was a vibrant facet of popular Jewish religion throughout late antiquity and the Middle Ages.[81] Much later, Jewish possession surfaces (or resurfaces) more certainly and more prominently in the accounts of *dybbuk* in the sixteenth century. However, despite the paramount importance of early Jewish beliefs on formative Christianity, the particular profiles of possession and exorcism in early medieval Christendom do not find extensive parallels in late antique Judaism. The Talmud is rife with demons, but these are monsters of the wilderness rather than indwelling pathogens which supplant a victim's personality. The time of Jesus seems to have coincided with an unusual upsurge in the prevalence of Jewish accounts of demon possession (at least in Roman-occupied Palestine), if the Gospel accounts are in fact reflective of general historical trends. Because of the New Testament's insistence on the special prominence of possession in first century Palestine, and because of the subsequent importance of the New Testament, this was the form of possession that became widely disseminated throughout Christian society.

Greece, Rome, and the New Testament

In the archaic and classical periods of the Greek world, "daimons" were ambivalent forces that mediated between the gods and humankind. Sometimes they were visualized as sentient beings, other times as impersonal forces. In many of the accounts, the *daimonic* is simply another facet of the divine: for example, for Homer, the "daimons" are the gods whom humankind would do well to obey,[82] while authors such as Hesiod and Euripides treat demons as the souls of the deceased.[83] As an impersonal divine force, *daimones* came to carry the sense of "fate," either good or bad. There is a neutral sense in Hesiod's "whatever be your lot [*daimoni*], work is best for you."[84] As with most appeals in any time or place to "luck," "destiny," "fate," or one's "lot," however, the general sense seems have been negative and consolatory: thus Odysseus and Oedipus both revile the *daimonos* that led them to their miserable states.[85] Pindar treats *daimones* as spiritual influences that can be either good or evil.[86] As late as the first century CE, Philo of Alexandria still holds a neutral position toward the moral nature of the daemonic: "Those whom the philosophers designate 'daemons,' Moses is accustomed to call angels. These are souls that fly through the air . . . souls, daemons, and angels are but variant names for one and the same underlying object."[87] As in Mesopotamian medicine, however the demons were envisioned (semidivine entities, disembodied souls of the deceased, etc.), they were at least potentially harmful to the individual, and could be warded off or supplicated through a variety of means.[88]

In the classical Greek world, priests or priestesses at oracle shrines would become "possessed" by the gods and assume an alien persona. People in such a trance may have seemed to be demonstrably infused by another being: for instance, a female may have spoken with a male voice, or a "possessed" man may have spoken of matters outside his common range of knowledge.[89] These were socially sanctioned trance states, rather than illnesses. There is some evidence that epileptic fits were considered forms of divine or daimonic possession also, most notably in the Hippocratic tracts "On the Sacred Disease" and "On the Maladies of Young Women."[90] "On the Sacred Disease" (fourth century BCE) endeavored to show that epilepsy was not caused by *daimones* (whether divine or demonic), but by the blockage of cerebral phlegmatic vessels. Wesley Smith, however, has argued forcefully that what we think of as demonic possession did not exist in ancient Greece and has only been read back into the sources erroneously. He notes that the first clear case of it in pagan literature (in Lucian of Samosata, in the second century CE) is of a Syrian exorcist from Palestine.[91] This implies that the phenomenon was a cultural borrowing and not an indigenous phenomenon: "the widespread and growing belief in possession around the beginning of the Christian era may have been a new development."[92] S. Vernon McCasland takes the absence of any reference to possession in Pausanias, who prolifically documented the routines at many healing shrines, to support this.[93] As Naomi Janowitz observes, when

Plutarch later (second century CE) theorized about the origins of demonological beliefs, he looked around to various foreign cultures: he "did not even consider the possibility that the contemporary daimonology was Greek in origin."[94] The emergence of possession and exorcism in Greece and Rome during the first few centuries CE possibly means that the rite was filling a growing social need, perhaps one left by the deteriorating religious and health care structures of centralized Roman authority in the late Empire.[95]

Healings, including exorcisms, were an integral component of Jesus's ministry. The New Testament consistently portrays illnesses of all types as battles in the ongoing spiritual war between the forces of light and of darkness. Demons suddenly appear in the New Testament not as the chaotic throngs of zoomorphic desert creatures long familiar in Egyptian and Mesopotamian lore but as invisible moral agents which, under the power and guidance of a single master, mount a concerted attack against the human species. It is the unity of this kingdom of evil that Jesus repeatedly emphasizes in his numerous encounters with demoniacs.[96] In fact, Jesus regularly reifies diseases as sentient beings, and sometimes casts them out no differently than he casts out spirits. Thus he "rebukes" a fever to depart and "rebukes" the wind to calm, using the same word with which he "rebukes" an unclean spirit (*επετιμησεν*).[97]

Jesus characterizes his own ministry as a "work" of exorcism and healing: "Listen, I am casting out demons and performing cures today and tomorrow, and on the third day I finish my work" (Luke 13:32). It is possible that it was his activities as an exorcist that attracted the jealousy of his contemporaries.[98] The synoptics relate five specific demoniac encounters, mostly derived from Mark: the Capernaum demoniac, the Gerasene (or Gadarene) demoniac, the Syrophoenician woman's daughter, the epileptic boy, and the blind and dumb demoniac in the Beelzebub controversy.[99] The Gospel stories portray the demoniacs—or the demons within them—as responding wildly to the very presence of Christ: "Whenever the unclean spirits saw him, they fell down before him and shouted, 'You are the son of God!' But he sternly ordered them not to make him known."[100] The apostles, Paul, and even itinerant strangers are described as performing exorcisms, both successfully and unsuccessfully. The general features of these brief narratives—such as the demon falling down at Jesus's approach and identifying him—would influence exorcism narratives throughout the Middle Ages. In the *Life of Hilarion*, for instance, St. Hilarion, who wishes only to remain anonymous, is plagued by demons announcing him publicly wherever he goes.[101] Additionally, the New Testament provides a number of more general statements about Jesus performing exorcisms and healings (such as Mark 1:34: "he cured many who were sick with various diseases, and cast out many demons"), statements which are again echoed throughout medieval hagiography.

Unlike other exorcists of his day, Jesus did not recite lengthy formulae or follow complicated procedures in casting out demons. He eschewed ancillary materials such as amulets, incense, knots, milk, or ashes. For him, a simple word of adjuration usually sufficed,[102] and he cast out demons through direct command (Matt. 17:18, Mark 1:25, 5:8) and prayer (Mark 9:29). He even cured a woman's daughter without being in her presence: he simply announced to the woman, after she came to him for help, that her daughter is already cured (Mark 7:30). Jesus's disciples were able to mimic his success by casting out demons in his name (Luke 9:49, 10:17). The New Testament emphasizes that the source of power behind all of these exorcisms, including those of Jesus, is the power of God, not the power of the exorcist or any powers inherent in the rites performed. Jesus claimed that the power to heal comes from the "Spirit of God" (*Spiritu Dei*, Matt. 12:28) or the "finger of God" (*digito Dei*, Luke 11:20). Thus the Gospel writers were less interested in tabulating the numbers of Jesus's successful healings than in portraying him as a qualitatively new divine presence: one sustaining an unprecedented, publicly acknowledged challenge to the forces of cosmic evil. The backdrop—and *sine qua non*—for these public dramas is a countryside teeming with demoniacs, paralytics, and other sufferers, who come long distances to appeal to Jesus's healing powers.

The ability to heal and cast out demons was among the preeminent selling points of early Christian evangelism, if writers of the apostolic and patristic periods can be believed.[103] The success of Christians in driving out demons was a crucial empirical test proving their religion to be the true one.[104] Justin Martyr, for instance, boasts that Christians prove their religion through the casting out of demons.[105] He justifies the universal rightness of the Christian faith by its ability to cast demons even out of pagans:

> Many demoniacs throughout the entire world, and even in your own city, were exorcised by many of our Christians in the name of Jesus Christ, who was crucified under Pontius Pilate; and our men cured them, and they still cure others by rendering helpless and dispelling the demons who had taken possession of these men, even when they could not be cured by all the other exorcists, and exploiters of incantations and drugs.[106]

Elsewhere he specifies that exorcisms conducted in the name of Christ are invariably successful; that those conducted in the names of prophets, patriarchs, or mortal kings invariably fail; and that those conducted in the name of the God of Abraham, Isaac, and Jacob may or may not be successful.[107] Irenaeus likewise attests that the efficacy of these exorcisms draws new recruits to the Christian religion.[108]

Since the success of Christian exorcisms was presented as confirming the truth of that religion, apologists necessarily felt threatened by the success of non-Christian exorcists. The ascetic sage and healer Apollonius of Tyana, a first-century figure whose memory was kept alive by numerous shrines and eulogistic writings, became a key figure in this controversy. Among the many works describing Apollonius's virtues and miracles, one of the few to survive is Philostratus's ambitious *Life of Apollonius of Tyana* (early third century).[109] Origen had berated Apollonius as a sorcerer, and it was Philostratus's purpose to defend Apollonius against such charges.[110] Philostratus includes two stories of possession. In the first, a woman comes to a group of Indian wise men who are discussing philosophy. She explains that her sixteen-year-old son is possessed by a demon (*δαιμον*), the spirit of a departed soldier. Her son seeks solitude and, she says, "his eyes, too, are more someone else's than his own."[111] The boy threatens violence to himself, speaking in the voice of a grown man, and the mother despairingly laments, "he does not recognize me."[112] In response, the sage Iarchas produces a letter of adjuration and tells the woman to deliver it to the boy. We are not subsequently told whether or not the written rebuke was effective.[113] In the context of Apollonius's travels to the East, this possession of the Indian boy—described in such detail—is presented as something of an exotic wonder.

Elsewhere, Apollonius himself encounters a demoniac, a young Greek man who laughs and cries seemingly without cause and who talks to himself. In Philostratus's narrative, Apollonius is the first to identify this person's behavior—which seems merely eccentric on the surface—as demonic. The drunken revelry of youth is simply the demon's clever cover. The demon howls in pain as Apollonius confronts him with his true identity and, as in Josephus's exorcism, Apollonius orders the demon to give some tangible sign of his departure. The young man's response is striking:

> The youth, as if waking up, rubbed his eyes, looked at the sun's beams, and won the respect of all the people gazing at him. From then on he no longer seemed dissolute, or had an unsteady gaze, but returned to his own nature no worse off than if he had taken a course of medicine.[114]

Such isolated passages describing non-Christian exorcism are invaluable, hinting at a wider range of social roles and contexts for exorcism than orthodox Christian sources allow. There is no consensus on how prevalent these phenomena—primarily available to us through Christian sources—were, on the whole, in Jewish and pagan societies of the first few centuries of our era. F. C. Conybeare assumes that "demoniac possession was a common feature in the ancient landscape."[115] Johannes Geffcken agrees that "pagans expelled evil demons as zealously as did the Christians"; but more recently, Aryeh Kofsky counters that Geffcken's claim "is not corroborated by literary evidence."[116] Sorensen argues that exorcism was originally "an unconventional activity in Greco-Roman society during Christianity's early centuries," but one which eventually "flourished to make the transition from superstition to institution."[117] That is, it became accepted and even promulgated by the educated. Rather than simply providing a more effective means of exorcism, Christianity itself may have been what spread possession and exorcism behavior throughout the Roman Empire and to regions beyond. Whatever forms of trance or possession a given region may have already had prior to the incursion of Christianity, they were molded over time to conform with the patterns of Christian possession as suggested in the New Testament and as elaborated in patristic era writings.

The Demons of the Egyptian Desert

Amidst the wealth of testaments, epistles, and gospels proliferating in the first few centuries CE, the canon of the New Testament had become relatively settled by the end of the second century.[118] Patristic authors struggled to articulate the underlying demonology of Old and New Testament passages throughout late antiquity, attempting to craft a model that was consistent yet sufficiently dynamic and flexible. Medieval commentators such as Peter Lombard continued to look back on authorities such as Jerome and Augustine with almost as much reverence as they paid to scripture. The explanations of beliefs and rites almost universally came later than the beliefs and rites themselves. The conceptual foundation for baptismal exorcism, for example, is often illuminated, even in modern theology, by reference to the learned commentaries of Augustine on demons, the devil, and original sin. However, over the past century—and especially over the past half century—it has become increasingly clear to what extent the educated writers of the patristic era were only part of the picture, and much recent work has concentrated instead on artifacts of popular religion. Popular practices were also instrumental in forming early Christian beliefs and custom, though these practices are much harder to reconstruct through the literate manuscript tradition. For instance, the development of archaeology was necessary before the amulet and incantation bowl tradition could be properly appreciated. It is now better understood to what extent there was a disconnect between commentators and theologians on the one hand, and on the other, the local healers and seers who were often in closer and more extensive contact with large numbers of illiterate Christians.

The magical traditions of Egypt and the surrounding Mediterranean cultures are especially well documented, and can serve as an instructive contrast for systematic patristic models of demonology. Most famously, the Greek Magical Papyri, though apparently recorded by scribes of a priestly class, reflect a range of popular religious responses to illness, theft, unrequited love, treachery, and other life crises.[119] Pagan, Jewish, and Christian elements often blend seamlessly in these popular rites and incantations. Written in Greek, demotic, and Coptic, the texts date from roughly the first through the sixth centuries. Numerous exorcisms in this tradition draw freely and syncretistically from various religions, relying on lengthy nonce formulas and on divine names (including Jesus, "Christ," Jahweh, and a host of pagan gods such as Zeus, Hermes, and Seth). Christian elements become more prominent in the later texts (fifth and sixth centuries), and what seem to be references to demon possession and popular exorcism begin appearing in the third century.[120]

It is sometimes difficult to sort out whether an apotropaic rite to keep demons away or an exorcism to cast them out refers to indwelling demon possession or to the countless other physiological afflictions that could also be conceptualized as demons. These afflictions include such things as fever, seizures, reptile bites, insomnia, and "one in whom there is a worm"; further supplications extend to all manner of protection and good fortune, such as rites for profit in business and safety aboard ships.[121] Often, the spirits being adjured are clearly not possessing agents who take over the mind: fevers of various sorts are directly adjured in a sixth-century (?) papyrus text designed to be used as an amulet.[122] (Fevers continue to appear near demon-related conditions in Anglo-Saxon medical books and are sometimes ascribed to "dwarves.")[123] The language of certain texts, however, is sufficiently provocative to suggest possession, as in the following rubric from a series of Coptic folk remedies: "For those who will be sick in their mind(s), if their mind(s) oppress them and they have a demon."[124] One ritual in the Papyri Graecae Magicae (PGM) collection promises "success and victory" and indeed alleges that when the wearer has the amulet, "you will always get whatever you ask from anybody." It states that the amulet will allow the user to open doors and to break chains and rocks, and then mentions almost as an after thought: "It also works for demoniacs. Just give it [to one] to wear, and the daimon will immediately flee."[125] A fourth-century papyrus codex provides the following exorcism:

> Excellent spell for driving out demons:
>
> Formula to be spoken over his head: Place olive branches before him and stand behind him and say, "Greetings, god of Abraham; greetings, god of Isaac; greetings, god of Jacob; Jesus the upright, the holy spirit, the son of the father, who is below the seven, who is within the seven. Bring Yao Sabaoth; may your power issue forth from N., until you drive away this unclean demon Satan, who is in him. I adjure you, demon, whoever you are, by this god, Sabarbarbathioth Sabarbarbathiouth Sabarbarbathioneth Sabarbarbaphai. Come out, demon, whoever you are, and stay away from N., hurry, hurry, now, now! Come out, demon, since I bind you with unbreakable adamantine fetters, and I deliver you into the black chaos in perdition."
>
> Procedure: Take seven olive branches. For six of them tie together the two ends of each one, but for the remaining one use it as a whip as you utter the adjuration. Keep it secret; it is proven.[126]

After the demon is expelled, an amulet is then hung around the neck to prevent reentry. One of the more involved rituals against demons is "A tested charm of Pibechis for those possessed by daimons."[127] Naomi Janowitz dissects this rite, noting it falls into four sections: (1) opening instructions ("Take oil of unripe olives with the herb *mastigia* and the fruit pulp of lotus, and boil them with colorless marjoram . . . "); (2) instructions for making an amulet ("On a tin lamella write . . . "); (3) a verbal exorcistic formula ("This is the adjuration: 'I conjure you by the god of the Hebrews, Jesus . . . '"); and (4) closing instructions for the subject ("And I adjure you, the one who receives this conjuration, not to eat pork . . . ").[128] The overall impression from these colorful, varied rites is that a great diversity of popular practices can thrive comfortably outside the more orthodox world of church councils and exegetical commentary for many centuries. Therefore, when we turn to the surviving records of early medieval England—though the Celtic and Germanic substrata of language, ethnicity, and culture are quite different from the late antique Mediterranean world—we would do well to recall that the monastic selection (and redaction) of texts leaves us with only a small part of the overall picture.

As the cradle of Christian monasticism, late antique Egypt also contributed another important strand of the Anglo-Saxon religious and literary background. Easily the richest and most varied demonological episodes of first-millennium literature appear in the writings of the "desert fathers"—the apothegmatic sayings collected from, or attributed to, the thousands of hermits and monks who set off into the deserts of Egypt (as well as Syria, Palestine, and around the southern and eastern Mediterranean), especially in the fourth and fifth centuries CE.[129] This tradition, though it contains a great diversity of ascetic practices and normative moral beliefs which do not always accord with the orthodox Christian doctrine as refined later in the Middle Ages, was profoundly influential on the formation of Christian monasticism. St. Anthony was among the pioneers of this harsh form of ascetic spirituality, and Athanasius's *Life of Anthony* (ca. 360), especially in its Latin translation by Evagrius of Antioch, became a primary source of demonological beliefs for the Middle Ages. Jeffrey Burton Russell explains that in a sense, the hardships of the desert and the ongoing combat with demons replaced for these spiritual seekers the agonistic role of martyrdom that had defined early Christian spirituality under Roman persecution. Suffering and even dying for Christ had been a pervasive element of self-definition within the early Christian centuries, and the adoption of Christianity as the state religion in 380 may have created a need which the beasts and demons of the desert—and of the human heart—were well suited to fill.[130] If the vivid stories related in Palladius's *Lausiac History*, John Cassian's *Conferences*, the *History of the Monks in Egypt* (often attributed to Rufinus of Aquileia), the anonymous *Sayings of the Elders* (*Verba Seniorum*), Suplicius Severus's *Dialogues*, and other writings of the period are to be believed, the demons were generously obliging in response to this need.

In the accounts of these desert fathers, demons throng around the saints in a relentless pageant of subtle temptation alternating with brazen, flamboyant assaults. All four of the major demonic functions outlined in the introduction here (demons as vices, as wild beasts, as characters in a broader mythological narrative, and as disease agents) are amply attested in this cycle, along with other functions less easy to define and characterize. Dark humor and cutting acuity, didactic pedantry and profound spiritual insight, brief aphorisms and extended narratives—all are blended into this fascinating and challenging cycle. Demons are there at every turn: "the desert was a vast trackless waste, and there were many demons in every part of it who made monks lose their way and destroyed them."[131] The male and female ascetics perceived themselves not as running from society but as hastening to the front lines of spiritual warfare: "an old man prayed God that he might see the demons. . . . So God opened his eyes and he saw the demons like bees around a man, grinding their teeth against him."[132] When an old man of Scetis casts a demon from a possessed person, the demon announces, "Look, it was you who cast me out, so upon you I shall come." The man answers, "Come, I'll gladly have you." After twelve years of constantly harassing the man of God, the demon is worn out at last because the man only eats twelve date pits a day. Seeing the demon departing, the old man taunts him, "Why do you flee? Stay a while longer."[133] A demon appears to one hermit as a seductive woman; when he is won over and tries to grab her, she disappears in thin air leaving only the sound of laughter behind her.[134] Things go otherwise when the devil appears as a woman to Abba Apelles: in an episode reminiscent of later tales of St. Dunstan, Apelles (who is at his forge) grabs a red hot iron from the fire and burns the devil's face and body with it.[135]

Among the key virtues for these saints is "discernment of spirits": the ability to recognize good visitants from evil ones (or else, read psychologically, the ability to recognize good thoughts and impulses from evil ones). Outside of valorizing virtues such as humility, obedience, resolve, and prayer, there is no systematic theology underlying these explorations of the human psyche and of human limits. One father crushes scorpions and snakes underfoot; another chastises himself with six months of sitting out, naked, in a mosquito-infested swamp, after reproving himself for killing a gnat that has bitten him.[136] The metaphors for guarding against demonic intrusion can be raw and unsettling:

> A brother renounced the world and gave his goods to the poor, but he kept back a little for his personal expenses. He went to see Abba Anthony. When he told him this, the old man said to him, "If you want to be a monk, go into the village, buy some meat, cover your naked body with it and come here like that." The brother did so, and the dogs and birds tore at his flesh. When he came back the old man asked him whether he had followed his advice. He showed him his wounded

> body, and Saint Anthony said, "Those who renounce the world but want to keep something for themselves are torn in this way by the demons who make war on them."[137]

The demons are uncomfortably intimate. In Palladius's *Lausiac History* (an early fifth-century work, dedicated to a certain Lausus of the Eastern imperial court), Pachon relates that demons came to him in the night: "the beasts, male and female, came out. They smelled me and licked me all over from head to foot."[138] These demon tales were available in the Middle Ages through widely disseminated Latin translations, and were accommodated for Latin Western spirituality through such figures as Jerome, Cassian, and Gregory the Great. Sulpicius Severus, balancing the harsh spirituality of the desert monks with the growing pastoral needs of metropolitan, sub-Roman Gaul, paints St. Martin of Tours as embodying the ideals of his Egyptian predecessors. Indeed, Sulpicius argues that Martin is even more holy (*potiorem merito*, "of greater merit") than the desert ascetics, because (says Sulpicius) it is easy to be ascetic in the desert, in the comparative absence of temptations and distractions.[139]

Anthologies of stories associated with the desert fathers—collectively known as the *Vitae Patrum* (or *Vitas Patrum*)—were popular in the Middle Ages, and their influence is discernible in Old English vernacular literature. English library catalogs from the earliest periods usually include some portion of the *Vitae Patrum* collection, such as a tenth-century Worcester Cathedral manuscript containing a life of Paul and one of Anthony, and the *History of the Monks* (*Historia monachorum*).[140] The work was recommended by name in the Rule of Benedict as appropriate monastic reading after supper.[141] The *Old English Martyrology* draws from the desert fathers, and there are vernacular translations of several stories from the *Vitae Patrum* collection.[142] Authors such as Ælfric struggled over how much material from these sometimes stark stories were appropriate for a lay audience.[143] A story known as "The Devil's Account of the Next World" preserves the setting of a narrative from the desert fathers, greatly elaborated with fantastic, wondrous lore. A devil captured by an anchorite in the Thebaid (a region in Egypt) is forced to expound upon the horrors of hell that await sinners. The devil tells the holy man that if a man spends even a single night in hell and is then permitted to escape, so calm would anything else be in comparison that he would sleep peacefully even if locked in a colossal iron room filled with fire, with men as strong as Samson stoking the flames (each with twelve locks of hair, and each lock filled with the strength of twelve men), and with a great multitude banging on the iron roof with hammers: "hweþere for eallum þyssum gedyne ne mæg seo sawl awacian seo þe wæs ær ane niht on helle" (despite all this racket, the soul would not wake up, for having spent a single night in hell).[144] Charles Wright has elucidated the Irish origin of the iron house motif and other facets of this cycle of texts, whose cosmology is traccable back to such apocryphal texts as 4 Ezra.[145] In fact, Ireland seems to have been the conduit through which much of the spirit of early Christian monasticism reached England, offering a complement and contrast to the Benedictine spirituality imported from Italy and the Carolingian Church. Many of the features associated with Paul's visionary tour of hell in the *Vision of Paul* found in Old English homilies (as well as the OE translation of the *Vision* itself) seem heavily influenced by Irish channels of redaction.[146]

These, alongside other exotic Eastern allusions and nonstandard theologies—such as those presumed in the *Solomon and Saturn* cycle, *The Phoenix*, the *Descent into Hell* cycle, and other Old English writings steeped in apocryphal lore—hint at the wide range of texts that traveled throughout the literate world in the early Middle Ages alongside mainstream pastoral and liturgical writings.[147] Such cycles preserve a baroque tapestry of peripheral demonological beliefs, such as the personification of letters as demons in *Solomon and Saturn I*.[148] If select Anglo-Saxon reformers struggled periodically to bring the island in line with current Roman mores of orthodoxy, the world of Old English literature continuously profited, in the meantime, by their inability to do so. The desert fathers are almost never themselves possessed by demons (as supplicants in the New Testament are possessed); instead, they combat spiritual demons of temptation, and they cure other locals possessed by demons. This is an important distinction, because it remains the literary paradigm still pervasive in continental Europe and in Anglo-Saxon England. The narratives of the desert fathers are diverse and dynamic; indeed, many appear to be authentic, firsthand accounts.[149] Anglo-Saxon hagiography deliberately attempts to mimic the social and contextual backdrop of the Near Eastern desert—the archetypal "wilderness"—complete with its accoutrements such as zoomorphic demons and suffering demoniacs, accommodated to the English landscape.

The Exorcist in Early Latin Christendom

The term "exorcist" is currently used to designate someone practiced in expelling or empowered to expel indwelling spirits from a demoniac. In the Middle Ages the saints, priests, and bishops called upon to heal the infirm were not usually called exorcists, even though the sick people they healed regularly included demoniacs. The term instead referred to a particular office within the ecclesiastical ranks, one which may have been closely associated in the formative period with driving out demons, but which had long devolved into a largely procedural function by the time of Anglo-Saxon England.

In early Christianity the power to cast out demons was a charismatic gift widely assumed to inhere generally in all followers of Christ (following the commissioning of the twelve, in Luke 9:1–2): "Then Jesus called the twelve together and gave them power and authority over all demons and to cure diseases, and he sent them out to proclaim the kingdom of God and to heal." In the mid-third century Cyprian of Carthage implies that anyone, according to the purity of his or her faith, is empowered to drive out demons.[150] The brief Pseudo-Clementine lesson "On Virginity" (perhaps from the early third century) urges "those who are brethren in Christ" to actively seek out and cure demoniacs by saying adjurations over them.[151] The tract cautions that exorcism should not be the mindless repetition of words or phrases, however eloquent and authoritative, but humility and sincerity are essential. The fear is that many who posture themselves as exorcists are more interested in showmanship than in true healing. The exhortation goes on to state that such poseurs "speak with terrible words, and affright people," but despite such bravado neglect to sustain an "earnest mind . . . with cheerfulness and all circumspection and purity, without hatred and without malice." Here exorcism is evidently a growing industry, not yet restricted to a class of priests or exorcists. In *Against Celsus*, Origen claims that the numerous Christian exorcists drive demons from people, "without any curious magical art or sorcerer's device, but with prayer alone and very simple adjurations and formulas such as the simplest person could use."[152] For him, invoking the name of Jesus should be enough. Origen also adds that generally speaking, "it is uneducated people who do this kind of work."[153]

Some church councils of late antiquity attempted to regulate "solemn exorcism" (the casting out of demons, as opposed to baptismal exorcism) by permitting only official church representatives to do it. Thus the Council of Laodicea, in the mid- to late fourth century, forbids lay exorcism: "They who have not been promoted [to that office] by the bishop, ought not to adjure, either in churches or in private houses."[154] This trend perhaps encounters some resistance in the *Apostolic Constitutions* (a mid- to late fourth-century collection of various writings on worship and discipline). Though the passage is open to diverse interpretations, on the whole it seems uncomfortable with the office of exorcist as a regular order. A passage in the eighth book considers the restriction of exorcism to a church office a misunderstanding of the spirit of charismatic power:

> An exorcist is not ordained. For it is a trial of voluntary goodness, and of the grace of God through Christ by the inspiration of the Holy Spirit. For he who has received the gift of healing is declared by revelation from God, the grace which is in him being manifest to all.[155]

The ability to heal is a gift from God, rather than a title bestowed by humans. At the same time, the passage goes on to restrict ordination to the higher orders, if the healer is to enter the church hierarchy: "But if there be occasion for him, he must be ordained a bishop, or a presbyter, or a deacon."[156] This text rejects exorcism as an exclusive church prerogative, while still granting it the respect and solemnity associated with higher orders. Elizabeth Leeper interprets the passage as an attempt to "bring an unsanctioned authority under firmer ecclesiastical jurisdiction," noting that, at the very least, it reflects "a developing hierarchy and the growing clericalization of the office."[157]

The official capacity to drive out demons, then, was at least in theory limited to a class of people appointed for that purpose, and the office of exorcist developed as a lower-level office (a "minor order," as opposed to the "major orders" which begin with subdeacon) in the ecclesiastical hierarchy. The church attempted to create what one commentator has called a "monopoly of exorcism," though it is unclear to what extent it was ever fully able to sustain such a monopoly.[158] The number of these early orders, which varied from region to region, eventually settled into a relatively unified progression that formed a hierarchy through which aspirants progressed on their way to the higher orders. In Rome the offices of doorkeeper, lector (or reader), exorcist, and acolyte were well established by the mid-third century, though their precise duties in the early church are not always obvious.[159] In the Gallican Church, exorcists were well established by at least the fourth century. The number of official orders in Gaul departed slightly from Roman usage, however: there was also an office of "singer" between doorkeeper and reader.[160] For Hrabanus Maurus, and in the Pseudo-Alcuinian *Debate among Boys* (*Disputatio puerorum*) and *Book of Divine Offices* (*Liber de divinis officiis*), as well as other sources, the exorcist appears immediately superior to the acolyte (contrary to the Hiberno-Hispanic ordering).[161] The diversity of nomenclature among different traditions, however, does not reveal much about the actual nature or prevalence of possession in a certain time or place. These are the signs of growth in an increasingly bureaucratic institution, one which has ossified the word "exorcist" in its corporate hierarchy largely because of the institutionalization of exorcisms within the prebaptismal scrutinies, and the need for exorcisms of vessels and materials used in a variety of other rites.

Adults could sometimes enter orders directly as an exorcist, while children had to enter as doorkeepers or lectors and wait until adulthood before promotion to exorcist.[162] Thus Martin of Tours, baptized at age twenty-two, entered the clergy directly as an exorcist. Epitaphs for exorcists in Rome are confined to the third and fourth centuries,[163] implying only a brief window in the importance of the office or a shift in demographics within the clerical ranks after that time. Louis Duchesne argues that exorcists were useful principally in the preparation of the catechumenate; as adult baptism became increasingly rare, however, the office became obsolete.[164] By ca. 615, according to at least one source (the Pseudo-Hieronymian *On the Seven Orders of the Church*), the exorcist had apparently decreased sufficiently in importance to be absent from the ecclesiastical sequence altogether.[165] It nominally remained one of the official minor orders of the Catholic Church, however, until 1972.

Even in the early Middle Ages, ecclesiastical control over solemn exorcism still continued to be brought up on occasion. The early tenth-century *Book of Divine Offices* reads:

> *Exorcismus* Graece, Latine dicitur sermo adjurationis sive increpationis: et inde *exorcista,* adjurator. Illorum officium est, ut ponant manus super daemoniacos, et per invocationem nominis Dei repellant daemones ab eis, dicentes: *Adjuro te, immunde spiritus, per Deum Patrem, et Filium, et Spiritum sanctum, ut recedas ab hoc famulo Dei.* Istud ministerium, ut canones dicunt, nemo debet usurpare, nisi qui idem officium habent, aut diaconus, aut subdiaconus, aut exorcista.[166]
>
> [The Greek word *exorcismus* in Latin refers to the reciting of an adjuration or rebuke: and from that, *exorcist,* the one who adjures. Their duty is to lay hands on demoniacs, and through the invocation of the name of God to repel demons from them, saying, "I adjure you, wicked spirit, through God the Father, the Son, and the Holy Spirit, that you depart from this servant of God." According to the canons, no one should take on this office except those who have the same entitlement, be he a deacon, subdeacon, or exorcist.]

In the ninth century, however, Amalarius of Metz (from whom the anonymous author of the *Book of Divine Offices* drew freely) had allowed a loose range of senses for the term "exorcist," noting that aside from the office of the minor orders, there is also the gift of the grace of God (*donum gratiae Dei*) which allows anyone of true faith to drive away the devil: "Si quis per orationes suas vitium diaboli potuerit expellere de homine, exorcista est" (if anyone can expel the vices of the devil from a person through prayer, that person is an exorcist).[167]

Yet all of these considerations were largely moot: throughout early medieval hagiography, there was little insistence that those people portrayed as casting out demons had to have any ecclesiastical imprimatur or official credentials. Since solemn exorcism was essentially considered a form of healing rather than a sacramental function, its practice could be shared, in various ways, with local (non-ordained) holy men. The author of the *Life of Cuthbert*, for instance, boasts that Cuthbert cast out demons even in his youth, prior to his ordination.[168] If many church authorities jealously guarded the ecclesiastical provenance over baptism, communion, confirmation of kings, and other rites, the ability to heal charismatically remained widespread both within and without the church orders.

Most of the time in the early Middle Ages the official ceremonies for receiving an individual into the lower orders were not extensive; the announcement of an office could be made summarily at a regular mass without higher authorization, signified only by prayer, laying on of hands, and delivery of the symbols of office. The *Gelasian Sacramentary* provides details concerning the initiation and duties of minor orders, in a section taken from the *Statuta ecclesiae antiqua*, a (perhaps) late fifth- or early sixth century Gallic composition which went on to enjoy great currency in the Middle Ages.[169] As symbols of office, doorkeepers were given the keys to the church, lectors were given books of readings, and acolytes were given candles and candlesticks. Appropriately, exorcists were ceremoniously handed a book (or literally, "booklet") containing exorcisms (*libellum in quo scripti sunt exorcismi*) and given instructions to memorize them:

> Exorcista quum ordinatur, accipiat de manu episcopi libellum in quo scripti sunt exorcismi, dicente sibi episcopo: Accipe et commenda, et habeto potestatem imponendi manum super energumenum, sive baptizatum sive catechumenum.[170]
>
> [When the "exorcist" is ordained, he receives from the hand of the bishop a book in which exorcisms are written, the bishop saying to him: "Accept and commit these exorcisms (to memory), and receive the power of laying hands on an energumen, whether already baptized or whether a catechumen."]

Two prayers follow the handing of the book to the exorcist:

> *Praefatio exorcistae.* Deum Patrem omnipotentem supplices deprecemur, ut hunc famulum suum nomine *Illum* benedicere dignetur in officium exorcistae, ut sit spiritalis imperator ad abiciendos daemones de corporibus obsessis cum omni nequitia eorum multiformi. Per.
>
> *Benedictio exorcistae.* Domine sancte, Pater omnipotens, aeterne Deus, benedicere digneris famulum tuum hunc nomine *Illum,* in officio exorcistae, ut per impositiones manuum et oris officium eum eligere digneris, et imperium habeat spirituum immundorum coercendo, et probabilis sit medicus ecclesiae tuae, gratiae curationum virtute confirmatus. Per Dominum.[171]
>
> [Prayer for the exorcist. Let us humbly pray to God the Omnipotent Father that He deem it worthy to consecrate his servant *N* in the office of exorcist, that he may be a spiritual leader in casting out demons from the bodies of the possessed with all their multiform wickedness. Through.
>
> Benediction for the exorcist. Holy Lord, Omnipotent Father, Eternal God, deem it worthy to bless this your servant *N* to the office of exorcist, that you may see fit to choose him through the imposition of hands and the service of prayer, and that he may have authority to compel unclean spirits, and that he may be a loyal healer of your church, confirmed in the power of the grace of healings. Through the Lord.]

These directions and ordination prayers remain intact throughout the Anglo-Saxon period.[172] The exorcists were evidently meant to memorize the exorcisms and then return the book. Peter Brown has mused upon this task of memorization as an impressive feat, but no extant series of exorcisms is all that long.[173] It is far simpler than memorizing the Psalms, for instance, a task required of all aspirants wishing to enter a monastery.[174] In any event, it is not the case that the prayers indicated as "exorcisms" in medieval liturgical books were all meant to be read over actively possessed persons. The majority of these prayers were procedural: that is, they were used in the preparation of holy water or oil, for instance, or read over baptismal candidates during their catechumenate.[175] The day to day life of an official "exorcist" in the early medieval church was in fact a fairly unglamorous and uneventful one, in comparison with what the title might suggest.

Even as the office of exorcist was declining in importance within the ecclesiastical hierarchy, cases of possession were rife throughout late antique Gaul, if the sources are credible. Late antique sources portray Christian healing shrines as bristling with the lame, the deaf, the paralyzed, the insane, and the possessed. The growing culture of relic veneration likely fueled the popularity of demoniac activity. Earlier generations of historians assumed that since possessions were widespread, it follows that Christian exorcism introduced a well-needed cure and represented, in that respect, a medical innovation responding to a preexisting need. This fails to recognize the participatory nature of exorcism as a rite: pre-Christian cultures were not engaging in possession behavior in a vacuum, waiting only to learn of the existence of exorcists. Some early sources specify that demoniacs were still an unfamiliar sight to Europeans. In a letter, Jerome writes of a certain Roman pilgrim who journeys to the Holy Land for the first time and is horrified by what she sees, at least in these particular iterations:

> Ubi multis intremuit consternata mirabilibus: namque cernebat variis daemones rugire cruciatibus, et ante sepulcra sanctorum ululare homines more luporum, vocibus latrare canum, fremere leonum, sibilare serpentum, mugire taurorum. Alios rotare caput, et post tergum terram vertice tangere, suspensisque pede feminis, vestes non defluere in faciem.[176]
>
> [She began to tremble, frightened at the many marvelous things there: for she perceived demons roaring in various afflictions, and people howling like wolves, barking with the voices of dogs, roaring like lions, hissing like serpents, and bellowing like bulls before the tombs of the saints. Others turned their heads around over their backs to touch the ground. There were women suspended by their feet, but their clothes did not drape down over their faces.]

Two centuries later, however—by the time of Gregory of Tours and Caesarius of Arles—public exorcism of possessed persons was evidently a routine and highly public phenomenon in Merovingian Gaul.[177] In the far south, Caesarius is reported to have performed numerous exorcisms, both in Arles and throughout the surrounding precincts.[178] This is a common hagiographic trope, of course. More telling, perhaps, are the offhand comments found in Caesarius's sermons, which vividly drive home how real a part of daily life this phenomenon apparently was in some places:

> Superiore dominica, fratres carissimi, dum missae celebrarentur, non parvum metum omni populo insaniens ille inerguminus generavit.[179]
>
> [Dearest brothers, last Sunday, when masses were being celebrated, that raging energumen caused not just a little fear in everyone.]

Since this would hardly make sense as literary trope—"last Sunday" is too specific—this can be justifiably read as a literal rather than a rhetorical statement. Caesarius's world was one in which demoniacs not only interrupted mass and frequented churches and shrines but also ubiquitously traveled the country roads and loitered in the forum.[180]

The sources in the north of Gaul paint a similar picture of widespread possession. Sulpicius Severus implies that the possessed are in no short supply in fourth-century Tours: whenever Martin approached the church, "uideres per totam ecclesiam energumenos rugientes" (throughout the whole church you could see energumens roaring).[181] In the *Life of Martin* Sulpicius paints Martin as able to call for a demoniac to be brought to him at his disposal—not because he wants to cure anyone but because indwelling demons must always tell the truth when confronted with questions from a holy man. Martin only wants to learn whether or not rumors about an army in the vicinity plotting to advance against Tours are true. The casual availability of demoniacs at will, without a need for additional background or explanation, is striking.[182] Gregory's observation of these miracles, or of what he perceives as miracles, is hard to dismiss as literary license. He cross-references the same miracles in different works, and in his *Books on the Miracles of Saint Martin* the reader can almost picture him at the shrine with writing implements in hand, waiting for the next miracle:

> Cum quinquaginta novem virtutes discripsissem et sexagesimam adhuc adtentius praestolarem, subito mihi sinistrum capitis timpus artatur doloribus.[183]
>
> [When I had recorded fifty-nine miracles and was attentively waiting for the sixtieth, my left temple suddenly felt painfully constricted.]

Of course, Gregory's pain is relieved once he prays to Martin—ironically, then, Gregory himself provides the sixtieth miracle for which he has been waiting. He soon closes the second book of *Miracles* having recorded an even one hundred miracles, but promises to add more books as more healings occur: "si adhuc meremur videre miracula, placet ea alteri coniungi libello" (if I am still worthy enough to see another marvel, it should appear in a separate book).[184] Gregory's account is vital and intimate.

The immediacy of Gregory's miracle-recording project reappears in the reign of Charlemagne. Einhard portrays Carolingian churches and healing shrines as crowded with demoniacs: a male demon, for instance, speaks through the mouth of a woman at Aachen before a horrified congregation. The woman and the demon rail at each other, both within the same body, alternating between a male and a female voice.[185] Einhard tells of another incident at Höchst, in which a sixteen-year-old girl is possessed by a demon named Wiggo. The demon is said to speak to the exorcizing priest in Latin, though the girl only knows German.[186] Einhard actively promoted a vision of Carolingian Germany as a unified, interconnected center of miracle activity, presenting it as a coherent and dynamic political entity on the one hand, and a locus of tangible, well-documented divine favor on the other.

Not all Carolingians interpreted the behavior of enthusiastic worshippers equally. If it suited Einhard's program to accept all accounts of healings as genuine conquests of faith over the forces of darkness, the early ninth-century Archbishop Agobard of Lyon, for one, speaks more cautiously. Bishop Bartholomew of Narbonne asks Agobard's opinion about numerous people suffering from the stigmata in the church of St. Firminus of Uzès, a place where "violent attacks" (*percussiones*) have also begun to occur, with "certain people falling down in the manner of epileptics or of those whom the common people consider to be, and call, 'demoniacs'" (caderent quidam more epilemticorum uel eorum quos uulgus daemoniacos putat uel nominat). Agobard, in a famous letter also signed by the priest Hildigius and the deacon Florus, seems overtly skeptical about the nature of these conditions and the motives of those who stand to profit from the whole affair.[187] Though he does not question the realty of diabolic agency or of demonic possession, Agobard concludes that these particular sufferers who rush back to make contributions at the church where they were cured "do this because they are deceived by their fears, having lost their better deliberation" (terroribus decepti hoc faciant, perdito consilio meliore).[188] In Agobard's categorization of types of possession, the devil can also infect the mind, causing auto-suggestive imitation of true possession:

> Alterum uero genus est, quo in quosdam homines praeualere uidetur diabolus, non tam ad percutiendum, quam ad inludendum, de quibus multos audiuimus et cognouimus a daemonibus, lapidibus et fustibus caesos et in nullo laesos, aliquos tamen et inlusos et laesos. In quibus nulla alia causa uidetur, qua id fiat, nisi aut inanitas fidei aut delectatio uanitatis.[189]

> [There is a second kind, in which the devil seems to overpower certain people—not so much to damage them physically, as to mock them. We have heard and are well aware that many people have been struck by demons with stones and sticks, but were not hurt. Others were mocked as well as hurt. In these cases, no other cause is apparent to make this happen, except either the absence of faith or indulgence in vanity.]

Agobard's successor, Amulo, was equally puzzled over how to distinguish genuine spirit possession from the mania he characterizes as popular superstition.[190] Amulo bears personal witness to what he obviously considers pseudo-possession: "vidimus namque aliquoties coram illo qui se daemoniacos advexaticios esse simularent" (We have personally seen, on a number of occasions, people acting as though [*simularent*] they were demoniacs vexed by demons).[191] He decries the deceit of counterfeit demoniacs, the gullibility of the uneducated, and the greed of self-styled exorcists.[192] This diversity of responses to occasional outbreaks of possession is strong evidence that they really were happening, and, moreover, that the church was divided somewhat over how to manage such occurrences. Between Einhard's sanguine list of miracles and the skeptical meditations of Agobard and Amulo, a more nuanced picture emerges of the multifaceted profile of possession in the Carolingian Empire.

Because there is a continuum of textual traditions between Merovingian Gaul, Carolingian Germany, and Anglo-Saxon England, it is easy to suppose that a similar culture of possession and exorcism existed in early medieval England as well. There is some evidence that it may have in seventh- and eighth-century Northumbria, but beyond that the documentary record becomes largely silent. Successful healing shrines (i.e., those that draw pilgrims from outside the immediate area) rely on some regional stability, secure routes of passage and communication, and a population not otherwise distracted in terms of time and resources. The Viking raids of the ninth through eleventh centuries disrupted many of the cults of post-Carolingian France and Germany, and perhaps prevented such cults from forming effectively in large parts of England. Furthermore, those shrines that did gain popularity in England specialized in the blind, the paralyzed, and the lame (if the hagiographic *topoi* are taken as reflective of actual events), but the possessed are conspicuously underrepresented or altogether absent in the (admittedly few) sources. To examine the usefulness and limitations of these sources in illuminating actual practice in Anglo-Saxon society, we turn now to the three main genres from which virtually all our evidence is gleaned: medicine and liturgy (chapter 2), and narrative sources (chapter 3).

NOTES

1. Until recently, prognostics have remained among the least studied facets of Anglo-Saxon letters. This is partly remedied now by Chardonnens, *Anglo-Saxon Prognostics*. For basic orientation, see Cockayne, *Leechdoms* (esp. vol. 3, pp. 149–283); Griffiths, *Aspects*, pp. 129–45; Hart, *Learning and Culture*; Liuzza, "Anglo-Saxon Prognostics"; and Hollis and Wright, *Old English Prose*, pp. 257–70.

2. For medieval China, see Guo, *Exorcism and Money*; concerning ritual exorcism, and for the interplay between ritual and non-ritual exorcism, see Davis, *Society*, esp. chap. 3. For the Arabic world, see Dols, *Majnūn*; for exorcism see esp. pp. 237–54, 274–96.

3. On disease constructs in Anglo-Saxon England, see Meaney, "Anglo-Saxon View"; Pettit, *Anglo-Saxon Remedies*, 1:xxxii–xxxiv; Pollington, *Leechcraft*, pp. 453–67; for further discussion, see below (chapter 2). For transmission, see Kitson, "Eastern Learning," pp. 57–71.

4. The second Merseburg Charm ("ben zi bena, bluot zi bluoda, lid zi geliden, sose gelimida sin" [bone to bone, blood to blood, limb to limb—thus may they be glued back together], Miller, "Old High German," p. 31) has traditionally been interpreted as intended for a horse's sprained foot, but Brian Murdoch notes that it could be for any sprain or broken bone, in animals or humans ("But Did They Work?," p. 365). The charm in *Atharva Veda* 4.12 is for "serious wounds" (probably cuts such as a sword slash): "Let thy marrow come together with marrow, and thy joint together with joint; together let what of thy flesh has fallen apart, together let thy bone grow over. Let marrow be put together with marrow; let skin grow with skin; let thy blood, bone grow; let flesh grow with flesh. Fit thou together hair with hair; fit together skin with skin; let thy blood, bone grow . . ." (Whitney, *Atharva-Veda Samhita*, p. 167).

5. Cryer and Thomsen, *Witchcraft*, pp. 32, 46. Exorcisms which attempt to diagnose the cause of the sufferer's misfortune are unusual: "He trod in some libation that had been poured forth, or / He put his foot in some unclean water, / Or cast his eye on the water of unwashed hands, / Or came in contact with a woman of unclean hands, / Or glanced at a maid with unwashed hands . . ." (Thompson, *Devils*, vol. 2, p. 137). A fascinating Akkadian diagnostical text is transliterated and translated into French in Labat, *Traité Akkadien de diagnostics*. So meticulous is the breakdown of symptoms in this work that various discolorations of right and left buttock are cataloged separately (pp. 131–33).

6. Abusch, "Demonic Image," pp. 35, 53n12. Some exorcistic texts are marked as secret—reserved only for initiates—because as the languages became increasingly fossilized through the ancient Near Eastern period, the texts became the provenance of a select group of scholars (Cryer and Thomsen, *Witchcraft*, p. 20; see also Abusch, "Demonic Image," p. 37).

7. Abusch, "Demonic Image," p. 29. The *āšipu* is distinct from the *asŭ*, the physician or herbalist.

8. Rubrics such as "From house to house they [evil spirits] break through, / No door can shut them out, / No bolt can turn them back" (Thompson, *Devils*, vol. 1, p. 53), "let loose in the street," or "running amok in the street" (Geller, *Forerunners*, pp. 31, 21) imply the need for ministering among the general populace, but it is likely that the class of professional exorcists reserved their services for only those who could afford them ("Unto the neighborhood of the palace may [demons] not draw nigh," Thompson, *Devils*, vol. 1, p. 109; see also Abusch, "Demonic Image," p. 29; and Cryer and Thomsen, *Witchcraft*, p. 14). For a fascinating collection of "letters from exorcists" (though most of them are probably better read as "letters from priests") preserved in royal archives, see Parpola, *Letters*, pp. 149–250. Abusch,

however, cautions that though the texts increasingly adopt the grand language of temple settings and accoutrements, this does not mean that they were not still performed in private homes ("Demonic Image," p. 36).

9. Cunningham, *Deliver Me*, pp. 14, 16.

10. Laying on of hands: "When I lay my hand on the head of the sick man, / May a kindly Spirit, a kindly Guardian stand at my side" (Thompson, *Devils*, vol. 1, p. 17; see also Geller, *Forerunners*, p. 21); sprinkling of water: "When I sprinkle the water of Ea on the sick man . . ." (Thompson, *Devils*, vol. 1, p. 19), "bring the holy water of Enki . . . sprinkle water on his bed" (Geller, *Forerunners*, p. 69). The water is apparently gathered from the confluence of two streams, and is consecrated before use in the rite (Thompson, *Devils*, vol. 2, p. 95). See also vol. 2, pp. 101, 109. Censors, torches, herbs, and sprigs of plant material are elsewhere mentioned (vol. 1, pp. 19, 137), as is the dressing of the supplicant in new robes (vol. 1, p. 135).

11. Abusch, "Demonic Image," p. 30. Abusch also outlines a remarkably detailed exception, however—a ceremony described in a letter from the exorcist Nabŭnādin-shumi to King Esarhaddon in early August, 670 BCE. Separate rites are provided for a ritual over the course of a night and the following morning (40ff.).

12. *Udug-hul*: for text references and discussion, see Cunningham, *Deliver Me*, p. 38. *Udug-sig*: Gudea Cylinders A iii 20 and B ii 9; Cunningham, *Deliver Me*, p. 38.

13. Avalos argues against K. van der Toorn's contention that illness is not linked with sin in Mesopotamian medicine (*Illness*, pp. 128–39), but he does not address the wide range of Mesopotamian exorcistic texts which simply refer to the luckless patient as a passerby. The word *muttaliku* ("wanderer") is frequently synonymous with "patient" in these documents (Thompson, *Devils*, vol. 1, p. xxviii). Thomsen calculates that in a certain exorcist handbook, a god is thought to be responsible for the illness in over half the cases, the spirits of the dead in about a fifth, and various demons in the rest (Cryer and Thomsen, *Witchcraft*, p. 32).

14. For instance, "May he not be held in bondage, / May his fetters be loosened" (Thompson, *Devils*, vol. 1, p. 15). See also Cunningham, *Deliver Me*, pp. 19–20. For the later development of "binding" in the curse scrolls of the first few centuries CE see Ogden, "Binding Spells," pp. 26–29. Though demons are said to "exist in" the victim's body (Geller, *Forerunners*, p. 61), they are also described as "enveloping" victims or "covering" them "like a garment" or "like a net" (pp. 31, 12, 81), and "snatching" them away (p. 31).

15. See Skemer, *Binding Words*.

16. Ælfric, *Passio Bartholomei* (Clemoes, *Catholic Homilies*, p. 441). On the thematic and theological use of binding and loosing in Old English, see Rendall, "Bondage," pp. 497–512.

17. Matthew 16:19, 18:18. See, for instance, Boniface's oath to Gregory II ("potestas ligandi solvendique," Letter 16; Tangl, *Die Briefe*, p. 29); Stephen of Ripon, *Vita Wilfrithi*, p. 39 (Colgrave, *Wilfrid*, p. 78).

18. *Lacnunga* 157 (Pettit, *Anglo-Saxon Remedies*, 1:108).

19. Murdoch, "*Peri Hieres Nousou*," p. 148.

20. Bede, *HE* 4.22, p. 402. Valerie Flint situates binding magic in its early medieval context in *Rise of Magic*, pp. 226–31.

21. Thus Augustine, *De civitate Dei*, 11.31 (Dombart and Kalb, *Sancti Aurelii*, 1:505). See also Bloomfield, *Seven Deadly Sins*, pp. 39–40; and Cunningham, *Deliver M*e, p. 26. Groups of seven demons survive into modern cases, and are sometimes given names (e.g., Asmodeus, Leviathan, Behemoth, Isacaaron, Balaam, Gresil, and Haman; see Oesterreich, *Possession*, p. 26; and Thompson, *Devils*, vol. 1, p. xlii–xlvii). Note also the passage from the *Old English Martyrology* cited above (introduction), in which "seven devils" are equated with

"all vices" (*OE Martyrology*, July 22 [Kotzor, *Martyrologium*, 2:156]). For a meditation on the number seven in the abstract, see Byrhtferth's *Enchiridion*, chap. 4 (Baker and Lapidge, *Byrhtferth's Enchiridion*, p. 208).

22. Strong man parable: Matthew 12:43–45, Luke 11:21–26; Mary Magdalene: Luke 8:2.

23. *Andreas*, lines 1311–12. For the number ambiguity, see Dendle, *Satan Unbound*, pp. 154–55n70.

24. Ælfric, "Dominica iii in Quadragesima": *gyfernyss*, *forlir*, *gytsung*, *yrre*, *asolcennyss*, *unrotnyss*, *idelgylp*, and *modignyss* (Pope, *Homilies*, vol. 1, p. 278). The Gregorian model of seven deadly sins was not the most popular model in Anglo-Saxon England; there, the division into eight sins (the Cassianic model) was far more common: e.g., Alcuin, "De virtutibus et vitiis"; Vercelli Homily 20; Ælfric, "Sermo de memoria sanctorum" and Letter to Wulfstan; Wulfstan, *De Christianitate*; the homiletic "De viii principalibus viciis" in London, British Library, MS Cotton Vespasian D.XIV; Byrhtferth, *Enchiridion* 4.2 (discussed in Bloomfield, *Seven Deadly Sins*, pp. 106–21). For the iconographic development of the motif, see Voelkle, "Morgan Manuscript M.1001," pp. 101–14 and plates xxxvii–liv.

25. Medieval Christian orthodoxy eventually settled on only three named archangels (those named in scripture: Gabriel, Raphael, and Michael), though lists of named demons and angels continued to circulate throughout the Middle Ages. A late medieval Irish prayer associates an archangel for every day of the week (Sunday, Gabriel; Monday, Michael; Tuesday, Raphael; Wednesday, Uriel; Thursday, Sariel; Friday, Rumiel; and Saturday, Panchel; text and translation in Nualláin, "Prayer," pp. 92–94; and see Jolly, "Prayers," p. 128n89). Anglo-Saxons (especially in the north, such as the Chester-le-Street community under Aldred) drew heavily from the sort of apocryphal lore, common in Ireland, that delighted in enumerated lists (Jolly, "Prayers," p. 129).

26. Foster, *Before the Muses*, p. 55. For discussion and details of a first millennium ritual, see Cryer and Thomsen, *Witchcraft*, pp. 72–74. The "evil eye" survives into medieval Latin belief as *fascinatio* and into Old English as *malscrung* (Meaney, "Anglo-Saxon View," pp. 23–24). Thus it appears in the "Nine Herbs Charm," for instance (*Lacnunga* 76 [Pettit, *Anglo-Saxon Remedies*, 1:64]).

27. Foster, *Before the Muses*, p. 55.

28. Many premodern remedies rely on expelling matter from the body: purgatives, laxatives, diuretics, emmenagogues, etc. An Anglo-Saxon remedy "wiþ feond seocum men" (against a fiend-sick person), for instance, gives a recipe for what it calls a *spiwedrenc* ("spew-drink," or purgative; more in chapter 2).

29. Bottéro, *Myths*, p. 32 ("isolé, et sans force").

30. A typical example runs thus: "An evil Spirit against his neck hath drawn nigh, / An evil Demon against his breast hath drawn nigh, / An evil Ghost against his belly hath drawn nigh, / An evil Devil against his hand hath drawn nigh, / An evil God against his foot hath drawn nigh" (Thompson, *Devils*, vol. 2, p. 29).

31. "Lorica of Gildas": Pettit, *Anglo-Saxon Remedies*, 1:40–56 (for *Lacnunga* version); Leofric Missal, no. 2479 (Nicholas Orchard, *Leofric Missal*, 2:437–38; see also Gerbert, *Monumenta*, 2:132). Pettit notes, "Such exorcisms and prayers enumerating parts of the body may have their roots in Irish tradition," citing specifically the *Antiphonary of Bangor*, fol. 30v (*Anglo-Saxon Remedies*, 2:71). On the exorcism of various parts of the body separately, see, for instance, Caciola, *Discerning Spirits* (pp. 259–62, for later medieval Catholic exorcism), and further references in Charles Wright, *Irish Tradition*, 99n210; and for meditation on the phenomenology implicit in this sort of ritual, see Versnel, "Essay," pp. 217–67.

32. *Juliana*: lines 289–315; *Solomon and Saturn I*: lines 84–140. In a prescription against *ælfsogoþa* ("elf-disease"?), the *Leechbook* book 3 even lists the soul as just another body part in a lengthy anatomical list (item 62; Cockayne, *Leechdoms*, vol. 2, p. 350)—a telling insight into popular theology of the early Middle Ages.

33. Text printed in Storms, *Anglo-Saxon Magic*, p. 315 (as "Fandorohel") and Jolly, "On the Margins," pp. 165–67 (as "Fondorahel"); for further discussion, see Jolly, "Prayers," pp. 118–19.

34. Cunningham, *Deliver Me*, p. 68.

35. Old Babylonian incantation: Cunningham, *Deliver Me*, p. 90; angry heart: Gudea Cylinders A x 22–23.

36. *Lacnunga* 76 (Pettit, *Anglo-Saxon Remedies*, 1:60–68).

37. *Leechbook* 1.45 (Cockayne, *Leechdoms*, vol. 2, pp. 112–14); see also *Leechbook* 2.64 (Cockayne, *Leechdoms*, vol. 2, p. 290), *Lacnunga* 18, 126 (Pettit, *Anglo-Saxon Remedies*, 1:10, 88).

38. Serpents: Cunningham, *Deliver Me*, pp. 90–91; worms: p. 106. The worm, not attested as a disease agent in original Sumerian documents, first appears as such in the Old Babylonian period (Cunningham, *Deliver Me*, p. 177). For its evolution in the Indo-European tradition, see Watkins, *How To Kill a Dragon*, pp. 519–24.

39. See Bonser, *Medical Background*, pp. 277–78. *Ana-wyrm*: *Leechbook* 1.46 (Cockayne, *Leechdoms*, vol. 2, p. 114); *deaw-wyrm*: *Leechbook* 1.50 (Cockayne, *Leechdoms*, vol. 2, p. 122); *flæsc-wyrm*: *Leechbook* 1.51 (Cockayne, *Leechdoms*, vol. 2, p. 124); *hond-wyrm*: *Leechbook* 1.50 (Cockayne, *Leechdoms*, vol. 2, p. 122); *rengc-wyrm*: *Herbarium* 65, 104 (de Vriend, *Old English Herbarium*, pp. 108, 150); *smea-wyrm*: *Leechbook* 3.39 (Cockayne, *Leechdoms*, vol. 2, p. 332) and also *Leechbook* 1.53 (Cockayne, *Leechdoms*, vol. 2, p. 126); *þeor-wyrm*: *Leechbook* 1.47 (Cockayne, *Leechdoms*, vol. 2, p. 118). One recipe distinguishes itself as good for a "small worm" (*smalan wyrme*: *Leechbook* 1.49; Cockayne, *Leechdoms*, vol. 2, p. 122). See also *Lacnunga* 26 (Pettit, *Anglo-Saxon Remedies*, 1:14). For discussion see Jolly, *Popular Religion*, pp. 128–30.

40. *Leechbook* 1.46 (Cockayne, *Leechdoms*, vol. 2, p. 114); *Leechbook* 1.48 (Cockayne, *Leechdoms*, vol. 2, p. 120); *Leechbook* 1.51 (Cockayne, *Leechdoms*, vol. 2, p. 124).

41. Braune, *Althochdeutsches Lesebuch*, p. 78.

42. Glosecki, *Shamanism*, p. 122.

43. Gager, *Curse Tablets*, p. 27.

44. See Tomlin, *Tabellae Sulis*. The vast majority of the British tablets are concerned with theft of property. There are Scandinavian analogues as well, such as what seems to be a curse for a rejected lover on a bone weaving tablet from (eleventh-century?) Lund, Sweden: "s[i] kuarar ikimar afaman m[i]n krat" (Ingemar son of Sigvor shall get my weeping; Moltke, *Runes*, p. 358).

45. Ogden, *Binding Spirits*, pp. 3–5.

46. Gager, *Curse Tablets*, p. 27; for overview of lorica tradition see Gougaud, "Étude sur les *loricae*," pp. 265–81.

47. Little, *Benedictine Maledictions*, p. 152; see also p. 125. The reference is to *Maldon*, line 242: "Abreoðe his angina . . ." (may his undertaking perish, *ASPR* 6.13). The treasure in the dragon's barrow in *Beowulf* lies under a curse (lines 3069–71). On Latin charter sanctions, see Little, *Benedictine Maledictions*, pp. 52–59. Such biblical passages as Deuteronomy 27 and 28 also kept cursing alive in the monastic consciousness.

48. See collected charters in Birch, *Cartularium Saxonicum*. The curse or sanction segments usually appear toward the end of the document, before the signatories. For vernacular

equivalents, see collected Old English charters in A. J. Robertson, *Anglo-Saxon Charters*. These curses have finally begun to draw attention, for instance in Danet and Bogoch, "'Whoever Alters This,'" pp. 132–65 (to be used, however, with caution); for similar documents in the cultural context of southern Gaul, see Bowman, "Do Neo-Romans Curse?" pp. 1–32.

49. *Leechbook* 1.64 (Cockayne, *Leechdoms*, vol. 2, p. 138).

50. Stol, *Epilepsy*, p. 52.

51. Breasted, *Ancient Records*, pp. 191, 192. The stele was inscribed as a propaganda piece eight or nine centuries after the alleged events and so it can only be of limited insight into the medical conditions of the Nineteenth Dynasty. It reflects instead the perception of illnesses in the fifth to fourth centuries BCE. Even so, it remains the earliest known clear-cut (to my mind) instance of demon possession in history, aside from the episode in 1 Samuel (see below).

52. Breasted, *Ancient Records*, p. 193.

53. Breasted, *Ancient Records*, pp. 194–95.

54. For a comparison of this narrative with the Lucan account of the "epileptic boy," see Klutz, *Exorcism Stories*, pp. 189–90. Robert K. Ritner situates the Bentresh Stela in its contemporary medical context in William Kelly Simpson, *Literature* (pp. 361–62), preferring the translation "ghost" for "spirit" (rendering *akh*). Ritner comments, "The spirit is famished and in need of attention, but not inherently evil" (p. 362).

55. Chajes, "Jewish Exorcism," pp. 387–88; Herrmann, "Les premiers," p. 306.

56. 1 Samuel 16:14.

57. 1 Samuel 18:11.

58. 1 Samuel 16:23.

59. Ben-Noun, "What Was the Mental Disease," pp. 270–82; McCasland, *By the Finger*, pp. x, 40–41. Ælfric treats Saul harshly in a passage that now appears as part of his homily "De auguriis" (Pope, *Homilies*, vol. 2, pp. 792–96, lines 36–128; on the origin and transmittal of this passage see Peter Jackson, "The *Vitas Patrum*," pp. 126–27).

60. Josephus, *Antiquities* 8.2 (Thackeray and Marcus, *Josephus*, p. 595). For discussion see Duling, "Eleazar Miracle," pp. 1–25; and Duling, "Solomon," pp. 235–52. The belief that exorcism was originally a gift bequeathed by Solomon survives in Anglo-Saxon England: a passage circulating in Bede (*Expositio super Acta Apostolorum* 19; PL 92: col. 983), Hrabanus Maurus (*De clericorum institutione* 1.10; PL 107: col. 304), and Amalarius of Metz (*De ecclesiasticis officiis* 2.9; PL 105: col. 1084–85) states, "Exorcista refert Iosephus regem salomonem excogitasse suamque gentem docuisse modos exorcismi" (Exorcist: Josephus says that King Solomon devised and taught his own people methods of exorcism). Aldred, in the tenth-century Chester-le-Street additions to the Durham Collectar, glosses the passage in Old English: "hælsere sægeð iosep ðone cynig salom' geðohte æc his cynn gelærde" (Lindelöf, *Rituale*, p. 194).

61. Klutz, *Exorcism Stories*, p. 63.

62. Josephus, *Jewish War* 7.6: "[the baaras] possesses one virtue for which it is prized; for the so-called demons [δαιμονια]—in other words, the spirits of wicked men which enter the living and kill them unless aid is forthcoming—are promptly expelled by this root, if merely applied to the patients" (Thackeray, *Josephus*, p. 559). The plant takes its name from the valley in which it grows and can only be extracted from the ground using a woman's urine or menstrual blood, in combination with the dog-and-rope trick that in later medieval tradition would be associated with the mandrake.

63. Intertestamental and pseudepigraphal literature allows insight into a wealth of

demonological and eschatological beliefs current in the Jewish community before, during, and shortly after the time of Christ, in such works as Tobit, 1 Enoch, Jubilees, the Book of Adam and Eve, and the Secrets of Enoch (complete English translations in Charles, *Apocrypha*, 2 vols.; for critical and contextual guidance, see Stone, *Jewish Writings*). Ranging from the third century BCE to the first century CE, these works provide enigmatic and sometimes baroque hierarchies of angels and demons. Erik Sorensen sees these works as explicitly attesting to Jewish practice of exorcism, and as contextualizing the role of exorcism in a postexilic society by providing more sharply defined characters and personalities for the demons (Sorensen, *Possession*, p. 223). His examples of possession in the pseudepigrapha are not convincing, however. In 1 Enoch 40:7 Enoch hears in a vision the archangel Phanuel "fending off the Satans and forbidding them to come before the Lord of Spirits to accuse them who dwell on the earth" (Charles, *Apocrypha*, 2:211). There is not much that implies possession here, and, in any event, Phanuel (the archangel in charge of hope and eternal life) does not govern medicine. It is the second archangel, Raphael, who is explicitly said to reign over "all the diseases and all the wounds of the children of men" (1 Enoch 40:9; Charles, *Apocrypha*, 2:211–12). In 3 Baruch 16:3–4, the Lord proclaims to Michael, "send forth the caterpillar and the unwinged locust, and the mildew, and the common locust (and) hail with lightnings and anger, and punish them severely with the sword and with death, and their children with demons" (Charles, *Apocrypha*, 2:541). Such references (these are two of Sorensen's three examples, on pp. 60–61; the third is simply an instance of Satan entering the serpent in Eden in the Book of Adam and Eve) are only weak analogues to demon possession, and (insofar as they can be taken as medical demons at all) bear a stronger resemblance to the external disease agents of Babylonian demonology than to New Testament corporeal possession. Sorensen must be correct, though, in the general time in which exorcism gained currency in Jewish communities, since it is apparently in place by the time of the New Testament. The Book of Adam and Eve, in its Latin translation, was for a time explored as a possible source or at least precursor for demonological concepts in the Old English *Genesis B* (McKillop, "Illustrative Notes," pp. 28–38; and especially F. N. Robinson, "Note," pp. 389–96).

64. Cryer and Thomsen, *Witchcraft*, pp. 137–38. For instance, the details given by Isaiah when healing the king in 2 Kings 20:4–11 parallel those which diviner-exorcists generally give in the Sumero-Babylonian tradition (e.g., whether or not the healing will work, the precise length of time it will take, and the interpretation of signs). The Lord directs Isaiah to apply a lump of figs to the king's boil.

65. Lesses, "Exe(o)rcising Power," p. 347.

66. Lesses, "Exe(o)rcising Power," pp. 346, 354, 359–61. See also Cyrus Gordon for an incantation that is apparently directed to a house and an indwelling demon simultaneously, again using the divorce formula ("Aramaic Exorcism," pp. 466–74).

67. Erica Hunter, "Aramaic-Speaking Communities," pp. 333–34.

68. Michael Morgan, *Sepher Ha-Razim*, pp. 51, 54. The *Sepher Ha-Razim* is a reconstruction, drawn from a handful of codices and Geniza fragments, of an early medieval Jewish magical handbook. Mordecai Margalioth, who initially proposed the reconstructed book and edited the collection, dates the original to the third or fourth century CE, based on references to Roman indictions, the purity of the midrashic Hebrew, parallels with the Greek Magical Papyri, and other factors (Michael Morgan, *Sepher Ha-Razim*, pp. 8–9). Alternatively, Ithamar Gruenwald dates the work to the sixth or seventh century (*Apocalyptic and Merkavah Mysticism*, p. 226). Naomi Janowitz devotes chapter 6 of *Icons of Power* to the *Sepher Ha-Razim*, analyzing its conceptual underpinnings and social context (pp. 85–108).

69. Josephus, *Antiquities* 8.2 (Thackeray and Marcus, *Josephus*, pp. 595–97).

70. Strack and Billerbeck, *Exkurse*, p. 535. The emperor in question may be Antoninus Pius (138–61 CE).

71. The rabbi does, however, banish a demon queen in *Pesachim* 112b (see McCasland, *By the Finger*, p. 80; Twelftree, *Jesus*, pp. 22–23).

72. Bilu, "Taming," p. 41. See also Chajes, *Between Worlds*, and Lieberman, "Concept," p. 99. Seidel modifies this claim, though, noting some appearances of the term as early as Geniza documents ("I see these Geniza terms as simply the expression of affliction, but without the extended narrative and expanded meanings of the later figure of the *dybbuk*," *Possession*, 89).

73. Chajes, "Jewish Exorcism," p. 388; Goldish, *Spirit Possession*, p. 99; Seidel, "Possession," p. 75.

74. Herrmann, "Les premiers," pp. 307–8. For the Psalms employed apotropaically in the Qumran record, see Puech, "11QPsAp[a]," pp. 377–408. Sorensen states that in the Qumran scrolls, "the language of demonic possession tends to be associated with ethical behavior" (*Possession*, 65).

75. 1Q20, section 20 (Vermes, *Complete Dead Sea Scrolls*, p. 455).

76. 4Q560, col. 1.1–5 (Penney and Wise, "By the Power," p. 632). Klutz considers this a clear instance of "fever" being metonymically envisioned as a type of demon, not unlike the fever rebuked in Luke 4:39 (*Exorcism Stories*, p. 76).

77. Sorensen, *Possession*, pp. 68–69; Penney and Wise, "By the Power," p. 628.

78. Penney and Wise, "By the Power," p. 628. The Hebrew and Aramaic fragments of early medieval medical texts in the Cairo Geniza are consonant, in many respects, with the attitudes toward illness and evil found in the Qumran scrolls, though the dating and provenance of many of the materials behind the Geniza collection are obscure (a handlist of medical fragments appears in Isaacs, *Medical and Para-Medical Manuscripts*). Jonathan Seidel associates the Jewish liturgical exorcisms of Geniza with the antidemonic psalms of Qumran: there is demon expulsion, but little in the way of "fact-finding" or interviewing a possessed person for information about an indwelling demon ("Possession," p. 79). The early Geniza exorcisms apparently belong to a highly scholastic tradition, one that (for the most part) downplays the herbal and medical particulars associated with most exorcisms of the ancient world (82). The exorcisms are, in many respects, familiar in form and spirit to incantation bowls and papyri of late antiquity and may indicate the continuity of these beliefs among Jewish communities throughout the early Middle Ages: "In your name, O Lord of Hosts, God of Israel, Enthroned on the Cherubim, the Explicit Name; by the seventy names of God Compassionate and Merciful, God who wounds and heals: Send healing and have mercy on Bunayna bint Yaman; and send her complete recovery. . . . I adjure you, spirits and demonesses, evil eye, evil affliction, evil satan, and all kinds of visitations: in the name of 'I Am That I Am,' who causes the entire world to quake; by the name that the sea heard and was split; that the fire heard and was quenched, that the boulders heard and were shattered, and that the stone heard and exploded—so shall you leave, depart, go far away, and shall not touch Bunayna bat Yaman from this day and forever, Amen, Amen, Amen, Selah . . . may she be healthy (and free of) any evil eye, evil spirits, evil plague, evil diseases, afflictions, chastisements, fever and chills, and any blasts and harmful spirits. I swear by you and adjure you in the name of Gabriel, Michael, and Raphael to move and depart from Bunayna bat Yaman, from her body, from her head, from her temples, and from the two hundred forty-eight organs that are in her" (Schiffman and Swartz, *Hebrew and Aramaic Incantation Texts*, pp. 115–16). As with the demons of Qumran, it is difficult

to know whether or not we should read "indwelling demons" into such exorcisms of illness. Joseph Naveh and Shaul Shaked discuss this problem as it relates to both the incantation bowl and Geniza traditions, urging caution with any particular supposition of how demons and illness are conceptualized in these sources (*Magic Spells*, pp. 34–36). An amulet description of a bone demon seems clear enough: "the spirit of the bones, that walks within the tendons and bones" (34). On the other hand, a disembodied demon that controls and causes various diseases could be adjured to leave the body by metonymy—without necessarily implying that the demon itself is physically in the body. If (as Seidel argues from analogy and interpretation), indwelling possession was a phenomenon in early medieval Jewish societies, then we can potentially turn to these exorcisms as a viable contrast against which to understand developing Christian beliefs of the same period.

79. Piska 4.7 (Braude and Kapstein, *Pĕsikta dĕ-Rab Kahăna*, p. 82). Johanan ben Zacchai flourished ca. 10–80 CE (528).

80. According to Seidel, "rabbinic discourse on exorcism acknowledges the performative, perhaps illusionist ritual power of the action but not necessarily its reality" ("Possession," p. 85). Seidel reads the Johanan ben Zakkai episode differently, however (85). For more on exorcism in medieval Judaism, see Bacher, "La légende," pp. 285–87; and Chajes, "Jewish Exorcism."

81. Bourguignon, foreword to *Spirit Possession*, p. 9; Goldish, *Spirit Possession*, p. 25.

82. Homer, *Iliad*, p. 19.

83. Hesiod, *Works and Days*, line 122 (Evelyn-White, *Hesiod*, p. 11). Euripides, *Alcestis*, line 1003 (Way, *Euripides*, p. 490). Pausanias describes the ghost (*daimona*) of one of Odysseus's sailors, who continued to haunt a temple in Eleia and demand a virgin every year from the local populace (Pausanias, *Description*, p. 40).

84. Hesiod, *Works and Days*, line 314 (Evelyn-White, *Hesiod*, p. 27).

85. Homer, *Odyssey*, p. 390; *Oedipus the King* 828 (Storr, *Sophocles*, p. 76). See Ferguson, *Demonology*, pp. 38–40.

86. See, for instance, the sense of evil fate in Pythian Ode 3.34 (Gildersleeve, *Pindar*, p. 72) and good fate in Olympian Ode 13.105 (55). On fate and *δαιμον* in Pindar, see Bowra, *Pindar*, pp. 173–75.

87. Philo of Alexandria, *Giants*, pp. 62–63. Ferguson shows that Philo's theology is already at odds with the rapidly shifting usage of the first-century Greek-speaking world, which is coming to treat demons as exclusively negative: "Occasionally Christians made reference to bad angels, as when the New Testament speaks of 'the Devil and his angels,' but the New Testament never speaks of demons in a good sense" (*Demonology*, p. 84).

88. Richard Gordon, "Imagining," pp. 187, 226.

89. Plutarch dismisses even this religiously sanctioned possession: "It is foolish, indeed childish, to believe god himself, like the ventriloquists . . . enters into prophets' bodies and uses their mouths and voices as his instruments" ("Oracles in Decline" 414E, p. 21).

90. Those works criticize what they regard as popular superstitions, or the attribution of seizures to spiritual rather than physiological causes (Sorensen, *Possession*, pp. 96–97n111).

91. Wesley Smith, "So-Called Possession," esp. pp. 404, 409. The passage in Lucian (*The Lover of Lies* [Harmon, *Lucian*, p. 345]) runs as follows: "'You act ridiculously,' said Ion, 'to doubt everything. For my part, I should like to ask you what you say to those who free possessed men from their terrors by exorcising the spirits so manifestly. I need not discuss this: everyone knows about the Syrian from Palestine, the adept in it, how many he takes in hand who fall down in the light of the moon and roll their eyes and fill their mouths with foam; nevertheless, he restores them to health and sends them away normal in mind, delivering

them from their straits for a large fee. When he stands beside them as they lie there and asks: "Whence came you into this body?" the patient himself is silent, but the spirit answers in Greek or in the language of whatever foreign country he comes from, telling how and whence he entered into the man; whereupon, by adjuring the spirit and if he does not obey, threatening him, he drives him out. Indeed, I actually saw one coming out, black and smoky in colour'" (345). Another interlocutor adds that such sights are common, and that he himself has seen hundreds of such cases, but it is clear that this third disputant is now talking about disembodied spirits, or ghosts, rather than indwelling demons or exorcisms proper. The entire dialogue, in any event, is written to expose such phenomena as popular superstitions. The "Syrian from Palestine" is not Jesus, since the dialogue clearly speaks of a contemporary.

92. Wesley Smith, "So-Called Possession," p. 425; for agreement see Chajes, "Jewish Exorcism," pp. 387–88, Sorensen, *Possession*, pp. 6–7.

93. McCasland, *By the Finger*, p. 66. Pausanias would be the most likely place to expect references to possession, but McCasland also points out the absence of references in Cicero and the elder Pliny: "the Greek and Roman writers themselves do not indicate a prevalence of demon possession and exorcism in the first century. These phenomena may have existed, but there is very slight evidence of them" (69). Sorensen also notices that when Pliny the Elder discusses magic and popular healing of first century Rome, he does not seem to know anything about exorcism (*Possession*, p. 7).

94. Janowitz, *Magic*, p. 33.

95. E. R. Dodds takes Wesley Smith's argument to task in "Supernormal Phenomena in Classical Antiquity" (pp. 195–96n3), but his counterevidence only addresses religiously sanctioned possession (the prophetic oracles), not the pathological possession of Middle Eastern tradition. Of Greco-Roman responses to possession as it was known in Palestine and Egypt, Dodds concedes, "All these texts are relatively late; and it seems likely that the practice of formal exorcism, as distinct from simple rites of purification, only developed *pari passu* with the growing fear of demons which characterized the Roman Imperial Age" (196). Sorensen also contests Smith's thesis (*Possession*, p. 75–117).

96. Matthew 7:21–23, and Luke 10:17–20, 11:14–22. See Ferguson, *Demonology*, pp. 19–22; Fridrichsen, "The Conflict," pp. 126–27; Ling, *Significance*, pp. 12–55; Jeffrey Burton Russell, *Devil*, pp. 237–39; and Yates, "Jesus," p. 39. It is worth recalling that since the Gospel of Mark was probably written about the time of the Roman-Judean War (ca. 66–70 CE), and the other three Gospels around the end of the first century, then they record the perceptions of Jesus's life and ministry not of Jesus's contemporaries but of those more than a generation after his death (Porterfield, *Healing*, p. 36).

97. Rebukes fever: Luke 4:39; rebukes wind: Mark 4:39; rebukes demon: Luke 4:35. Twelftree posits that Luke is here embellishing on Mark's narrative, which has no such direct rebuke: "He came and took her by the hand and lifted her up. Then the fever left her, and she began to serve them" (Mark 1:13; Twelftree, *Jesus*, p. 138; see also Klutz, *Exorcism Stories*, pp. 75–77).

98. Thus Hollenbach: "it is directly in connection with this activity [exorcism] that all the prominent public authorities manifest extreme hostility toward him" ("Jesus, Demoniacs, and Public Authorities," p. 569).

99. Capernaum demoniac: Mark 1:21–28, Luke 4:31–37; Gerasene: Matthew 8:28–34, Mark 5:1–20, Luke 8:26–39; Syrophoenician woman's daughter: Matthew 15:21–28, Mark 7:24–30; epileptic boy: Matthew 17:14–21, Mark 9:14–29, Luke 9:37–43; Beelzebub controversy: Matthew 9:32–34 and 12:22–30, Luke 11:14–23 (cf. Mark 3:22–27). A further

narrative from Luke involving a crippled woman with a spirit (Luke 13:10–17) may be included also, depending on how literally one takes the "spirit of infirmity" involved in that case. In that episode, however, Jesus addresses the woman rather than the spirit (Twelftree, *Jesus*, pp. 55–56, 138). For greater precision in distinguishing how illness and the demonic are related in each of the Gospels, and across the New Testament canon, see Thomas, *Devil*.

100. Mark 3:11–12; see also Luke 4:41. Cf. Mark 5:6–7.

101. Jerome, *Vita Hilarionis*, chaps. 33–37, 42 (PL 23: cols. 46B–48B, 50C–51A).

102. E.g., Matthew 8:16: "he cast out the spirits with a word, and cured all who were sick." He also lays on hands (Luke 13:13). See Ferguson, *Demonology*, pp. 8–11; McCasland, *By the Finger*, p. 6; and Twelftree, *Jesus*, pp. 157–65. Janowitz lists some common techniques of first-century exorcisms: looking upwards, sighing or groaning, making hand gestures, spitting, invoking the deity, and speaking nonsense words or letter strings (*Magic*, p. 39).

103. Acts 19:11–17. Among the most comprehensive collections of references to demon possession in classical and early Christian sources (especially those in Greek) is Tambornino, *De Antiquorum Daemonismo*. A series of early references is conveniently collected and translated in Cotter, *Miracles*, pp. 75–127. See also Brown, "Rise and Function," p. 96: "Exorcism was the classic cure associated with the holy man [of late antiquity]"; and Flint "Demonisation," p. 326: "there is much to be said for the idea that, as it progressed in the pagan world, Christianity owed most of its first successes to its clear victories over the demons" (and see p. 341). See also Kee, *Miracle*, pp. 252–86; Porterfield, *Healing*, pp. 43–44, 63–65; and Sorensen, *Possession*, pp. 148–53, 173–77. Sorensen cautions, however, that claims of Christian exorcism leading to conversion come mostly from sophisticated literary and theological writings (178n23). Barrett-Lennard provocatively draws attention to the lack of references to possession or exorcism in Christian papyrus letters before the fourth century: "this contrasts sharply with the situation in relation to our literary and liturgical sources" (*Christian Healing*, p. 137). This suggests a top-down inculcation of adopting the rhetoric of possession, rather than a grassroots upsurge consisting of authentic descriptions. Elizabeth Leeper writes, "exorcism did not gain its chief importance as an impromptu evangelistic tool to attract and convert the pagan; rather, exorcism found its niche within the institutional church as a rite for Christians" ("Exorcism," p. 182).

104. Caciola, *Discerning Spirits*, pp. 228–29. Porterfield observes, "Christian exorcism, healing, and concern for the poor and sick developed in a diversified market of religious and medical services. . . . Christians competed well in this arena" (*Healing*, p. 48). According to Hector Avalos, the health care system offered by Christians was cheaper and more accessible than that offered by rival deities and the intricate rites attached to them (Avalos, *Health Care*, pp. 93–95 (on fees); 99–107 and 111–14 (on geographical and temporal accessibility).

105. Justin Martyr, *Dialogue with Trypho* 30, 76 (Falls, *Dialogue*, pp. 46, 119); cf. *1 Apology* 18 (Falls, *Dialogue*, p. 53).

106. Justin Martyr, *2 Apology* 6 (Falls, *Saint*, p. 126).

107. Justin Martyr, *Dialogue with Trypho* 85 (Falls, *Dialogue*, p. 132).

108. Irenaeus, *Against Heresies*, 2.32.4: "Some do certainly and truly drive out devils, so that those who have thus been cleansed from evil spirits frequently both believe [in Christ] and join themselves to the church " (Alexander Roberts and Donaldson, *Apostolic Fathers*, p. 409).

109. On the context and background of the *Life of Apollonius*, see Graham Anderson, *Philostratus*, and Dzielska, *Apollonius*.

110. Origen, *Contra Celsum* 6.41; Philostratus, *Life of Apollonius*, ed. and trans. Conybeare,

p. x. Following the appearance of the *Life of Apollonius*, Sossianus Hierocles composed a similar defense of Apollonius in the late third century, stating that the pagan sage was as effective an exorcist as Christ. This was in turn attacked by Eusebius in his short treatise *Against Hierocles*, chap. 30 (des Places, *Contre Hiéroclès*, pp. 162–64; see also Kofsky, *Eusebius*, pp. 165–214).

111. Philostratus, *Life of Apollonius* 3.38, trans. Jones, p. 301.

112. Philostratus, *Life of Apollonius* 3.38, trans. Jones, p. 301.

113. Similar distance exorcisms, also performed through the delivery of a written text, appear in several medieval Christian contexts, such as the *Life of Eugendus*. In a letter addressed to the demon Eugendus writes the appropriate adjuration, which is folded, sealed, and sent via messengers back to the possessed woman—though it apparently has its intended effect before the couriers are even able to deliver it (*Vita Eugendi* 144; Martine, *Vie*, pp. 392–94). Sulpicius Severus also reports a practice of letter-exorcisms in *Dialogi* 1.20 (Halm, *Sulpicii Severi*, p. 172).

114. Philostratus, *Life of Apollonius* 4.20, trans. Jones, p. 363.

115. Conybeare elaborates, "the exorcist driving demons out of afflicted human beings by use of threats and invocations of mysterious names was as familiar a figure in old Pagan society as he was in the early church" (Philostratus, *Life of Apollonius*, ed. and trans. Conybeare, p. xv).

116. Geffcken, *Last Days*, p. 57; Kofsky, *Eusebius*, p. 165.

117. Sorensen, *Possession*, pp. 2–3.

118. But the canon is still very much an ongoing problem for Eusebius throughout the *Ecclesiastical History*—for instance, in the early third century. Amidst the apocryphal and pseudepigraphal texts of late antiquity, the (probably) third-century Testament of Solomon, most likely from Egypt, provides an especially notable inventory of demons. Solomon, as narrator, has a pageant of demons brought before him, including Ornias, Beelzebul, Onoskelis, Asmodeus, Lix Tetrax, seven spirits of the heavenly bodies (Deception, Strife, Fate, Distress, Error, Power, and The Worst), Obyzouth, Enepsigos, and many dozens more in various elemental and zoomorphic forms. A three-headed-dragon demon comes forth, claiming dominion over three evils: he makes infants blind while still in the womb, he makes them deaf and dumb, and he makes people "fall down, foam (at the mouth), and grind their teeth" (Charlesworth, *Old Testament*, 1:973). On the provenance, Klutz writes: "several lines of evidence converge in a fashion that would seem to point to Egypt, both for the *Testament*'s earliest literary sources and for its final stage of redaction" (*Rewriting*, p. 35). The Anglo-Saxons would know Asmodeus through the book of Tobit, and were well familiar with Solomon's legendary power over the demons.

119. Hans Dieter Betz made significant portions of this tradition widely accessible in his 1986 translation of the Greek Magical Papyri, but Marvin Meyer notes that Betz omitted texts that were predominantly Christian (Meyer and Smith, *Ancient Christian Magic*, p. 27).

120. Sorensen, *Possession*, p. 116.

121. These instances, all fairly typical, come from a single text (Ann Arbor, University of Michigan, Coptic Magical text 593; Meyer and Smith, *Ancient Christian Magic*, pp. 306–7).

122. Vienna, Austrian National Library, Coptic MS 337; Ranier 197 (Meyer and Smith, *Ancient Christian Magic*, pp. 44–45). Another sixth-century papyrus is directed generally against evil spirits: "[Christ! I adjure] you, O lord, almighty, first-begotten, self-begotten, begotten without semen, [. . .] as well as all-seeing are you, and Yao, Sabao, Brinthao: Keep me as a son, protect me from every evil spirit, and subject me to every spirit of impure, destroying demons—on the earth, under the earth, of the water and of the land—and

every phantom. Christ!" (Cairo, Egyptian Museum, MS 67188; Meyer and Smith, *Ancient Christian Magic*, p. 47).

123. Thus Cameron: "*Dweorh* has almost always been translated as 'dwarf,' which may be its primitive meaning, but there is ample evidence in other Old English medical texts that it also means 'fever,' apparently fever accompanied by delirium or convulsive seizures" (*Wið dweorh* charm, *Anglo-Saxon Medicine*, p. 152). For the text of *Wið dweorh*, see Pettit, *Anglo-Saxon Remedies*, 1:72–74.

124. Ann Arbor, University of Michigan, Coptic Magical text 136 (Meyer and Smith, *Ancient Christian Magic*, p. 88). This rite is sandwiched between one for a woman whose womb hurts and another for ridding the house of vermin.

125. PGM XII.281–82 (Betz, *Greek Magical Papyri*, p. 164).

126. PGM IV.1227–49 (Meyer and Smith, *Ancient Christian Magic*, pp. 43–44).

127. PGM IV.3007–86 (Betz, *Greek Magical Papyri*, pp. 96–97). Betz explains that Pibechis was a legendary Egyptian magician.

128. Janowitz, *Magic*, pp. 41–42. Wilfred Lawrence Knox argues that this is a composite rite, stitched together from Jewish exorcistic formulas originally intended for different purposes ("Jewish Liturgical Exorcism," pp. 191–203).

129. The classic introduction to this phenomenon is Chitty, *Desert a City*. On demonology in this tradition, see Brakke, *Demons*; and Crislip, *From Monastery to Hospital*, pp. 78–81.

130. Jeffrey Burton Russell, *Satan*, p. 166.

131. Norman Russell, *Lives*, p. 109.

132. Benedicta Ward, *Wisdom*, p.64.

133. Stewart, *World*, p. 25.

134. Norman Russell, *Lives*, p. 57 (Latin version at PL 21: col. 399D). See also Benedicta Ward, *Wisdom*, pp. 6–7: "A woman's body is a fire, and from it comes the remembrance of other women."

135. Norman Russell, *Lives*, p. 93 (PL 21: col. 433C).

136. Scorpions and snakes: Norman Russell, *Lives*, p. 106 (PL 21: col. 448A); gnat: Palladius, *Lausiac History* 18, p. 59. The Latin translator of this latter anecdote apparently finds it too petty to spend so much bother for a gnat—or at least not sufficiently moralistic—so instead of being molested by a gnat, that version has Macarius molested by the *spiritus fornicationis* (PL 73: col. 1113C).

137. Benedicta Ward, *Sayings*, p. 5 (Latin version in *Verba Seniorum* at PL 73: cols. 772C–D). See Palladius, *Lausic History*, p. 22 for an analogous metaphor: just as a dog will stop coming to a meat market if no one there throws it any scraps, so will the demons leave Abba Moses alone if he stops wavering in his resolve (PL 73: col. 1120D).

138. Palladius, *Lausiac History* 23, p. 81. Latin version: "Egressae ergo ferae in illa hora, et masculus et femina, me a pedibus ad caput usque odorati sunt, circumlingentes" (PL 73: col. 1130D).

139. Sulpicius Severus, *Dialogi* 1.24 (Halm, *Sulpicii Severi*, p. 177).

140. Rosenthal, *Vitae Patrum*, p. 53 (and see 53–63 more generally for awareness of the *Vitae Patrum* corpus in Anglo-Saxon England).

141. Benedict of Nursia, *Rule of Benedict*, chap. 42 (for an Anglo-Saxon instance—CCCC 57—see Chamberlin, *Rule*, p. 51).

142. For some devil tales from the *Vitae Patrum* in Old English (from London, British Library, MS Cotton Otho C.i, vol. 2, fols. 137v–143v), see Assmann, *Angelsächsische Homilien*, p. 195–207. These are now translated into modern English; see Dendle,

"Old English 'Life of Malchus.'" In the early Latin Middle Ages, many of the texts of the *Vitae Patrum* tradition were attributed to Jerome.

143. Ælfric, preface to the translation of Genesis (Wilcox, *Ælfric's Prefaces*, p. 116). For more references, see Rosenthal, *Vitae Patrum*, pp. 57–62.

144. Oxford, Bodleian Library, MS Hatton 115, fol. 145v (Scragg, *Vercelli*, p. 177). See also Fred Robinson, "Devil's Account," pp. 362–71; Scragg, "'The Devil's Account," pp. 107–10.

145. Charles Wright, *Irish Tradition*, pp. 23, 175–214.

146. Charles Wright, *Irish Tradition*, pp. 106–74.

147. Most recently, see Powell and Scragg, *Apocryphal Texts*.

148. For the demonology of *Solomon and Saturn I*, see Dendle, "*Solomon and Saturn*"; Thomas Hill, "The Devil's Forms," pp. 164–76; and Thomas Hill, "Tormenting the Devil," pp. 157–66.

149. The genre is generally pervaded by the rhetoric of travel literature ("first I visited so and so, when I encountered this holy man . . ."), but in fact the pioneers of the genre did visit these communities. Rufinus of Aquilea and Jerome both visited Nitria in the Egyptian desert; Palladius spent a year there before visiting Evagrius of Pontus at Cellia. John Cassian spent some fifteen years in Egypt before writing his *Collationes* and *Institutiones*.

150. Cyprian of Carthage, "Epistle 1.5" (*Ad Donatum*, trans. Wallis; Alexander Roberts and Donaldson, *Fathers of the Third Century*, p. 276).

151. Alexander Roberts and Donaldson, *Ante-Nicene Christian Library*, p. 379.

152. Origen, *Contra Celsum* 7.4, pp. 397–98.

153. Origen, *Contra Celsum* 7.4, p. 398.

154. Canon 26 (Percival, *Seven Ecumenical Councils*, p. 147). The canon was promulgated in collections such as Fulgentius Ferrandus's *Breviatio*, p. 142: "Vt non exorcizent illi qui necdum ab episcopo sunt prouecti" (they should not perform exorcisms who have not yet been promoted by a bishop; PL 67: col. 957A).

155. *Apostolic Constitutions* 8.3 (Alexander Roberts and Donaldson, *Fathers of the Third and Fourth Centuries*, p. 493).

156. *Apostolic Constitutions* 8.3 (Alexander Roberts and Donaldson, *Fathers of the Third and Fourth Centuries*, p. 493).

157. Leeper, "Exorcism," p. 321.

158. Coulange, *Life*, p. 223. On the evolution of the office of exorcist in the early church, see Leeper, "Exorcism," pp. 274–331.

159. Duchesne, *Christian Worship*, p. 346. Eusebius cites a letter from Cornelius, bishop of Rome (ca. 251–53 CE), giving the breakdown of offices: at that time there were fifty-two exorcists, lectors, and doorkeepers total, though he does not subdivide that total for these minor orders (Eusebius, *History of the Church* 6.43, p. 216). A brief letter addressed to Cyprian of Carthage from Lucianus on behalf of *universi confessores* (also from the mid-third century) mentions an exorcist among the witnesses: "Lucianus wrote this is in the presence of the clergy, both an exorcist and a lector" ("Letter 16": "praesente de clero et exorcista et lectore, Lucianus scripsit"; PL 4: col. 0269A). Edmund Keller notes that it was "very likely" Cornelius's predecessor, Pope Fabius, who introduced the order, but does not give reasons ("Glimpses," p. 290).

160. Munier, *Les Statuta*, p. 174; Reichel, *Complete Manual*, p. 195.

161. Hrabanus Maurus, *De clericorum institutione* 1.3–12 (PL 107: col. 299B); Hrabanus Maurus, *Disputatio puerorum* (PL 101: col. 1132B). See Roger Reynolds, *Ordinals*, pp. 122–23.

162. Duchesne, *Christian Worship*, pp. 347–49.

163. Duchesne, *Christian Worship*, p. 349.

164. Duchesne, *Christian Worship*, p. 350. Documents differ over how long a candidate remained an exorcist before advancing, ranging from a single day to a month or even ten years (see Duchesne, *Christian Worship*, pp. 349–50).

165. *De septem ordinibus Ecclesiae*; Roger Reynolds, *Ordinals*, p. 124.

166. Pseudo-Alcuin, *Liber de divinis officiis* 36 (PL 101: col. 1234D).

167. Amalarius of Metz, *De ecclesiasticis officiis* 2.9 (PL 105: col. 1084D–1085A).

168. Anon., *Vita Cuthberti* 1.7 (Colgrave, *Two Lives*, p. 72).

169. Article 95 (Munier, *Les Statuta*, p. 97).

170. H. A. Wilson, *Gelasian*, p. 145.

171. H. A. Wilson, *Gelasian*, pp. 147–48.

172. E.g., Leofric Missal 2309–11 (Nicholas Orchard, *Leofric Missal*, p. 394); Lanalet Pontifical, fol. 72b (Doble, *Pontificale Lanaletense*, p. 51); Egbert Pontifical, fol. 24r (Banting, *Two Anglo-Saxon Pontificals*, pp. 19–20); Sidney Sussex Pontifical, fol. 3r (Banting, *Two Anglo-Saxon Pontificals*, p. 158); Samson Pontifical (CCCC 146, pp. 111–12); CCCC 163 (p. 273); London, British Library, MS Cotton Vitellius E.XII (fol. 147r–v).

173. Brown, "Saint," p. 191. The longest series of exorcisms is probably that in the tenth-century *Romano-German Pontifical* (running about thirty pages in a modern edition; Vogel and Elze, *Le Pontifical Romano-Germanique,* pp. 193–224). Most are substantially less: exorcisms run for some twenty pages in the Leofric Missal (fols. 308r–318r) and ten pages in the Lanalet Pontifical (fols. 162r–167r), including procedural exorcisms of salt, water, etc.

174. Altogether, the entire sequence of exorcisms in the Leofric Missal has a lower word count than Vulgate Psalm 118 alone. Of course, recital of the Psalms would receive continuous reinforcement in the monastic offices.

175. More on this below (chapter 2).

176. Jerome, "Letter 108" (PL 22: col. 889).

177. Brown, *Cult*, p. 106.

178. See esp. *Vita Caesarii* 1.5, 2.18–19, 2.20, 2.29, 2.30 (Morin, *Sancti Caesarii Episcopi Arelatensis*). For Caesarius as healer and exorcist, see also Klingshirn, *Caesarius of Arles*, pp. 159–70.

179. Caesarius, "Sermon 79" (Morin, *Sancti Caesarii*, p. 325). He goes on to console the congregation and—issuing a timeworn palliative still used of snakes and spiders—assures them that demons have more to fear from Christians than vice versa.

180. Mass: *Vita Caesarii* 2.20; roads: 1.5, 2.29; forum: 2.30 (Morin, *Sancti Caesarii Episcopi Arelatensis*).

181. Sulpicius, *Dialogi* 3.6 (Halm, *Sulpicii Severi*, p. 204).

182. Gregory of Tours, *Vita Martini* 18: "daemoniacum ad se exhiberi iubet" (Halm, *Sulpicii Severi*, p. 127).

183. Gregory of Tours, *Libri de virtutibus sancti Martini Episcopi* 2.60 (Krusch, *Miracula et opera*, p. 179).

184. Gregory of Tours, *Libri de virtutibus sancti Martini Episcopi* 2.60 (Krusch, *Miracula et opera*, p. 180).

185. Einhard, *Translatio et miracula sanctorum Marcellini et Petri* 4.16 (Waitz, *Translatio*, p. 263).

186. Einhard, *Translatio et miracula sanctorum Marcellini et Petri* 3.14 (Waitz, *Translatio*, p. 253).

187. Agobard of Lyon, *De quorundam inlusione signorum* (or *Ad Bartholomeum*) 1 (Van Acker, *Agobardi Lugdunensis*, p. 237).

188. Agobard of Lyon, *De quorundam inlusione signorum* (or *Ad Bartholomeum*) 12 (Van Acker, *Agobardi Lugdunensis*, p. 243). Furthermore, he notes that Satan seems to target "boys, and girls, and the dull-witted" (pueros, ac puellas, et hebetes; Van Acker, *Agobardi Lugdunensis*, p. 242), not people who are "faithful . . . and endowed with reason" (fidelis . . . et ratione praeditus; Van Acker, *Agobardi Lugdunensis*, p. 243).

189. Agobard of Lyon, *De quorundam inlusione signorum* (or *Ad Bartholomeum*) 7 (Van Acker, *Agobardi Lugdunensis*, p. 240).

190. Amulo of Lyon, "Epistle 1" (*Ad Theodboldum*; PL 116: cols. 77B–84B).

191. Amulo of Lyon, "Epistle 1" (*Ad Theodboldum*; PL 116: col. 81D).

192. Amulo of Lyon, "Epistle 1" (*Ad Theodboldum*; PL 116: col. 81B). In Constantinople, the Council of Trullo (692) decreed against the faking of possession (Canon 60; Percival, *Seven Ecumenical Councils*, p. 392).

Chapter 2

Medical and Liturgical Responses

"Ha, so simple is it?" the hermit said. "A potion!"—*The Tiger's Whisker*[1]

SOMETIMES MEDIEVAL WRITERS APPEALED to "demons" to account for anomalous disturbances that defied common experience or ready explanation: for instance, a woman in Lantfred's *Translation and Miracles of St. Swithun* who dislocates her jaw while yawning is said to have been seized by a demon.[2] Demonic attribution was never systematic, uniform, or exhaustive, and it formed part of a broader conceptual scheme in which any detrimental or misunderstood behaviors—or indeed any of life's misfortunes in general—could be imputed to any of a number of potential causes. Few thinkers attributed every human evil directly to the devil or to demons, though any particular evil could potentially be considered the work of demons in the subjective assessment of a medieval observer.[3] Behavioral disorders which caused people to act with the outward appearance of volition, but in a manner contrary to their usual social commitments and ideals (and in the Middle Ages, this could include heretical speech no less than seizures), readily invited the diagnosis of "demon possession." Christian monastic literature had always spoken comfortably of sin and spiritual struggle in medical terms; this blended effectively with popular medical traditions that routinely anthropomorphized disease agents. The body and mind of the "possessed" thus became contested sites for the ongoing development of conceptual models regarding identity, sites which challenged healers to demonstrate medical efficacy and church representatives to assert spiritual authority.

Among the most consistently demonized of medical conditions were the more intractable muscle-control and behavioral disorders against which premodern palliatives and sedatives were of little use.[4] Therapy (including amulets, incantations, herbal remedies, and exorcisms) was generally aimed at creating a sense of psychological control over the situation, both for calming the patient and affirming social order within the community. There are frequent references in medieval sources to beating, binding, and other extreme measures in treatment of the possessed. For the medieval writer, however, these details carried sensationalistic impact as well as symbolic significance, and so it would be imprudent to take them invariably at face value. Wilfrid Bonser, the author of the first comprehensive study of Anglo-Saxon medicine, was unduly persuaded by such descriptions:

> If exorcism was of no avail and the devil was obstinate, more drastic measures were taken. Attempts to punish the demon led to harsh treatment of the victim whom he had possessed. It seems strange that experience should not have demonstrated that this treatment, which could but aggravate the mental disease, was wrong.[5]

Bonser is here referring specifically to a prescription in the *Leechbook* directing the physician to beat a *monaþ-seoc* patient (a "month-sick" patient, or "lunatic") with a dolphin-hide whip (*mere-swines fel*).[6] The curious material suggested for the whip smacks more of exotica than routine procedure, however. The mentally ill or possessed could have faced a wide range of communal responses depending on individual circumstances, but there is no strong evidence for systematic abuse of the possessed in Anglo-Saxon England.[7] Throughout the early medieval period hagiography portrays possession as an unfortunate condition that befalls the luckless far more often than the guilty, and the victim's caregivers are invariably presented as compassionate and empathetic.

Ronald Finucane paints the medieval healing shrine—perhaps with some melodrama—as something of a horror scene, complete with "wretched cripples writhing on the floor," "the stench of poverty and disease," and "the screams of fettered madmen straining at their bonds."[8] For extreme cases of pathological violence or thrashing convulsions, in which danger to self or others was a significant possibility, patients were of course restrained in the Middle Ages, as they are today. The thirteenth-century Friar Bartholomaeus Anglicus, after localizing the causes of madness to the lateral ventricles of the brain, prescribed binding the patient only so that "they hurt not them selfe & other men."[9] This, however, applied to only a small minority of mentally disturbed patients. In Sulpicius Severus's *Dialogues* an anchorite of the Egyptian desert seized by a demon is fettered hand and foot, from necessity (*necessitate*).[10] Einhard says he had to be persuaded to bind the raging priest Waltbert, which in the end he only does reluctantly, after the mad priest threatens someone with a knife.[11] Felix of Crowland speaks of a youth so violent and uncontrollable that he has to be bound; in fact, it is the intensity of the violence that Felix stresses as the most notable symptom of this condition.[12] Here, then, the binding seems to result from the unusually severe nature of the particular case. The more severe the illness, after all, the holier is the saint who manages to cure it. As noted in the introduction, the rhetoric of "binding" and "loosing" is an ancient trope, firmly rooted in the Christian tradition, which readily lends greater symbolic resonance to the detail that the demoniac is brought "bound" to the healer.

While early medieval hagiography tended to portray saints in conflict with lay healers, and sermons regularly contrasted Christ as the true "healer," in many ways medical and devotional works shared many similarities in spirit, method, and even manuscript contexts. Medical explanations of diseases were sometimes held as alternatives to spirit agency; at other times the two stood in virtual apposition, as though they were two ways of describing the same process.[13] Local physicians or pastors (if they were not the same person) might make themselves equally available to those in need of healing. They could respond in a variety of ways, from a simple prayer or incantation to a complicated series of rituals, many of them folkloric and so strongly reminiscent of pagan practices that they occasionally attracted the censure of reformers such as Ælfric and Wulfstan. Two broad textual traditions record some of the possible responses to individuals in distress, in the form of practical directions: medical books prescribe herbal remedies and ritual gestures, while liturgical books provide formal procedural exorcisms. These are overlapping genres in many ways. The recipes of the medical books rely heavily on *materia liturgica* such as holy water, and the exorcisms of liturgical books are, it can be argued, simply a different presentation of directions and prayers without being inherently different in kind. Medical books contain a number of familiar liturgical prayers, and liturgical books often contain series of benedictions for popular use that may appear to be magical "charms" to the modern observer. Finally, most manuscripts from both genres owed their origin and continued preservation to ecclesiastical houses.[14]

In this light, perhaps the most helpful way to visualize the relationship between medical and liturgical responses is to view the official exorcisms of the church (as found in the Gelasian, the Gregorian, and then the Romano-German pontifical traditions) as simply a subset of the wider matrix of possible responses, which more broadly includes the entire range of prayers, adjurations, ritual gestures, and applications of materials available to early medieval priests and healers. It was, to be sure, an important subset: there are many more liturgical books than medical ones from the early Middle Ages, reflecting the needs and interests of those centers where books were produced. We should not mistake, however, the fact that there are more copies in Anglo-Saxon England of the supplemented Hadrianum (a Gregorian-type Sacramentary) than there are of the *Leechbook* book 3 to mean that throughout England the liturgical response was the most prevalent. The ecclesiastical contexts of book production and preservation were, quite obviously, more conducive to the survival of liturgical books. Yet taken together, the medical and the liturgical evidence can offer a more complete picture of the landscape of healing in Anglo-Saxon England, with the understanding that each might have had greater appeal than the other in different communities and contexts.

Medical Responses

Throughout the Anglo-Saxon period patients were chiefly cared for by the family, in the home.[15] The nuclear family seems to have been the basic family structure, with the expectation that children would move out upon marriage.[16] Only wealthier classes are consistently represented as being surrounded by "households," with servants and perhaps extended family: for the average Anglo-Saxon herder or farmer, the immediate family and neighbors (probably in many cases, the better part of the village) formed what we might now call the support structure. Hospitals as we know them were a postconquest development.[17] The Rule of Benedict directs that there should be a separate infirmary in every monastic community. This was common practice in larger houses long before the reforms of the tenth century more vigorously attempted to regularize monastic practice. Bede, for instance, mentions that both Whitby and Lindisfarne have access to a sickroom or separate building (*hospitale*, OE *cumena-bur*) for the infirm.[18] These areas were presumably intended for use of the religious community rather than the general public, though some accounts portray the monasteries as munificent and accommodating to all manner of guests.[19]

Bede states that Queen Æthelthryth had a personal physician, and the *Life of Alfred* mentions that King Alfred was attended by multiple physicians (*omnibus medicis*).[20] Physicians as a separate class, however, may or may not have existed outside of royal houses. The occasional mention of a "physician" (*medicus*) probably referred to the person in the community locally considered as the most knowledgeable about healing, without implying that that was the person's sole occupation.[21] The amount of knowledge such a person had and the precise techniques employed no doubt differed widely from village to village. Access to books was mostly restricted to the clergy, and, beyond that, access to herbals and medical books was mostly restricted to more important scribal centers. Lay healers, therefore, necessarily drew on orally transmitted traditions and experience to treat patients. Medical recipes frequently called for liturgical procedures, in which case the local priest would have had to be included. Nonetheless, we should be careful not to read directions too strictly or literally. The recipes offer some flexibility: a series of rituals against *ælf-sogoða* in the *Leechbook* book 3 seems to presume that a priest is the reader and the celebrant (it calls for *oleum infirmorum* and the recital of liturgical prayers), yet the item ends, "gif þe ne lyste hat hine selfne oþþe swa gesubne swa he gesibbost hæbbe ⁊ senige swa he selost cunne" (if you prefer not, then have the person himself or whatever closest of kin he may have do it, and may that person make the sign of the cross as best he or she knows how).[22]

Anglo-Saxon accounts refer on several occasions to physicians and clergy in close proximity, working with one another to treat patients.[23] All references to physicians in the historical documents are to male physicians, but it is likely that women practiced midwifery and were largely in charge of female conditions.[24] It is also probable that women practiced a separate range of informal medicinal arts, as a sort of shadow-class parallel to male physicians (as women are known to have done on the continent).[25] In any event, this would help account for certain small herb boxes (or thread boxes) which have been found in the graves of some Anglo-Saxon women. Since the boxes contained such minute quantities of plant and mineral material, Audrey L. Meaney speculates that they may have been more symbolic than practical in nature—for instance, the particular emblems of a healer. Unidentified plant remains were found in such a thread box at Sibertswold, Kent, and caper spurge in another at Barton-on-Humber.[26]

A number of medical manuscripts from Anglo-Saxon England survive, and contain many hundreds of recipes and remedies for a wide variety of ailments. Unfortunately, the ailments are usually only mentioned by name, not described in terms of symptoms, and so the modern reader often has to guess what a given remedy is for. The *Herbarium of Apuleius* and its companion text the *Medicine from Quadrupeds* (*Medicina de quadrupedibus*) survive in a handful of manuscripts, some beautifully illustrated. The texts are categorized by ingredients and list all the ailments that a particular plant or animal product can alleviate. The Old English translation adheres closely to the Latin original, so it is not certain to what extent this text reflects contemporary Anglo-Saxon practice.[27] A fascinating manuscript from around 1000 CE that has come to be known as the *Lacnunga Book* (London, British Library, MS Harley 585) contains a large selection of material in Latin, Old English, and fossilized snippets of Old Irish and Greek. This manuscript provides tantalizing glimpses into what are presumably earlier strata of Germanic and Celtic pagan beliefs, though (as Karen Louise Jolly has demonstrated) the texts in their current redaction are thoroughly Christian.[28] Some of the items are in Old English verse, including the "Nine Herbs Charm" and "For a Sudden Stitch." Though it begins with remedies for head ailments, the *Lacnunga Book* quickly abandons the head-to-foot ordering of most medieval medical compilations. A great deal of interesting lore is preserved in the manuscript, and in fact the principles of selection suggest more of a concern with lore, exotica, and highly stylized charms than with the more systematic and exhaustive lists of herbs and ailments one might expect from a working practitioner.[29] Edward Pettit, the manuscript's most recent editor, has likened the book's structure to a working "notebook" and suggested that its intended owner was likely "Christian, but probably not a model of orthodox piety."[30]

The oldest and (what many consider) one of the more promising manuscripts for recovering authentic Anglo-Saxon practices is Bald's *Leechbook* (London, British Library, MS Royal 12.D.XVII), preserved only in a manuscript from the mid-tenth century but possibly compiled during the reign of Alfred. The first two books of this work form a unit (the first on external ailments, the second on internal ones), largely based on the wide range of Byzantine and Roman medical recipes available in Latin in the early Middle Ages, many of them arranged and adapted for practical use. The careful, exhaustive nature of the compilation makes it an impressive work of scholarship. *Leechbook* book 3 is an independent unit that records remedies for which there are no known continental exemplars, and that relies heavily on indigenous northern European ingredients. Cameron considers it "the closest we can get to the native medicine of northern peoples" at this time.[31] In addition to these vernacular sources, Anglo-Saxons may have had access to some of the numerous Latin medical treatises circulating widely in the early Middle Ages, including epitomes and redactions of Caelius Aurelianus, Pliny, and Isidore.[32] Debbie Banham argues, however, that prior to a sudden influx in the eleventh century of medical knowledge based on continental exemplars—as found in a new generation of texts such as the *Practica Petrocelli*, the *Passionarius Galieni*, and the Pseudo-Galenic *Liber tertius*—Anglo-Saxon medical knowledge remained relatively isolated from mainstream European medical trends.[33]

Anglo-Saxon collections are rich repositories of folkloric as well as professional medical beliefs. In addition to the major collections, popular rites and recipes also appear in separate quires or odd leaves (as "For Unfruitful Land," now bound with London, British Library, MS Cotton Caligula A.VII), as additions to otherwise unrelated books (for instance, the CCCC 41 charms added to a copy of the OE Bede; or "Against a Wen," added to the psalm commentary and homilies of London, British Library, MS Royal 4A.XIV), miscellanies (the "Theft of Cattle" charm included in London, British Library, MS Cotton Tiberius A.III), and a variety of other contexts. This was clearly a vibrant and important tradition, and not so easily dismissed as church reformers might have liked. Practical books include rituals to help make a field produce better yields, rituals against elves and worms, antidotes for ill-defined poisons and venoms, herbal remedies against all manner of infirmity, prayers for protection and guidance, procedures for finding lost cattle, and practices for guarding against the temptations of the devil. Christian prayers appear side by side with vestigial pagan references to Woden and dwarves, and both are interspersed with a variety of gibberish charms pasted together from various languages. Jolly has shown how these collections were the culmination of a long process of amalgamation between popular folkloric beliefs and ecclesiastical codification, and that their coexistence in these manuscripts argues against too strict a categorical separation between folk belief and orthodox doctrine.[34]

Through such evidence, therefore, we know that the Anglo-Saxons had at least some doctors and at least some medical books, but it is impossible to determine to what extent the doctors used those books in treating patients or to what extent an average Anglo-Saxon villager had access to either. The books are monastic productions with many items copied from classical exemplars. Some evidence points to the existence of lay physicians: Charles Singer shrewdly observes that virtually all manuscript illustrations of Anglo-Saxon physicians picture them as untonsured.[35] On the other hand, we know that many within the clergy practiced medicine, and it is presumably these who consulted the medical books.[36] It seems unlikely, given the small number of medical manuscripts and the need to administer medical attention in most cases out of convenient range of a library, that the physical books themselves could have formed any part of regular Anglo-Saxon medicine outside of minster centers.[37] The books drew from the common repository of popular medicine, however, and probably influenced popular medicine in turn.

While their interpretation remains problematic, medical books are valuable sources of potential information regarding what conditions the Anglo-Saxons may have recognized as inherently demonic in nature, and what sorts of remedies local practitioners may have brought to bear on such cases.

Conditions Recognized as Possession

Greco-Roman medicine recognized such aberrant mental states as mania, phrenitis, and melancholia, behavioral categories still operative in the Middle Ages even if not used precisely or consistently.[38] Perhaps the most obvious terms for "demon possessed" in Old English are *deofolseoc* and *feondseoc*, which appear in Old English translations for phrases such as *vexatus* and *obsessis daemones*.[39] A diversity of terms and variants such as *wedenheort*, *witleas*, *monaþseoc*, and *wod* imply a semantic range more complicated than one in which the mad are all "devil-sick" (*deofolseoc*)—however incapable we are of reconstructing the precise differences.[40] The *Herbarium* implies that *gewitleaste* and *deofulseocnes* are essentially the same: "Wið gewitleaste, þæt is wið deofulseocnysse" (Against witlessness, that is, against devil-sickness).[41] Elsewhere the *Herbarium* equates *gewitleaste* with the Greek *phrenesis* and provides further detail:

> Wið þa adle þe Grecas frenesis nemnað, þæt is on ure geþeode gewitlest þæs modes, þæt byþ ðonne þæt heafod aweallen byþ.[42]
>
> [Against the sickness that the Greeks call "phrenesis": that is, in our language, "madness of the mind"—which is when the head is overheated.]

Audrey Meaney tentatively constructs a rough classification in which "imbalance and 'evil humours' affected the human constitution, parasitic worms the flesh, and evil spirits the mind."[43] Alternately, Basil Clarke proposes four loose categories of Old English medical terms referring to mental disturbance and related behavioral or neurological conditions: those referring to epilepsy (*fyllewærc*, *fylleseocnes*, *bræcseoc*), to a fever or delirium (*brægenes*, *hwyrfness*), to intellectual derangement (*gewitleast*, *gewolding*), or to lunacy (*monaþseocnes*).[44] Bede explains that the apparent link between lunacy and the moon arises not from inherent natural properties but from demonic influence:

> Lunatici dicuntur quorum dolor in ascensione lunae crescebat, non quod inde vere fieret, sed ob daemonum fallaciam.[45]

[They are called "lunatics" in whom a pain would arise at the rising of the moon, not because it actually originates from that but through the deceit of demons.]

Monaðseoc appropriately glosses *lunaticus* in Ælfric's Glossary and in Antwerp, Plantin-Moretus, MS 32, thus retaining the original association with the moon.[46] Clarke harbors no illusions about the ultimate success of systematizing the conceptual categories in the surviving lexical data, however, as the glosses—as in so many cases—often confuse matters as much as they clarify them. Use of the glosses introduces an entirely new host of textual and contextual problems.

The textual history of Latin-Old English glosses (sometimes compiled into *glossæ collectæ*) is complicated, with common sources and intertwined routes of influence. For our purposes, however, we can look at the earlier glossarial tradition as a group (the Épinal-Erfurt Glossary, the Corpus Glossary, and the Leiden Glossary) and then compare these with glossaries from late Anglo-Saxon England (London, British Library, MS Cotton Cleopatra A.III; the Harley Glossary; and Ælfric's Glossary). Drawing from a common ancestor, the Épinal and Erfurt Glossaries are two independent copies of the same material. That ancestor, according to J. D. Pheifer, editor of a modern edition of the glossaries, was from the last half of the seventh century—probably around 670 or 680 CE.[47] This situates the ancestor in the earliest period of written English, a period contemporaneous with our only cases of exorcism from Anglo-Saxon England (the late seventh and early eighth centuries). Pheifer places the Épinal Glossary very close to its ancestor—within a generation or two, perhaps around 725.[48] Furthermore, this glossary group is dialectically close to our region of primary interest (Northumbria and Anglia—more on this in chapter 3), retaining a number of Anglian features.[49] In the late eighth or early ninth century, a new compilation of material derived from the same archetype as Épinal-Erfurt was produced in England: the Corpus Glossary (CCCC 144). This incorporated most of the Épinal-Erfurt material, while adding an equal amount of new material. Taken together, these glossaries provide invaluable guides to what some compilers in early Anglo-Saxon England considered vernacular lexical equivalents for concepts in the Latin source texts.

In this light it is interesting how sparsely words for madness, possession, and the demonic appear in these glosses. The earliest surviving strand, Épinal-Erfurt, does not gloss *energumenus*, *daemoniacus*, *freneticus*, *insanus*, *lunaticus*, or *mania* (or their variants). The only vernacular equivalents present are *uuoda* for *ephilenticus* and *uuoendendi* (Erfurt *uuodenti*) for *lymphatico*, all derived from glosses on Aldhelm.[50] The Corpus Glossary includes one further vernacular gloss in addition to these two: *wodan* for *inerguminos*.[51] Another early compilation, the late seventh- or early eighth-century Leiden Glossary, yields some interesting Latin equivalents (such as *demones* for *manius*, and *demoniosum* for *arreptitium*), but it contains no vernacular entries for madness or the possessed.[52] Overall, in these early texts vernacular glosses for possession and madness are rare. Where they appear, the term *wod* seems to be the catchall Old English equivalent for the various Latin terms for madness (and these are mostly found in glosses on Aldhelm). Also, when used, *wod* is linked with behavioral conditions, but is not explicitly linked with demons or spirits in the vernacular.

Material from the Épinal-Erfurt-Corpus strands is incorporated later into BL Cleopatra A.III, a manuscript of the mid-tenth century whose three glossaries, which cut off at the letter *P*, reflect a wide variety of sources. The first of the glosses retains some of the familiar readings (e.g., *wedende* for *lymphatico*), and adds a significant number of new Old English equivalents:

freneticus: bræcseoc	[frenetic: break-sick
furias: wuhunga	the Furies: rages
inerguminum: þære gewitseocan	energumen: the wit-sick
inerguminos: wodan	energumens: the mad
insanum: þone weddendan	insane: the raving (or mad)
frenesis: weding	frenesis: raving (or madness)
lunaticos: bræcseoce	lunatics: break-sick][53]

Wod and its variants (*weding*, *weddendan*) still predominate, and if we "back translate" *inerguminum*, *insanum*, and *frenesis* to their lemmas, there is implied equivalence or semantic overlap between the three words. There are further nuances: *bræcseoc* (epilepsy) understandably renders *lunaticos* (gloss derived from Matt. 4:24)—*bræcseoc* may often simply refer to recurring or cyclical seizures, and *lunaticos* implies cyclicality with intermittent periods of abatement—but the identification of *bræcseoc* for *freneticus* is less obvious. In the likely source text of the original gloss, Aldhelm's *De virginitate*, the glossed word appears in a famous passage in which mad, lustful Dulcitius attempts to rape Chionia, Irene, and Agape, but instead finds himself groping and kissing sooty pots and pans in the darkness. He is said to be "quasi limphaticus uel freneticus" (like a crazed or frenzied person).[54] Here, then, *bræcseoc* apparently means something more like "violent, furious, uncontrolled" than the more conventional reference of "breaking-sickness" to fits, either in recurrence or periodicity. Other terms for fury also appear in BL Cleopatra A.III, such as *wuhunga* (rage, fury, madness), glossing *furias*. Finally, *inerguminum* is translated by *gewitseocan*, capturing the sense of "irrational, insane," if not necessarily "taken over by a spirit."[55] The Old English terms in this collection thus either refer broadly to madness in general (*wodnes*), or else focus on the effects of the type of sickness (*gewitseoc*, "sick in reason"; and *bræcseoc*, "sickness causing falls or seizures") rather than on putative causes or agents of the condition (*deofolseoc*, *feondseoc*). The role of demons or the devil as sentient, indwelling agents is not especially evident in the lexical roots of vernacular terminology here.

The Harley Glossary, roughly contemporary with BL Cleopatra A.III or slightly later (late tenth or early eleventh century), contains an even greater diversity of terms, introducing "elves" and implying a clearer connection between madness and violence.[56] The inclusion of multiple glosses for many lemmas, with Latin and Old English mixed, results in a complicated matrix of interrelated concepts. This glossary only survives up through the letter *F*, a letter which reveals significant detail in its attention to fury and rage:

> freneticus: demoniaticus, insanus, amens, gewitleasa
> frenesis: insanitas
> funeste: funere pollutus, cruente, insaniente, wedende
> furor . . . reþnes, wodendream
> furis: insanis, erras, bacharis
> furia: insania, amentia, vel dea wodscipe, reþnes
> furias: insania, vel deas, iras, reþscipas vel hatheortnessa
> furalia [read furiale]: seua, reþe
> furiosus: iracunda, rabidus, insanus, amens
>
> [frenetic: demoniac, insane, senseless, witless
> frenesis: insanity
> destructive: polluted with death, blood-thirsty, insane, mad
> fury . . . savagery, mad ecstasy
> you are raving: you are insane, you stray, you rave wantonly
> fury: insanity, senselessness, or the goddess of raving, rage
> the Furies: insanity, or goddesses, wrath, raging or "hot-heartedness"
> furious: ferocious, savage
> furious: ireful, enraged, insane, senseless][57]

The vernacular *wod* is now joined by *reþe*, *reþnes*, and *reþscipas* ("cruelty," "savagery," and "harshness"), and *hatheortnessa* (rage, anger, passion); *wod* also appears in a separate item in the Harley Glossary explicitly for demoniacs: "demoniaticus: insanus, amens, vel woda."[58] Madness and "breaking-sickness" are now more clearly linked with demoniacs: after the lemma *caducus* ("falling sickness," but also "vain, futile") appears "demoniacus, a cadendo dicitur bræcseoca vel inanis" (demoniac: said to be from "falling"; breaking-sickness or hollow).[59] Also, of especial interest in the Harley Glossary is a marginal note to "Comitiales, id est garritores" (Epileptics, that is to say, chatterers; perhaps referring to trembling or teeth grinding);[60] alongside this in the right margin has been added, "vel dies mensi, vel ylfie, vel monaþseoce vel dagas" (or a day of the month, or "elf-y," or "month-sick" or days).[61] The OE adjective *ylfie* is unique to glosses, and seems especially associated with this traveling gloss on *comitiales* (epileptics) from chapter 52 of Aldhelm's *De virginitate*.[62] *Ylfie* may be related to OE *gydig* (modern English "giddy") through a Common Germanic root.[63] *Gydig* is another word attested only in the glossaries in Old English, and one which also travels exclusively with the glosses for Aldhelm's *De virginitate* (for the word *lymphaticum*).[64] In the Middle English period *gidi* is common, with a semantic range including "insane, crazy; possessed by a devil; foolish, stupid, senseless; dizzy; uncertain, unstable."[65] Alaric Hall suggests that, along with *ylfie*, *gidi* could well have been in common use during the Old English period and is not simply a glossary neologism (as many elf words, such as *dun-ælfa* and *land-ælfe*, are believed to be).[66] Here then in the Harley, its marginalia, and related glossaries, is a lively vocabulary for mental derangements linked with a diversity of spirit beings, with particular attention (if this is not an accident of the letters which survive in Harley) to anger and fury.

At the turn of the eleventh century, Ælfric compiled a glossary for use with his Latin Grammar.[67] Unlike the mostly alphabetical glossary compilations examined so far, Ælfric's is a class gloss, clumping words together in groups with related meanings. This is especially useful because it shows at once the general range of things that Ælfric considered forms of mental illness. Furthermore, Antonette diPaolo Healey argues that despite Ælfric's use of sources such as Isidore's *Etymologies*, his purposes are practical and he is likely transmitting words that were active in everyday use:

> Ælfric . . . takes great care in winnowing his material to preserve only that vocabulary which is most useful for the beginning student of Latin. The approximately 1300 Latin words and their Old English translations are, for the most part, basic and familiar terms. . . . While we cannot attribute a record of normal usage to most glossaries, exceptions do occur, and one of them is Ælfric's *Glossary*. The evidence of the Latin vocabulary seems then to support the evidence of the English vocabulary: for this particular glossary, at least, we do not have a learned vocabulary but rather the vocabulary of ordinary life in the monastery.[68]

Following terms for sickness in general (*untrum* for *infirmus*, and *adlig* for *aeger*), there is an entry for paralysis, one for leprosy, and then those for (mostly) mental illness begin:[69]

lunaticus: monaðseoc	[lunatic: month-sick
daemoniacus: deofolseoc	demoniac: devil-sick
energuminus: gewitseoc	energumen: wit-sick
morbus: adl	sickness: sickness
pestis: cwyld	pestilence: pestilence
amens vel demens: gemyndleas	senseless or mad: senseless
rabidus vel insanus: wod	raging or insane: mad
sanus: hal	healthy: healthy
rabies: wodnys	rage: madness
incolomis: gesund	uninjured: sound
freneticus: se ðe ðurh slæpleaste awet	frenetic: he who remains awake, without sleeping

frenesis: seo untrumnys	frenesis: infirmity (or weakness)
lethargus vel letargicus: ungelimplice slapol	lethargy or lethargic: immoderate sleeping]

I have included the entire block (including *morbus*, *pestis*, *sanus*, and *incolomis*) to contextualize the items more completely and, perhaps, to give a greater sense of Ælfric's flow of thought. (Following these items, the glossary proceeds to more terms related to sleeping and wakefulness, then to good and bad character traits.) We should recall Ælfric's main purpose: to familiarize students of Latin with the vocabulary they will eventually be encountering in texts such as the Bible, the liturgy, and saints' lives. Furthermore, he is not a doctor concerned with exact synonyms or nuanced parallels; his point is to find a (usually) single-word equivalent or something close enough to it for pedagogical expedience, and then to move on.

With these points in mind, we learn from Ælfric that *monaðseoc* (here *lunaticus*) still retains its association with cyclical recurrence or lunar influence, as it did for Bede. (For Ælfric, *monaðseoc* can also refer to a woman's menstrual cycle.)[70] One manuscript of Ælfric's Glossary (Oxford, St. John's College, MS 154) also equates it with *fellseoc* (falling-sick), another term usually associated with epileptics.[71] *Gemyndleas* apparently refers to primarily intellectual derangement (*amens*, *demens*), as does *wod* (*insanus*). *Wod* is also still strongly linked with rage (*rabidus*, *rabies*). On the other hand, Ælfric associates *frenesis* simply with *untrumnys* (illness, weakness, infirmity), a very general term with no specific reference to the mind or to behavior. Ælfric's conceptualization is far removed from Isidore's *phrenesis*: an *impedimento mentis* (hindrance of the mind) that involves gnashing the teeth.[72] *Freneticus* also does not seem to be a madness or behavioral disturbance, as Ælfric translates it, so much as a sleep disorder: "se ðe ðurh slæpleaste awet" (he who remains awake, without sleeping). The subsequent item in the glossary continues this line of thought: *lethargus* means sleeping too much. These are natural concerns, presumably, for those undertaking the rigorous schedule of monastic life—especially for novitiates or for boys. There is also a spiritual dimension to insanity, as in the gloss of *gewitseoc* for *energuminus*, and *deofolseoc* for *daemoniacus*, but overall this is not the dimension of madness that Ælfric emphasizes.

Interestingly, Ælfric employs a slightly different terminology in his narrative accounts of the possessed: for instance, he frequently uses *ofsettum* (oppressed, afflicted) and *gedrehtum* (troubled, tormented), words that do not appear in the glosses in demonic contexts.[73] These are more general terms, like *untrumnys* for *frenesis*. Ælfric, then, presents a range of terms for mental disorder, vices, and behavioral pathologies, but (outside of *deofolseoc*) chooses terms that do not make specific reference to demons (e.g., *awyrgedan gastas*). For him, perhaps, the connection does not need spelling out: in his *Passion of Simon and Jude* Ælfric indicates that the *wittseocum* (*energuminus* in his glossary) are those who have "devils" (*deoflu*), and he places *ofsettan deofulseocan* in direct apposition in his homily on the assumption of John.[74]

In fact, *deofolseoc* itself only appears late in the glossary record, beginning in the late tenth century: in Ælfric (above); the Abingdon glosses of Brussels, Royal Library, MS 1650 ("energuminos: gewitlease, diouelseoce; energuminum: deouelseocne"); Oxford, Bodleian Library, MS Digby 146 ("inerguminos: amentes, gewitlease, deofelseoce; inerguminum: deofelseoce"); and Antwerp, Plantin-Moretus, MS 32 ("demoniacus: deofelseoc").[75] *Deofelseoce* in this late context also glosses Latin *larbatos*—one of the types of sick people brought to Anatolia for healing in Aldhelm's *De virginitate*.[76] The original meaning of *larvatos* (bewitched, enchanted, haunted) seems to have caused some confusion among glossators, who provide as equivalents *æfærede*, [*e*]*nerguminos*, *infirmos*, *deofelseoce* (frightened, energumens, sick, devil-sick); *woðe* (mad); *hreofe* (scabby, leprous); and *unfægere* (ugly).[77] *Feondseoce*, in the meantime, does not appear in any of the glosses, though it appears in the medical literature and in narrative contexts.

Eleventh-century glosses also appear in a manuscript of Aldhelm's *De virginitate* from Abingdon, which has since been fragmented and must be pieced together from four separate manuscripts (Antwerp, Plantin-Moretus, MS 47, Salle iii.68; London, British Library, MS Additional 32246; Antwerp, Plantin-Moretus, MS 190, Salle iii.55; and Brussels, Royal Library, MS 1650).[78] Goossens places the glossing hands in the first half of the eleventh century.[79] In this series *freneticus* is glossed with *awoffod* (delirious, insane) and with *brægenseoc* (brain-sick), an elegant term but one unattested outside of Aldhelm glosses.[80] Moreover, in this series the association of madness (fury) with possession becomes more explicit in both the Latin and the Old English glosses of *furiis*: along with *gyde*, the term is glossed with *malignis spiritibus* and *mid awyridum gastum*.[81]

The overall story the glossaries tell, from early to late, is one of increasing complexity and nuance in the various terms used for madness—beginning with simple variations on *wod* in the eighth century, and arriving at a diverse class of terms in the eleventh and twelfth centuries. Furthermore, the glosses devote an increasing amount of attention to terms specifically implying demonic posssession (*energumen*, *demoniaticus*, *deofolseoc*) through the tenth, eleventh, and into the twelfth centuries—perhaps implying that these words were gaining in currency, or (though it seems rather less likely) implying that they were increasingly in need of glossing for the beginning student. Though glossary evidence is only partial evidence, the story it tells is one of increasingly nuanced conceptions of madness, and of a perception of madness increasingly linked with demons. It remains curious, then, that the only time and place in which demon possession seems most securely attested in Anglo-Saxon England—seventh- and early eighth-century Northumbria and Anglia (see chapter 3)—produced glosses that show the weakest conceptual links between behavioral disorders and demons. By way of supplement to this fragmentary evidence, the medical texts themselves can provide some symptomatic details of what might have invited a diagnosis of possession or demonic influence.

The *Leechbook* book 1 contains half a dozen or so recipes for mental disorders (*feondseocum*, *bræcseocum*, *weþenheorte*, *ungemynde*), clustered together in two chapters fairly close to one another.[82] This section also contains recipes to ward off charms, fever, elvish "influences" of some sort (*ælf-siðenne*, translation uncertain), and rabies (*wede hundes slite*, "the bite of a mad dog"). Jolly discusses these as "mind-altering afflictions" (which is presumably what lends them their demonic associations), commenting, "spiritual forces must be invoked to counteract ailments involving the mind or soul."[83] The *Leechbook* book 3—the medical text most confidently associated with early medieval northern Germanic practices—contains at least five more recipes for the mad or possessed (*monaþseoc*, *gewitseocne*, *ungemynde*, *deofulseoce*, *wedenheorte*), although there are so many related, poorly-understood items in the same section of the manuscript that precise selection becomes somewhat arbitrary.[84] There is, however, a clear association here between madness and diabolic instigation: four of these recipes contain instructions against the devil's temptations (*feondes costungum* and *deofles costunga*).[85] Furthermore, there are sundry items against elves, "night-goers" or possibly "nightmares" (*nihtgengan*), "elf sickness" and "water-elf sickness" (*ælfadle*, *wæterælfadle*), and a very poorly understood "elf-sogoth" (*ælfsogoþa*).[86]

Some scholars have read indwelling possession states into the elf charms (by analogy with Christian demon possession) because of their positioning in these text clusters. To be sure, the exorcisms incorporating both herbal and ritual material treat elves and demons in largely the same way, as in the following passage from the prescription for *ælf-sogoþa* in the *Leechbook* book 3:

> Wyrc þonne drenc: font wæter, rudan, saluian, cassuc, draconzan, þa smeþan wegbrædan niþewearde, fefer fugian, diles crop, garleaces iii clufe, finul, wermod, lufestice, elehtre, ealra emfela, writ iii crucem mid oleum infirmorum ⁊ cweð: *pax tibi.* Nim þonne þæt gewrit, writ crucem mid ofer þam drince ⁊ sing þis þærofer: *Deus omnipotens, pater domini nostri iesu cristi, per Inpositionem huius scripturæ et per gustum huius expelle diabolum a famulo tuo, N . . .*
>
> [Then prepare a drink: font water, rue, sage, sedge grass, "dragon-wort," the lower part of smooth greater plantain, feverfew, a cluster of dill, three cloves of garlic, fennel, wormwood, lovage, lupine—all in equal amounts. Make the sign of the cross three times, with the Oil for the Sick, and say, "Peace to you." Then take that writing (the rite has previously indicated a prayer to be written out), make a cross with it over the drink, and sing this over it: "Omnipotent God, Father of our lord Jesus Christ, through the application of this writing and through a taste, expel the devil from this your servant, N . . ."][87]

The item concludes, "þes cræft mæg wiþ ælcre feondes costunge" (this procedure is effective against every temptation of the devil). The language of liturgical exorcism is here blended with an herbal remedy, all in response to someone suffering something identified as *ælf-sogoþa* at the beginning of the instructions, but the "devil's temptations" or perhaps "devil's afflictions" at the end. With such rites in mind, Bonser concludes, "When Christianity came, the elves of heathendom were equated with demons, and therefore elf-shot and flying venom were thought to be the same as demoniacal possession (*deofolseocnes*)"; while Nils Thun concludes summarily, "[elves] themselves penetrate into the body of the victim like other evil spirits."[88] For Richard North, "OE *ylfi[g]e* seems to mean 'demoniacally possessed.'"[89]

But such readings have been called into question recently. Alaric Hall has shown, for instance, that G. Storms introduced the concept of possession in his reading of "Gif hors ofscoten sie" through Storm's translation of "Sy þæt ylfa þe him sie" as "Whatever elf has taken possession of it"[90] The elf charms, Hall concludes, "offer no hint as to how *ælfe* inflicted illness—certainly neither projectiles nor possession, both assumed in the past, seems necessarily to be implied."[91] Elves appear to be associated rather with sharp, sudden internal pains, and perhaps also reflect cutaneous conditions and jaundice. On the whole, the tradition of reifying, anthropomorphizing, and mythologizing diseases and disease agents should caution us against reading these putative elf-disease exorcisms as the literal casting out of demons from possessed persons: the sufferers and healers could have visualized a wide range of conditions as "enemies" in need of expulsion. Grattan and Singer could be right after all that "[t]he Teutonic peoples originally knew nothing of possession by demons which is so characteristic of the New Testament."[92]

Whatever role they may have played prior to conversion, by the time of our sources, disease agents such as poisons, elves, dwarves, and worms exhibit significant conceptual overlap with demons. It is surprising, therefore, that the demons themselves are explicitly named so infrequently in these remedies as indwelling possessors. The *deoful* and his "temptations" are mentioned a few times, and despite the appearance of the word "demon" in a few Latin passages (all of them demonstrably imported, such as in the *Lorica of Gildas*), the most common vernacular equivalents of "demon" or "unclean spirit" (*awyrgeda gast*, *unclæna gast*) are conspicuously absent.[93] Apparently the native dwarves and elves of pre-Christian folklore continued to occupy slightly different conceptual registers than the demons teeming in the landscapes of the saints' lives.[94] For instance, precategorical demonic influence might be spoken of differently in one context than in another: the same underlying semantic concept (or range of concepts) might be called "elves," "dwarves," or "poisons" in the context of practical healing, and "demons" or "unclean spirits" in the more elevated (perhaps) context of narrative literature such as saints' lives and Gospel translations. A modern analogue might be something like *Coriandrum sativum*, which Americans commonly call "coriander" when referring to the seed or to the plant's use in Indian cooking, but "cilantro" when referring to its use in Mexican cooking. The distinct cultural backgrounds of the two cuisines have become embedded in linguistic usage—perhaps as the distinct cultural backgrounds of the native Germanic and Latin Christian traditions regarding pathogens continued to show in independent usage between medical and literary (narrative) contexts.

Consistent with this general view of the demonic as precategorical and elemental, the Old English translation of the Gospels treats demons not so much as distinct sentient beings but as abstract illnesses or illness states. By far the most common phrase in the Vulgate for demoniacs is that the person "has a demon" (e.g., Matt. 9:32: "demonium habentem"), the demon being referred to either by *daemonium* or *spiritus inmundus*. Sometimes, the vernacular translation (the Old English Gospels) adheres to the original in saying that the demon is driven out of the subject: in Mark 7:26, for instance, "daemonium eiceret" is translated as "he ðone deofol . . . adrife."[95] In the vast majority of cases, however, the Old English departs from biblical phrasing in identifying what is being expelled not as the demon (*deofol*) but as the illness (*deofolseocnes*). Thus, for instance, the translation of Luke 7:33 ("daemonium habet") is "deofolseocnysse he hæfð," and, in Mark 16:17, "daemonia eicient" becomes "deofolseocnessa ut drifað."[96] Even the seven demons expelled from Mary Magdalene in Mark 16:9 are not devils but "devil-sicknesses": "he ut adraf seofon deofolseocnyssa."[97] This tendency is the norm for all three synoptic Gospels.[98] These disease agents thus seem to be visualized less as individual demons and more as generalized, impersonal forces.

If the demons presumed in the medical books do not bear much initial resemblance to the indwelling antagonists of the Gospels and of medieval saints' lives, the treatments ostensibly prescribed for such conditions are even more removed from the rarefied world of monastic letters.

Herbal and Ritual Treatments

Early medieval medical books respond to mental illness—however that is conceptualized—with a number of approaches. (I am reminded of what Brian Murdoch has noted of Old High German epilepsy formulas: "There are few better indicators of a complete medical helplessness than a very wide variety of eccentrically different remedies for a given condition.")[99] In the Old English *Herbarium of Apuleius* plants such as *clufwyrt* (buttercup) and *pionia* (peony) are to be worn as amulets against *monaþseocnes*.[100] The accompanying text on medicine derived from animals prescribes wolf's flesh against devil-sickness.[101] By far the most common type of prescription calls for some mixture of herbs to be worn or ingested—usually the more the better. These recipes contain more or less the same range of herbs, listed in various combinations with more of an eye to inclusiveness than discrimination, interspersed occasionally with fascinating diagnostic tips and procedural directions.[102] The *Herbarium*, for instance, lists *deofolseocnes* as a condition treatable by four plants: *mucgwyrt*, *smerowyrt*, *mandragora*, and *priapiscus*.[103] The directions in the two chapters of the *Leechbook* book 1 for the mentally ill, mentioned above, prescribe some thirty plant products in all,[104] which are to be used in conjunction with religious ritual. The following passage gives a sample:

> *Wiþ feond seocum men*. Þonne deofol þone monnan fede oððe hine innan gewealde mid adle. Spiwedrenc: eluhtre, bisceopwyrt, beolone, cropleac, gecnua tosomne. Do eala to wætan. Læt standan neahterne. Do fiftig lybcorna on ⁊ halig wæter.
>
> *Drenc wiþ feond seocum men*, of ciricbellan to drincanne: gyþrife, glæs, gearwe, elehtre, betonice, attorlaþe, cassuc, fane, finul, ciric-ragu, cristes mæles ragu, lufestice. Gewyrc þone drenc of hluttrum ealað. Gesinge seofon mæssan ofer þam wyrtum. Do garleac ⁊ halig wæter to ⁊ drype on ælcne drincan þone drenc þe he drincan wille eft. ⁊ singe þone sealm *Beati inmaculati* ⁊ *Exurgat* ⁊ *Saluum me fac Deus*, ⁊ þonne drince þone drenc of ciricbellan. ⁊ se mæsse preost him singe æfter þam drence þis ofer, *Domine Sancte Pater omnipotens*.
>
> *Wiþ bræcseocum men*: cost, gotwoþe, eluhtre, betonice, attorlaðe, cropleac, holecersan, hofe, finul. Asinge mon mæssan ofer wyrce of wiliscum ealoð ⁊ of halig wætere. Drince þisne drenc æt æghwilcum niwe nigon morgenas ⁊ nane oþre wætan þæt þicce ⁊ stille sie, ⁊ ælmessan selle ⁊ him arena god geornlice bidde.
>
> *Wiþ weden heorte*: bisceopwyrt, elehtre, banwyrt, eofor-fearn, giþrife, heahhioloþe. Þonne dæg scade ⁊ niht, þonne sing þu on ciricean letanias—þæt is, þara haligra naman ⁊ pater noster. Mid þy sange þu ga þæt þu sie æt þam wyrtum ⁊ þriwa ymbga ⁊ þonne þu hie nime gang eft to ciricean mid þy ilcan sange, ⁊ gesing xii mæssan ofer ⁊ ofer ealle þa drencan þe to þære adle belimpaþ on weorðmynde þara twelfa apostola.[105]
>
> [*For a fiend-sick person*. When the devil imbues a person or controls him from within with sickness. A drink to cause vomiting: pound together lupin, *bisceopwyrt*, henbane, cropleek. Add ale, to make a liquid. Let stand for a night. Add in fifty *lyb*-grains and holy water.
>
> *A drink for the fiend-sick*, to be drunk from a church bell: corn-cockle, hound's-tongue, yarrow, lupin, betony, *attorlathe* (a corydalis?), sedge, iris, fennel, church lichen, cross-of-Christ lichen,[106] lovage. Prepare the drink from clear ale. Sing seven masses over the herbs. Add garlic and holy water, and drip this drink into every drink that he drinks thereafter, and sing *Beati inmaculati* and *Exurgat* and *Saluum me fac Deus*,[107] and then he should drink that drink from a church bell, and after that drink the mass priest should sing over him, *Domine Sancte Pater omnipotens*.

For people with breaking-sickness: costmary, ground-elder, lupin, betony, *attorlathe*, cropleek, *holecersan* (holly-cress?), ground ivy (*Glechoma hederacea*), fennel. Masses should be sung over them; work into a drink of British ale and holy water. He should drink this drink anew for nine mornings and no other drink that is thick or still. And he should give alms and earnestly pray for God's favors.

For those mad in spirit: *bisceopwyrt*, lupin, *banwyrt*, common polypody (*Polypodium vulgare*), corn-cockle, elecampane. When day turns to night, then sing the litanies in church: that is, the names of the holy and the *Pater Noster*. While singing, go to where the herbs are and go around them three times. When you pick them, go back to the church while singing the same thing, and (then) sing twelve masses over them and over all the drinks to be used for this illness, in honor of the twelve apostles.]

The flower lupine (or lupin) is the only plant to appear in all six recipes in this section, followed by four mentions apiece of *bisceopwyrt* and *gythrife*. It is tempting to look more closely at these oft-mentioned plants, to see whether their potential pharmacological effects may respond in some way to symptoms presumably associated with demonic possession or mental disturbance (e.g., seizures, anxiety, or psychosis).

A major obstacle in evaluating the physiological effects of these herbs, however, lies in identifying them with any precision.[108] Lupine—probably *Lupinus albus*—seems a fairly safe identification for *elehtre*, but after that the waters muddy quickly. The *Dictionary of Old English* lists a number of possible meanings for *bisceopwyrt*, including betony and marshmallow (*Althaea officinalis*; this is Bierbaumer's preference); yet in the glosses *bisceopwyrt* also translates vervain (*hierabotane*) and soapwort (*struthion*). *Gyþrife* is probably corn cockle (*Agrostemma githago*), a plant which is poisonous to horses and livestock. Bierbaumer lists two identifications for *hindheoloþe*: hemp agrimony (or water hemp, *Eupatorium cannabinum*) and wood germander (or wood sage, *Teucrium scorodonia*). Besides determining the proper names of the plants, other obstacles include the various effects of soil and climate on plant composition, the shifting geographical range of plant species, and possible alterations in the species over the intervening thousand years. Finally, nomenclature was not necessarily consistent in all parts of Anglo-Saxon England, and even within a given region, different individuals probably employed different semantic taxonomies for the vast repertoire of medicinal herbs.

Some of the herbs indicated for devil-sickness and its cognate ailments could conceivably have significant psychotropic properties.[109] Mandrake (*Mandragora vernalis* or *officinarum*) and henbane (*Hyoscyamus niger*) contain the powerful alkaloids hyoscyamine and scopolamine. In small quantities these are sedatives, but greater doses can lead to hallucinations, manic episodes, and death. The *Herbarium* prescribes mandrake for *deofulseocnysse*: three pennies' weight are to be drunk in warm water.[110] Yet it is unclear whether this recipe was used with any regularity in England, since mandrake does not grow there naturally. The *Lacnunga* shows awareness that these herbs could induce sleep; as sedatives, they are potentially effective pain relievers and perhaps surgical anesthetics.[111] If *ælfþone* is woody nightshade (*Solanum dulcamara*), as Nils Thun argues, then that places it in a family with known narcotic, antispasmodic, and analgesic properties (though these are more prominent in black nightshade, *Solanum nigrum*).[112]

None of these potentially mind-altering plants, however, is repeated more than once in the cluster of recipes concerned with devil-sickness, and they all appear somewhat lost in long lists of herbs which characterize many of the recipes. Other herbs, such as *solsece* (deadly nightshade or belladonna), *hymlic* (hemlock), and *tunsingwyrt* (hellebore), are at no time indicated for mental illness, though they appear in the medical record for the treatment of other ailments. Wormwood and henbane are among the herbs prescribed against *ælfcynne* and *nihtgengan* and "those who have intercourse with the devil" (þam mannum þe deofol mid hæmð) in one item from the *Leechbook* book 3, but here the herbs are not ingested: they are boiled in sheep's fat, prayed over, strained, and smeared on the face.[113] In the item translated above ("Wiþ feond seocum men"; *Leechbook* 1.63), henbane is included in the "spew-drink" to cause someone to vomit up the devil. Thus while these psychogenic and poisonous herbs are often associated with witchcraft in Early Modern lore, we are likely to be disappointed if we try to correlate them with the demonic conditions in early medieval medical texts too neatly.[114] On the contrary: while some of the suggested ingredients would make for rather indifferent fare (e.g., *cassuc*), the impression on the whole in these remedies is one of sober, systematic application of plant ingredients, some of which may conceivably induce tranquility (as many modern herbal teas purport to do), couched in comforting ritual procedure.

Fennel, frequently cited in prescriptions for *feondseocum men*, *bræcseocum*, *ungemynde*, *ælfcynne*, and other mental conditions, has been shown to have an antispasmodic effect and is used as a digestive aid.[115] The *Leechbook* book 3 recommends celandine root for a "wit-sick" person (*gewitseocne man*); the alkaloid chelidonine is a weak analgesic and a sedative.[116] In one gloss *bisceopwyrt* translates the Latin *hierabotane*, or vervain (*Verbena officinalis*). Used since the time of the Egyptians for various purposes, vervain's tranquilizing and analgesic qualities—though rather mild—have been confirmed in recent studies.[117] A variant of catnip (OE *nepte* or *nefte*) is listed as an herb against the devil and mindlessness ("wið deofle ⁊ ungemynde"); the nepetalactone isomers it contains are similar to certain natural human sedatives (valepotriates, found in valerian) and have been shown to have a (very mild) tranquilizing effect in our species—precisely the opposite of its effects on cats.[118] The most commonly prescribed herb for *deofulseocnesse* is lupine (OE *elehtre*), probably *Lupinus albus*. Lupine could conceivably serve as a mild neurotransmission inhibitor through the action of its alkaloids (sparteine, cytisine, and lupinine), and thus possibly reduce the seizure threshold or lessen the impact of a seizure in epilepsy.[119] Furthermore, this is a plant unusually high in manganese, a trace element which has been correlated with higher seizure thresholds in both humans and laboratory animals.[120]

These observations on potential therapeutic value, however, stem from careful experimental and clinical studies using controlled doses of samples with consistent chemical compositions. It is much more tenuous to assume that an early medieval practitioner could consistently rely on a sample to contain significant quantities of the right substances. Even if some of these herbs can be singled out as containing certain constituents that can cause some relief for specific conditions, for the most part, it is hard to assess what the pharmacological effect would be of the three dozen or so herbs prescribed for conditions associated with madness, possession, or the devil. A review of the literature shows that the constituents of these herbs do more to ease digestion and facilitate nutrient absorption than they do to reduce potential neurological or muscle-control disorders.

Liturgical Exorcism

The saints' lives imply ongoing tension between saints and secular physicians throughout the Middle Ages. This is probably exaggerated for rhetorical effect, especially given the intermixture of lay and clerical participation presumed throughout the medical texts.[121] It is not a stretch, however, to imagine that churches and minsters liked to monitor the activities of local healers, both to assure that invocations were properly Christian and to ensure that ecclesiastical authority remained implicitly understood in community practices. As we saw in chapter 1, the casting out of demons was an important dimension of the church's growing presence and authority in the countryside in the early centuries of Christian expansion. If demons were actively being cast out in Anglo-Saxon England, however, the official exorcists of the church may not have been the ones most frequently performing that task, or may not have occupied the principal role in the ceremony. The narrative sources never portray the exorcists in that role, and liturgical books reserve the right for higher orders.

The existence of Anglo-Saxon "exorcists" as independent officers of the church is deduced primarily from liturgical ordination rubrics, rather than from direct references to specific people. Only a single Anglo-Saxon exorcist is known to us by name: a certain "Pinewald, exorc" witnessed a charter dated 692—a donation of ten hides of land by King Æthelred of Mercia to Worcester Cathedral.[122] Exorcists were usually too low a rank to appear as signatories in official documents.[123] *Exorcista* remained a lower clerical order, and perhaps (as in the modern era) a somewhat nominal one—the function of solemn exorcism (i.e., driving demons out of demoniacs, as opposed to procedural exorcisms such as the preparation of liturgical materials), as far as the liturgical record indicates, was becoming the province of priests and bishops. A passage often attributed to Isidore of Seville states that exorcists perform exorcisms, but this may be a meditation on the word rather than a factual description.[124] The early medieval *Statuta ecclesiae antiqua* imply a lively role and a busy schedule for exorcists: "omni die exorcistae energumenis manus imponant" (every day the exorcists are to lay hands on demoniacs).[125] However, Ferrandus's sixth-century *Breviario* (a collection of canons) advises, "Vt non exorcizent illi qui necdum ab episcopo sunt prouecti" (they should not perform exorcisms who have not yet been made bishops).[126] By the period of Anglo-Saxon letters, solemn exorcism may have become restricted to the major orders in many ecclesiastical centers. Thus the Lanalet Pontifical explicitly mentions the *episcopus* (bishop) as performing exorcism, and the Romano-German Pontifical specifies the *sacerdos* (priest).[127]

If "exorcists" were not the ones usually called upon to perform solemn exorcism and were only occasionally needed for prebaptismal ceremonies or perhaps ordeals, it is unclear what exactly an exorcist like Pinewald did most of the time. Certain texts do not presuppose that their readers know much about the matter, either. A scene in Bede's *Ecclesiastical History* presumes knowledge of exorcistic prayers in the original Latin ("dicebat presbyter exorcismos" [the priest recited exorcisms]), but the Old English translation of this passage avoids the term *exorcismos* and explains the procedure from scratch: "Song he se mæssepreost 7 rædde orationem, þa ðe wið þære aðle awritene wæron" (the mass priest then sang and recited a prayer, of a sort which were written for this sickness).[128] The Old English translation of Bede is perhaps from the reign of Alfred, and if so, was intended for a clerical audience perceived by Alfred himself to be in a state of intellectual decline. For smaller communities, in which the priest was probably responsible for most parochial and devotional functions, the broader spectrum of ecclesiastical orders and functions may have been less familiar.

There are numerous Anglo-Saxon variants of a text known as the "Ordinals of Christ," a popular type piece from the early Middle Ages presenting the ecclesiastical hierarchy in terms of Christ's own precedents, and articulating the symbolic significance of the various ranks.[129] The "Ordinals" portray Christ as having himself embodied the functions of all ecclesiastical orders. Christ was a doorkeeper when he descended into hell and broke open its gates, and he was a lector when he entered the temple of the Jews and interpreted Scripture, etc. Christ was also an exorcist, as the *De vii gradibus aecclesiae* variant of the "Ordinals" in the Anderson Pontifical tells us:

> Exorcista fuit quando eiecit septem demonia de Maria Magdalenae.
> Exorcistae ex Greco in latinum "adiurantes" vocantur.[130] Invocant enim

> super catecuminos et super eos qui habent spiritum inmundum nomen Domini Iesu adiurantes per eum ut egrediatur abeis.[131]
>
> [He was an exorcist when he cast seven demons from Mary Magdalene. "Exorcists," from the Greek, are called "adjurers" in Latin. They invoke the name of God over catechumens and over those who have unclean spirits, adjuring that they leave through Him.]

None of the entries in this Anglo-Saxon manuscript for the other six orders provides an explanation of the term or refers to a Greek origin, as they do in Latin analogues.[132] Ælfric translates *exorcista* in his first letter to Wulfstan as *halsiend* (adjurer), and characterizes him as "se þe ræt ofer þa witeseocan men and ofer þa untryman" (he who reads over the insane and the ill).[133] In his letter to Wulfsige, Ælfric briefly explains the duties of the seven church ranks:

> Exorcista is on englisc: se þe mid aðe halsað þa awyrgedan gastas, þe wyllað menn dreccan, þurh þæs hælendes naman, þæt hy þa menn forlæton.[134]
>
> ["Exorcist" is, in English, "he who by an oath adjures those wicked spirits who try to afflict people, through the name of the Savior, that they leave the people alone."]

In both of these passages Ælfric describes the duties of each of the seven offices, but in both places "exorcist" is the only one of the seven to include no mention of any specific duties in the church or for the mass. This is then perhaps an idealized definition of an exorcist drawn more from literary portrayals of exorcism than from that office's practical utility in day-to-day life. At the very least, we know that exorcists aided in the preparation of catechumens for baptism, administering the exorcisms as part of the prebaptismal "scrutinies." On the continent exorcists had diversified their activities to include a variety of routine functions by this time: for instance, in the Carolingian Proto-Pontifical exorcists were assigned the task of dismissing from the church those who were not to take communion, such as catechumens (a task previously assigned to deacons).[135]

If the role of exorcists in quotidian affairs of the Anglo-Saxon church is never explicitly laid out, the role of exorcisms (whether performed by exorcists, priests, or bishops) is much better documented. There are different types of exorcisms in early medieval liturgical documents, implying a diversity of church needs in different times and regions. The Hadrianum Sacramentary that Charlemagne received from Pope Hadrian I in response to his request for an official Roman service book proved wholly inadequate for Carolingian pastoral needs: it contained papal prayers for a limited number of feast days, but none of the occasional and votive prayers that were so integral to the church-populace relationship in Charlemagne's kingdom.[136] The Gallic votive prayers that had long gained widespread use were thus added (along with other material) to form what is known as the Supplemented Hadrianum. This book could now guide priests in presiding over weddings and funerals, conducting field ceremonies, and performing exorcisms. The Leofric Missal is an early and important version of the Supplemented Hadrianum.[137] It contains blessings for fruitful fields and for starting out on a journey, prayers for war and for peace, and orisons to repel storms. The Durham Collectar (or Durham Ritual) is a miscellany containing some fascinating votive prayers—such as blessings of bread and trees, and, taking a rather practical shortcut, "ad omnia quae volveris" (for anything you may wish for).[138] The exorcisms preparatory to judicial ordeal in the Durham Collectar have drawn especial attention, in part because they appear both in Latin and Old English. Thus exorcisms appear in these votive collections as part of a broader spiritual landscape in which appeals to God were encouraged for all manner of adversities, both public and private.

A case can be made that a great many medieval Christian prayers, with varying degrees of abstraction or precision, are implicitly apotropaic or exorcistic in that they call on God to defend against or to remove evil and spiritual persecution. For our purposes, it will be necessary to focus on prayers that most clearly and unequivocally call on the rhetoric of expelling demons, or which have manuscript rubrics specifically indicating that they are to be used for energumens. With this in mind, then, we can identify three primary types or functions of exorcism in the early medieval liturgy: (1) exorcism of inanimate materials, (2) prebaptismal exorcisms, and (3) solemn exorcisms. The first two classes can be thought of as procedural, in that they are routinely performed as part of the functioning of the church in its normal activities. The third, solemn exorcism, is occasional, in that it would only be called for when a priest was faced with a demoniac (e.g., for someone raging, falling, foaming at the mouth, or striking out). Solemn exorcism might then require consecrated materials and might thus implicitly require the first type of exorcism as well (in fact, as we will see, it might draw as needed from either of the first two types).

1. The term "exorcism" itself is most often found in the liturgy applied not to people but to inanimate objects such as the salt, water, and oil—the *materia liturgica*—to be used in baptism, mass, and various other ceremonies.[139] This calls for an exorcism that usually directly addresses the creatures "of" the objects ("Exorcizo te, creatura aquae"), followed by a benediction which usually addresses God. Similar purification rituals accompany the objects to be used in judicial ordeal, such as iron.[140] Sometimes these elements themselves seem to be addressed as though they are infested—as though demons literally dwell in them and need casting out—while the wording in other passages implies that the element addressed is simply "adjured" (the literal sense of *exorcizo*) to do something in particular, e.g. water is directed to, "efficiaris in eo qui in te baptizandus erit fons aquae salientis in vitam aeternam" (become in this person about to be baptized a

spring of water flowing to eternal life).[141] *Creatura aquae* (creature of water) might be visualized as a spirit inhering in the water, or might refer to no more than the water itself as a created substance (in which case "created water" might capture the sense somewhat better than "creature of water"). Jolly offers for such exorcistic contexts, "*creatura* . . . might be understood less literally and more liturgically as 'substance' or 'element.'"[142]

The exorcism of inanimate objects raises interesting questions of agency. A similar rhetoric appears in the medical formulas as well:

> [Contra dolorum dentium]: (Cristus) super ma[r]rmoreum sedebat; Petrus tristis ante eum stabat, manum ad maxillum tenebat; et interrogebat eum Dominus dicens, "Quare tristis es, Petre?" Respondit Petrus et dixit: "Domine, dentes mei dolent." Et Dominus dixit: "Adiuro te migranea uel gutta maligna per Patrem et Filium et Spiritum Sanctum et per celum et terram, et per XX ordines angelorum, et per LX prophetas et per XII apostolos et per IIIor euangelistas et per omnes sanctos . . . ut non possit diabolus nocere ei."[143]
>
> [Against tooth pains: Christ was sitting on a stone; Peter stood sad before him and held his hand to his jaw. The Lord questioned him, saying, "Why are you sad, Peter?" Peter responded and said, "Lord, my teeth are hurting me." And the Lord said, "I adjure you, migraine or malignant drop (or 'malignant bit'), by the Father and Son and Holy Spirit and by the heaven and the earth, and by the twenty orders of angels and by the sixty prophets and by the twelve apostles and by the four evangelists and by all the saints . . . that the devil not be able to harm him."]

Though invoking the Trinity and numerous other spiritual powers, it is the offending *migranea* or *gutta maligna* that Jesus addresses directly, commanding the illness that the devil not be allowed to afflict the sufferer further. Neither God nor the devil is directly addressed. If read literally, the narrative scene becomes somewhat absurd (with Jesus calling not only on the Father and on himself, but also on the saints and on the Gospel writers for his own power and authority), but evidently the narrative backdrop that provides context is only secondary. The voice of Jesus blends with that of the practitioner administering the cure. By contrast, in solemn exorcism it is not the animate subject (the demoniac) who is abjured. God and the devil are the principal players there, while the subject ostensibly remains an entirely passive nonparticipant—a substrate or "vessel," rather than (as with *creatura aquae*) an active agent.

2. In addition to these adjurations of inanimate materials are prebaptismal exorcisms, which even today form an integral part of the baptismal rite. These adjurations over the catechumens are intended for both the community (to reinforce vividly the conception that anyone not yet baptized is still under the devil's

dominion) and the individual (to help make the transition from unbaptized to baptized more definitive and emotionally compelling). Unlike solemn exorcisms, prebaptismal exorcisms in conjunction with the other elements of the baptismal rite are in effect "speech acts": they create the desired effect or state of affairs (baptism) through their very pronouncement, in context. It is inconceivable that a correctly performed prebaptismal exorcism will not work—that it will fail to accomplish the task of cleansing and preparing the catechumen's soul. Having undergone the complete sequence of scrutinies and baptismal rites, the initiate is, by definition, baptized. This contrasts with solemn exorcism, which on various occasions is well known to fail, entirely independently of whether or not it is performed correctly. In medieval liturgical books the vast majority of exorcisms to be read over a person (rather than over an object) are prebaptismal exorcisms, and it is worth pausing to consider the significance of prebaptismal exorcism in Anglo-Saxon England.

The length and complexity of the catechumenate, during which an individual learns basic Christian doctrines and prepares for baptism by fasting and prayer, was much abridged in Anglo-Saxon England.[144] In continental practice the catechumenate begins with the Making of the Catechumen prayer (Ad catechuminum faciendum), reserved exclusively for the third Sunday in Lent. On Holy Saturday the catechumens are anointed with oil and saliva, and are required to renounce the devil ("Abrenuntio . . .") and affirm the creed ("Credo . . . ").[145] Infant candidates are dipped three times in the font and signed at last with the chrism. M. Bradford Bedingfield notes that many of the intricacies of the continental source texts are lost in the Anglo-Saxon manuscript tradition. The Missal of Robert of Jumièges, for instance, is abridged to the point of blurring the distinctions between the various stages of the catechumenate.[146] A series of procedures which in the Gelasian tradition requires a month can here be done in a day, for all the manuscript evidence tells us: "there is no indication, either in the order of sections or in the rubrics, that the ceremonies are not to be performed all at once."[147] There could be a variety of possible explanations for this (e.g., that the celebrants knew the full ceremony well enough, or that the book was intended to complement other books), but there is other evidence as well that points to English baptismal practice deviating from continental rites.

Traditionally, the stages of the catechumenate and baptism were linked to the Paschal cycle, beginning in Lent. However, the correspondence between the ceremony and any particular feast day is largely lost in the Anglo-Saxon tradition: "we see clearly a single ceremony, performed at any time, not explicitly tied to a particular time of the year."[148] The concern was that a child—especially a sick one—should be able to receive baptism quickly.[149] The Laws of Ine thus insisted that a child be baptized within thirty days of birth.[150] This anxiety is heightened by the eleventh century: in the Northumbrian Priests' Law, the child was to be baptized within nine days.[151] Since bishops were sometimes notoriously scarce in many areas of Anglo-Saxon England, confirmation could take place at a later time. Thus the Anglo-Saxon church developed mechanisms intended to minimize the instances of unbaptized children dying before the rite could be administered, resulting in baptism services that were much abbreviated and that could be administered in a single day where necessary. The process is truncated to the point that the essential core of the catechumenate (instruction in Christian fundamentals) can be postponed altogether until after baptism.

For much of the prebaptismal ceremony, the priest directly addresses God and the devil, rather than the catechumen. In the Missal of Robert of Jumièges, the series of prayers Ad caticuminum faciendum begins with the command, "Recede diabole ab hac imagine dei increpatus ab eo et da locum spiritui sancto" (Depart, devil, from this image of God, rebuked by Him, and make room for the Holy Ghost).[152] Following two prayers, the priest exorcizes the salt ("Exorcizo te creatura salis . . .") and places a pinch of it in the candidate's mouth. He signs the candidate with the cross while reciting a series of prayers that addresses God, at first, and then the devil:

> Audi maledicte satanas adiuratus per nomen aeterni dei et saluatoris nostri filii eius cum tua uictus inuidia tremens gemensque discede. Nihil tibi sit commune cum seruo dei iam caelestia cogitanti. renuntiatori tibi ac saeculo tuo et beatae inmortalitatis uictori. . . . Exorcizo te inmunde spiritus in nomine patris. et filii et spiritus sancti ut exeas et recedes ab hoc famulo dei. ipse enim tibi imperat maledicte dampnate qui pedibus super mare ambulauit et petro mergenti dexteram porrexit.[153]
>
> [Hear, accursed Satan, adjured by the name of eternal God and of our Savior the Son of God; depart along with your envy, trembling and groaning, conquered. May there be nothing in common between you and this servant of God, even now meditating on the heavens, about to renounce you and your world and gain blessed immortality. . . . I adjure you, unclean spirit, in the name of the Father, the Son, and the Holy Spirit, to leave and depart from this servant of God. He himself commands, accursed one, damned one, who walked on the water with his feet, and extended his right hand to Peter when he sank.]

At this point there are separate prayers for males and females, citing diverse scriptural passages (and thereby providing distinct role models for men and women). The sign of the cross is then made over the candidate's head, followed by a reading from Matthew and the recital of the Lord's Prayer and the creed. There is another adjuration in which Satan is addressed directly, where he is called upon once again to leave the candidate: "praecipio tibi ut exeas et recedas ab hoc famulo Dei" (I order you to leave and depart from this servant of God).[154] The priest touches the candidate's nostrils and ears with spittle, saying, "Effeta quod est adaperire in odorem suauitatis; tu autem effugare diabole" ("Effeta": that is, be opened, to the odor of sweetness; and you, devil, flee).[155] The priest makes the sign of the cross with holy oil on the candidate's breast, and calls upon him or her to renounce the devil, all his works, and all his pomps ("Abrenuntias Satanae?" Resp: "Abrenuntio . . . "). Following another sequence of prayers, the candidate is immersed three times in the font and given a vestment and a taper. The confirmation can take place immediately, if there is a bishop present to perform the rite.[156] There are separate prayers for a sick infant, and an additional sequence for "Making a Catechumen from a Pagan" (Ad caticuminum ex pagano faciendum).[157] The prayers and directions in this manuscript draw from the well-known stock of continental liturgical instructions (as found in the Gelasian and Gregorian Sacramentary traditions), though from one manuscript to another there are significant differences in point of detail: which prayers are included, their order, etc. The Leofric Missal contains many of the same prayers as the Missal of Robert of Jumièges, though in a somewhat different order. The priest's warning to Satan not to be deceived ("Nec te latet"), for instance, comes before the creed and the renunciation of the devil in the Missal of Robert of Jumièges, but after them in Leofric.[158]

The ceremonies preparing catechumens for baptism, and the baptism itself, presuppose that the individual is under the provenance of the devil in some sense (through original sin) and requires exorcism: "Se deofol bið adræfed þurh ures Drihtnes mihte of þam hæþenan men þonne hine man fullað" (The devil is driven out, through our Lord's power, from heathens when they are baptized).[159] Not everyone presenting him- or herself for baptism is literally possessed by a demon, of course—certainly not in the same sense as those raging wretches in need of solemn exorcism.[160] One might well imagine, in fact, that the intricate, methodical ceremonies of the catechumenate and baptism would be postponed for someone exhibiting severe symptoms of dissociation or convulsions, or for someone actively resisting the procedure by any overtly disrespectful attitude. Such an awkward state of affairs could explain, in part, the need for a separate prayer found in both the Gregorian and Gelasian traditions: "Inpositio manuum super energuminum caticuminum" (Laying on hands over possessed catechumens).[161] Although the catechumen is considered to be in the devil's control in some way, inasmuch as all unbaptized people are, the exorcism of the devil in this context more resembles the purification rituals of liturgical vessels than the dramatic, adversarial confrontations between demoniacs and saints recorded in narrative accounts. Just as vessels require blessing before they can be used in the mass, here the candidate becomes a "vessel" to be cleansed, in order to be filled with the Holy Spirit. In short, prebaptismal exorcisms are not dynamic, interactive, and adversarial; they are procedural.

Henry A. Kelly argues that from at least the time of Augustine, prebaptismal exorcism was considered more allegorical than literal by some commentators:

> At first, the ceremonies corresponded very closely to reality, but soon symbolic or fictive elements were introduced or perceived, which had the effect of making the service more figurative and less realistic. This was particularly true of the exorcisms. The notion that all sinners were literally possessed by demons did not find much favor with the Fathers, and when they were confronted with baptismal ceremonies that presupposed it, they were forced to interpret them allegorically.[162]

For many medieval commentators, however, there was no conflict between allegorical and literal meanings of baptism and its attendant exorcisms. Baptism removes pollution, the taint of the kingdom of evil.[163] However the substance of that taint is visualized, the symbolic gestures of the rite create an atmosphere of reverence and demarcate liturgical activity as holy rather than mundane.[164] In his early dialogue *On the Happy Life* (386 CE), written in preparation of his own baptism, Augustine makes a distinction between two senses of "unclean spirit"—one referring to medical demons and the other to the moral state of a soul living in sin:

> . . . spiritus immundus, quantum intelligo, duobus modis appellari solet: vel ille qui extrinsecus invadit animam sensusque conturbat, et quemdam hominibus infert furorem; cui excludendo qui praesunt, manum imponere vel exorcizare dicuntur, hoc est, per divina eum adjurando expellere: aliter autem dicitur spiritus immundus, omnis omnino anima immunda; quod nihil est aliud quam vitiis et erroribus inquinata.[165]
>
> [. . . "unclean spirit," as I understand it, is usually spoken of in two ways: either, it is that which invades the soul from outside and confuses the senses and stirs a certain kind of fury in people; those in charge who drive the spirit out are said to "lay hands on" or "exorcize" it—that is, to expel it by adjuring it through holiness; or else, every single unclean soul—which is nothing other than a soul defiled by vices and errors—is called an "unclean spirit."]

Though this distinction is not prominently observed either in early medieval theology or homiletics, it accords with the sacramental treatment of catechumens as distinct from that of energumens. The "demon" expelled in prebaptismal rites represents the corruption of the fallen, post-Edenic world in general, and does not imply physical illness or mental dissociation.

The Carolingian liturgical reforms focused primarily on mystical and eschatological aspects of baptismal cleansing.[166] Peter Cramer sees Bede especially as a key figure in revitalizing the Augustinian approach to baptism, which stresses allegory at every turn and interprets liturgical actions as imitations of scripture.[167] In that same vein, Wulfstan sees baptism principally in terms of a black-and-white change of state, from the domain of darkness to that of light, and so naturally he emphasizes the demonological dimension of baptismal ceremonies. The various actions of the baptismal rite are interpreted as signs (*getacnunge*): for instance, the salt symbolizes wisdom ("sal enim sapientiam significant"), and the wax taper symbolizes the holy spirit.[168] Every element of the ceremony is systematically read as allusion, analogy, or figure. Through the *exsufflatio*—the ritual breathing of the priest on the candidate—the evil spirit is not expelled but is merely "shown" to be already expelled: "per insuflationem sacerdotis monstratur inmundus spiritus expelli" (through the priest's insufflation the evil spirit is shown to be expelled).[169] The kind of spirit being expelled is clear, though. These are not the demons of raving and madness but the symbolic representations of the stain of original sin:

> Exorcizatur etiam idem malignus spiritus, ut exeat et recedat ab illo plasmate quod iamdudum per peccatum primi hominis possidebat.[170]
>
> [Indeed the evil spirit is adjured that it leave and withdraw from this creature because it had control over him for a long time now through the sin of the first man.]

The devil is primarily in the candidate, that is, to the extent that he is in all humankind, subsequent to the transgression of Eden:

> se deofol wyrð aflymed fram þære menniscean gesceafte, þæt is, fram þam menn ðe ær wæs þurh Adam forworht.[171]
>
> [the devil is expelled from the human being—that is, from the person who had formerly been undone by Adam.]

The exorcisms are symbols of leaving behind an old way of life and thinking, and of embracing a new one. Wulfstan is at pains to explain that driving out the devil essentially means adopting a new code of conduct: the new Christian is now to "wiðsace anrædlice deofles gemanan: þæt is, þæt he forsace ⁊ forbuge his unlara" (resolutely abandon the devil's company: that is, that he forsake and avoid the devil's perverse teachings).[172] While demonology is emphasized throughout Wulfstan's explication of the baptismal rite, it is introduced mostly to illuminate moral and theological considerations. This allegorical approach is characteristic of the broader Anglo-Saxon homiletic tradition. Ælfric, for instance, similarly describes baptismal exorcism as figural: "ðonne se preost cristnað þæt cild, þonne adræfð he þone deofol of þam cilde: for þan ðe ælc hæþen man bið deofles" (when the priest anoints the child, he drives the devil from the child: because every heathen is of the devil).[173]

Allegory was rarely in direct conflict with literal interpretation in the early Middle Ages; if anything, each perspective was seen as reinforcing the other. The primary focus of Ælfric and Wulfstan was pastoral rather than medical, and perhaps there is no particular reason for us to expect them to enlighten us concerning demon possession in late tenth- and early eleventh-century England. It can be said, however, that if those homilists did know of contemporary cases of possession and exorcism—especially cases with which their audience might have been familiar—then they passed up on potentially outstanding examples with which to reinforce their points.

3. Beyond these procedural exorcisms, some Anglo-Saxon books also contain prayers specifically indicated for the demon possessed—that is, solemn exorcisms proper.[174] The Leofric Missal contains three "prayers for those vexed by demons" (Orationes super eos qui a daemonio vexantur) and four prayers "for a baptized energumen" (Super energumino baptizato).[175] The Lanalet and Anderson Pontificals (liturgical books for use by a bishop), moreover, contain a series of performance instructions (*ordines*) for exorcisms, which accompany their prayers.[176] On the other hand, many other books (such as the Missal of Robert of Jumièges, the Egbert Pontifical, the Sidney Sussex Pontifical, the Winchcombe Sacramentary, and the Durham Collectar) are more abbreviated, carrying no specific provisions for curing a demoniac.

The *ordines* in the Lanalet Pontifical are invaluable in allowing us to reconstruct how the compiler envisioned an exorcism unfolding. The bishop is to begin by fasting for three days, "cum elemosinis et orationibus" (with alms and prayers).[177] Three prayers are then provided to exorcize and bless the water, followed by two for the salt. While the salt is being mixed into the water, three more adjurations address the element (or perhaps the spirit within it) directly, alternately addressing it as "creature of salt" and "creature of water." After this, six chapters of the Gospels are read over the water (*super iliam*)—Matthew 26:2–27:66, Mark 14:1–15:47, and John 18:1–19:42—representing three pairs of chapters each from Matthew, Mark, and John. The chapters do not contain any of Jesus' exorcisms; instead, each relates his Last Supper, Trial, and Crucifixion. The complete Passion of Christ, then, is read three times in a row. Now the blessed water containing the separately blessed salt is to be used in the preparation of all the subject's meals and drinks:

> Ex hac aqua preparetur ei omnis usus in cibo et in potu sed et balneum ut interius exteriusque illa inrigetur.[178]
>
> [From this water is to be prepared for him his food and his drink and even his bath—for all purposes—so that he may be nourished (*inrigetur*, lit. "moistened" or "irrigated") both inside and outside.]

Following this, the material and gestural components essentially stop, and the celebrant is directed, with one last instruction, to recite a series of prayers. These go on for some six manuscript pages (fols. 164v–167v). Reciting them out loud at a leisurely pace, I time them as taking some ten to fifteen minutes in total. The first begins:

> Domine sancte pater omnipotens aeterne deus pater domini nostri ihesu christi qui illum refugam tyrannum gehennae deputasti, qui

unigenitum tuum in hunc mundum misisti, illum refugam leonem contemtum, uelociter adtende et adcelera ut eripias hominem tuis formatum manibus a rapina et demonio meridiano.[179]

[Holy Lord, omnipotent father, eternal God, father of our Lord Jesus Christ who condemned the fugitive tyrant to Gehenna, who sent your only-begotten son to this world, having disdained the fugitive lion: attend quickly, and hasten to snatch this man—created by your own hands—from plundering and from the noonday demon.]

And the last concludes:

Te supplex deprecor domine ut ad inuocationem nominis tui ab huius famuli tui uexatione inimicus confusus abscedat et ab eius possessione anima liberata ad auctorem suae salutis recurrat liberatoremque suum diabolico foetore depulso et odore suauissimo spiritus sancti percepto sequatur. Per.[180]

[I humbly pray, Lord, that at the invocation of your name, the Enemy, confounded, will withdraw from troubling this your servant, and that, in possession of a freed soul, (your servant) may return from him to the author of his salvation, and—the devilish foulness being driven off, and the sweetest scent of the Holy Spirit being perceived—he may follow his liberator. Through.]

The pontifical proceeds immediately after this to judicial ordeals. This exorcism stands out for its intensity and relentlessness, once the actual recital of prayers over the demoniac has begun. It is interesting that the preparatory procedures (the three days of prayer and fasting, and the blessing of salt and water) do not have to be performed in the presence of the demoniac. Indeed, conceivably, the bishop does not necessarily have to wait until confronted with a demoniac at all: these preparations can all be done well in advance, and then the holy water used when and if there is occasion. Presumably, though, the spirit of the text is to perform all the directions once a case has come forward, so that the celebrant can spend the three days praying specifically for the given individual (this is how Felix describes Guthlac as doing it, for instance).[181] If so, then the overall rhythm of the rite involves an intricate preparation of materials in the presence of the energumen (perhaps with his or her family), followed by an emotionally charged—but controlled—display of power and authority over the offending spirit or spirits. The rite does not require or presume any response, rebuttal, or participation at any stage on the part of the demoniac.[182]

The user of the Leofric Missal would find a similar range of prayers, and though the prayers are given without performance instructions, they are subdivided for more particular ranges of circumstances. For all possessed people ("eos qui a daemonio vexantur"), the sequence begins with a total of some two hundred and fifty words in two prayers, followed by a brief statement as the celebrant signs the demoniac with consecrated oil: "Vnguo te de oleo sanctificato, ut salueris in nomine patris et filii et spiritus sancti in secula seculorum. Amen" (I anoint you with holy oil, so that you will be saved in the name of the Father and Son and Holy Spirit, throughout all the ages. Amen).[183] Then one of three prayers is selected, depending on the condition of the subject: a possessed catechumen (*energuminum caticuminum*), a possessed child or infant (*parvulo energumino*), or a possessed person already baptized (*energumino baptizato*).[184] Following this is a dramatic sequence, as in Lanalet (in fact the same core of material appears, more or less, in both), although it is not explicitly clear from the rubrics whether this entire block of material (fols. 310r–312v) is meant to be recited for all three of the circumstances mentioned previously, or only for the last. Following this sequence, many more adjurations and exorcisms begin on fol. 312v, but here they are meant for baptismal preparations rather than for demoniacs: "Ordo super electos ad caticuminum faciendum."[185] It is possible, of course, that a user of the book might freely draw exorcisms from the baptismal procedures as part of a solemn exorcism: he would find them in roughly the same part of the book, and they are rhetorically indistinguishable from one another in many respects.

Many of these exorcisms were in fact very fluid in use and context. While no prayers in the Missal of Robert of Jumièges are given explicit rubrics indicating that they are to be used against the possessed, portions of solemn exorcisms appear in that book under different headings. Moreover, the Medelam tuam deprecor—which in the Gregorian Sacramentary is associated with emergency baptism for the sick ("Oratio ad baptizandum infirmum"), and appears in that capacity in the Missal of Robert—becomes an exorcism to be read over demoniacs in the Leofric Missal ("super eos qui a daemonio vexantur").[186] Similarly, the internal performance rubric "ut hunc famulum tuum .ill. eruas ab hac inualitudine" (that you may deliver this your servant .N. from this illness) becomes in Leofric, "ut hunc famulum tuum ill. eruas ab hac uexatione diaboli" (that you may deliver this your servant .N. from this vexation by the devil).[187] Specific passages can also be shuffled around for distinct occasions, such as a certain adjuration ("In cuius uirtute") which appears twice in the Leofric Missal—once as part of the baptismal ceremony and once for solemn exorcism.[188] The text has been stitched into the Medelam tuam deprecor, to apply a prebaptismal exorcism to a demoniac.[189] Two more prayers, which are assigned specifically for a possessed catechumen in the Leofric Missal and in the Sacramentary tradition in general, appear in the Lanalet Pontifical as available rather to treat all demoniacs.[190]

The prayers for solemn exorcism are often found alongside prebaptismal exorcisms in the manuscripts, forming clusters in which the parts can apparently be easily interchanged if desired. Other prayers have lost their rubrics altogether and so it has become uncertain what performance context is intended: the series of prayers that is labeled Exorcismus contra demonum in the Lanalet Pontifical has no title or rubric whatsoever in the Anderson Pontifical.[191] As far as one can tell from the manuscript presentation in the Anderson Pontifical, the exorcisms of water and salt that begin this section seem to still fall under the preceding rubric, "Oratio contra fulgora" (Prayer against lightning). Possibly, the priests and bishops who used these books regularly knew what they contained and what each prayer was for, and if so, rubrics were redundant. More obviously, however, the rhetoric of exorcism drew from a common pool of tropes for casting out demonic influences or presences, and this could be applied to any of a number of circumstances.[192]

Paleographic considerations can help us further understand the significance of exorcisms in Anglo-Saxon manuscripts. It was important to a scribe of the Leofric Missal, for instance, to get the text right: the Latin prayers were corrected against a copy of the Gregorian Sacramentary (for an example, see erasure and interlinear addition in prayer 2478). On the other hand, in Anglo-Saxon manuscripts none of the rites of solemn exorcism are glossed extensively in the vernacular, in the way that, for instance, the masses for the sick (*infirmis*) are glossed in the Missal of Robert of Jumièges.[193] Exorcisms had often been translated into Old English, along with entire series of exorcism directions—but only for the materials to be used in judicial ordeal.[194] Finally, the grammatical endings of words referring to the subjects of exorcism in the Lanalet Pontifical are potentially significant: the scribe has gone through the solemn exorcisms and added plural endings above the singular, a practice frequently encountered in early medieval liturgical manuscripts (for instance, *famulo dei* becomes *famulis dei*, and *oculos tuos* becomes *oculos uestros*).[195] Such alterations imply that the subjects of these exorcisms may have been groups of people rather than individuals. This seems to fit the context of catechumenal exorcisms, in which candidates usually undergo the various ceremonies as a group, rather than solemn exorcism, which is presumably an individual, ad hoc affair more often than not. There is no specific mention of either energumens or catechumens in the text, and the opening rubric ("Incipit exorcismus contra demonum") leaves the possibility open for either one. If that is the case, then prayers which in earlier texts and traditional sources are specifically for demoniacs have here been appropriated for a prebaptismal context (or even, perhaps, for the infirm more generally, if illness by its very nature is considered demonic).

Such sequences of prayer and gesture encourage us to visualize a systematic, carefully choreographed regimen of liturgical exorcisms employing previously prepared materials (which needed up to three days' preparation) and being conducted under the supervision of a priest or bishop. A major obstacle in presuming that these written exorcisms were actually employed for demoniacs, however, lies in the notable disparity between liturgical and narrative sources. The liturgy calls for a formal procedure conducted under controlled conditions (e.g., with access to church accoutrements such as salt, incense, and tapers), while the exorcisms described in narrative sources seldom paint such a portrait.[196] On the contrary: the narrative accounts describe exorcisms as charismatic rather than procedural, and their essence is spontaneity, simplicity, and immediacy.[197] When Aldhelm summarizes the passion of St. Anatolia for his prose *De virginitate*, for instance, he changes the exorcism in that narrative from a formal procedure to a brief, improvised encounter:

> etenim filium consulis inergumenum rigidis catenarum nexibus asstrictum expulso habitatore, dicto citius curauit.[198]
>
> [Anatolia cured the son of a consul—an energumen closely bound in tight fetters—having expelled the indweller quicker than it takes to say it.]

In Aldhelm's ostensible source the demon is only cast out following a debate between the saint and the demon, and the recitation of a formal adjuration: "Impero tibi in nomine Domini mei Jesu Christi, immunde spiritus, exi ab homine isto" (I command you in the name of my Lord Jesus Christ, evil spirit, to depart from this person).[199] In Ælfric's account of St. Gallicanus, the saint cures demoniacs merely by looking at them: "swa hraðe swa he beseah on ða witseocan menn swa wurdon hi aclænsode fram þam unclænan gastum" (as soon as he looked upon "wit-sick" people they were cleansed of unclean spirits). Cuthbert is said to cure demoniacs *uerbo tantum* (with barely a word).[200] The tendency to focus on immediacy rather than protracted procedure is clearly a function of hagiographic agenda; it does after all serve to paint an individual figure as particularly blessed and powerful. Furthermore, there is a powerful impulse in the narrative patterning of medieval hagiography to mimic New Testament descriptions of miracles. The contrast between narrative and liturgical evidence, however, is striking. Liturgy and hagiography both operated within the sphere of their own generic constructs, and, in all likelihood, neither provides a reliable portrait of how those perceived as demonically possessed were actually treated when brought to a local priest in Anglo-Saxon England. The presence of exorcisms in liturgical books does not by itself imply their frequent use, nor the forms they took when they were actually employed.

There are other precedents for liturgical ceremonies which show significant disparity between their regular formulaic presentation in manuscripts and their varied patterns of actual application. Despite the elaborate rituals of excommunication described in liturgical texts, F. D. Logan finds that these rituals were never once explicitly said to be used in the fifteen thousand cases he cites from English ecclesiastical courts in the High Middle Ages.[201] The simple phrase "excommunico te" (I excommunicate you) apparently sufficed. Additional practices attending the ceremony may have varied, without being recorded in the court records. By this time there was perhaps a gap between the conservative written record and actual practice.[202] The shape and form of excommunication in Anglo-Saxon England is a similar matter of great uncertainty: Elaine Treharne writes, "In the Anglo-Saxon period, documentary evidence for excommunication is patchy, reflecting the lack of uniformity in its practice; it was not systematically defined until the twelfth century."[203] She deduces that while it was probably more frequently practiced than is sometimes thought, it was less regular a procedure than the eleventh- and twelfth-century manuscript formulas—which reflect a deliberate attempt to codify and regularize—might imply.[204] Therefore, the appearance of excommunication formulas in an Anglo-Saxon copy of the Romano-German Pontifical (London, British Library, MS Cotton Tiberius C.I, fols. 195v–197r), for instance, does not imply its regular or widespread use. "The practice of excommunication before the twelfth century," Treharne writes, "is localized rather than uniform."[205] Similarly, the texts for judicial ordeals were copied in numerous Anglo-Saxon and continental manuscripts, though actual cases of its application were, many believe, rare.[206] The solemn exorcisms preserved in early medieval manuscripts may have been widely used, or perhaps, as with excommunication rites and ordeal texts, the manuscript witnesses may give a misleading picture of the currency or actual application of exorcisms.

We know then that Anglo-Saxon manuscripts contain exorcisms, but given that they could well be (and in some cases demonstrably were) used for other liturgical situations, or were used for other illnesses unconnected with personality displacement or neurological disorders, it is hard to know how much insight they provide regarding Anglo-Saxon demon possession. Presumably exorcisms were used more by some than others, and they were more likely to be used in districts with greater access to manuscripts. If the prayers were memorized—as the ordination instructions for "exorcist" specify—then that person would carry in his memory the particular exorcisms available at the time and place of his ordination. This availability would vary greatly from the library of one church or monastery to another.[207] Furthermore, the rites would certainly be adapted to particular circumstances: for instance, in a longer, more difficult exorcism, sections could be repeated or additional prayers, psalms, and Gospel readings could be included.[208] The modern Roman Ritual still allows for adaptive exorcism.[209]

On those occasions when solemn exorcism was administered, did it work? There is abundant anecdotal evidence that the performance of ritualized healing practices—especially within a religious context—can have significant therapeutic value to a member of the community.[210] Indeed, some modern therapists and psychoanalysts still consider the demon-possession model a useful tool, if that is part of the patient's cultural experience.[211] There is a strong cultural dimension to how an individual responds to trauma. A thirty-one-year old Ethiopian refugee whose baby had been smashed to death during her flight from Ethiopia continued to carry the infant corpse for several days. Upon reaching Israel at last, she was treated for dissociative disorder and psychosis. The haloperidol was ineffective; it was only after a religious leader was consulted and purification rituals were conducted to cleanse her of contact with a corpse that normal functioning was regained.[212] Likewise, Ferracuti, Sacco, and Lazzari record cases of possession in modern Rome in which patients diagnosed with schizophrenia reported that psychiatric treatment and neuroleptics had no effect, but that religious rituals (Roman Catholic exorcisms) brought "some improvement."[213] On the other hand, Hale and Pinninti were finally able to relieve a Hindu man of ghost-possession delusions through administration of neuroleptics, after Hindu, Muslim, and Christian priests had all tried various exorcisms unsuccessfully.[214] Cultural and biochemical factors can both play important roles, and we should be careful not to completely reduce possession to either a social ritual or a neurological condition.

In modern analyses of folk healing in traditional societies, short-term behavior improvements elicited through powerful, dramatic ceremonies reinforced through the concerted efforts of the healer, family, and community are well documented.[215] Exorcism works by inducing sensory arousal and creating a heightened dissociative state, an excitatory phase which is concluded eventually with emotional collapse. During the excitatory phase, the subject enters a trance-like state and is able to access varying layers of the subconscious to release what Obeyesekere calls "primary process" (e.g., libidinal, oral-erotic, aggressive, and prerational) material.[216] Verbal interrogation or exposition on the part of the exorcist, who serves as a guide during this procedure, tracks the escalating conflict publicly to create a communal narrative of what is happening (in mythological rather than psychological terms, which allows the dialectic to unfold un-self-consciously). Through the role-playing that occurs during this stage of liminal consciousness, the public narrative emphasizes that the individual is subordinate to a more powerful authority figure or divine presence. The temporarily intensified relationship between the possessed and the exorcist is the prevailing worldwide therapeutic constant, rather than any particular practices or underlying theoretical principles.[217] The exchange is a "controlled explosion and interchange of violence," as Peter Brown puts it, and, in this light, the exorcist's greatest weapon is his calm in the face of this violence: he "shows his power, by being able to bring into the open and ride out so much pent-up rebellion and anger."[218]

Though he covers a period slightly later than ours, Finucane paints a vivid picture of how exactly "miraculous" cures can be understood to work, as recorded in the miracle registries of Norman England. His study is of posthumous miracles at saints' tombs, rather than interactive exorcisms by living people, but his insights into how healing miracles are perceived in a culture receptive to them are nonetheless instructive. Saints' lives often imply or directly state that the cure is immediate and the supplicant walks away completely cured. Finucane found, however, that the vast majority of patients became aware of an improvement in their condition only gradually—an improvement which they retrospectively attributed to whatever supplications they made to a given saint. He states: "The instantaneous faith-healing miracle was rare."[219] On one occasion the recorder of Wulfstan's posthumous miracles was even surprised to encounter such an instantaneous cure: he states that it happened "not, like others, in starts and stops and after delays, but all at once" (non per interualla et certas interpolationes temporum sicut alias . . . sed simul et semel).[220] Moreover, partial recoveries were often accepted as miraculous cures. A man falsely accused of theft in Lantfred's *Translatio et miracula Swithuni*, for instance, has his eyes and ears mutilated and his hands and nose severed. The eyes and ears are restored to health at the saint's shrine—leaving him much happier but, presumably, still without hands or nose.[221] Finally, after the cured or partially cured supplicant returned later to repay the saint with a votive offering and to inform the shrine's registrar of the cure, it was easy—indeed, quite natural—to exaggerate the extent of the initial ailment and of the relief brought.[222] All of this should serve to make us wary about the number and nature of miraculous cures reported in medieval sources, and even more so of those for less tangible ailments such as behavioral disorders.

Most modern psychiatrists and many medical anthropologists generally accept that exorcism can materially help minor psychiatric disorders, but not so for major ones or for neurological conditions such as epilepsy or Tourette's Syndrome.[223] No amount of ritual will bring permanent relief for serious conditions rooted in neurochemical imbalance. What cannot be determined beyond this core of biological pathologies is the extent to which possession behavior was also present in Anglo-Saxon England as an accepted and even encouraged outlet for the pain and frustration of day-to-day life that assuredly beset any age. Some cultures encourage people to come forth and pour out their natural human anxieties in a dramatic ritual of rage and resistance ("functional possession"). In these cases exorcism will, eventually, work in the vast majority of cases, because the cure itself is an imbedded component of the ritual: it is the final act of the drama. In any event, the drama can be repeated if the psychosocial conditions causing it continue to place pressure on the individual. That Anglo-Saxons had epileptics, severe psychotics, and people with Tourette's Syndrome is certain. These are organic conditions with strong cross-cultural profiles (more in chapter 4). If Anglo-Saxons had a sizeable number of demoniacs actively adopting possession behavior beyond these (and a few other organically rooted) dysfunctions, however, the documentary record preserves little trace of it. While the medical and liturgical genres suggest, by their inclusion of remedies and prayers, the existence of demoniacs, narrative literature is the only genre that purports to describe actual cases of them in any detail. It is thus to the narrative literature that we now turn.

NOTES

1. Courlander, *Tiger's Whisker*, pp. 9–10.

2. Lantfred, *Translatio et miracula Swithuni* 33 (Lapidge, *Cult*, p. 322). The reason provided is that the woman neglected to make the sign of the cross over her mouth upon yawning. Giselle de Nie identifies the suddenness of a condition as one of the factors that suggests demonic influence to Gregory of Tours: "A not inconsiderable number of the ailments that Gregory describes are specified as having come about suddenly. In these cases, Gregory mentions or seems to assume the agency of the devil, a demon or some shade or ghost . . . sudden nervous illnesses of contraction and paralysis are also associated with a 'diabolical influx (*incursio diabolica*)'" (Nie, *Views*, pp. 231–32).

3. Dendle, *Satan Unbound*, p. 21; and Dendle, "Plants," p. 50.

4. Clarke, *Mental Disorder*, p. 62; Finucane, *Miracles*, pp. 72, 107–9; Stanley Jackson, "Unusual Mental States," p. 292; Meaney, "Anglo-Saxon View," p. 17.

5. Bonser, *Medical Background*, p. 258.

6. *Leechbook* 3.40 (Cockayne, *Leechdoms*, vol. 2, p. 334). We await a definitive critical edition of the *Leechbook*. I have used Cockayne as my base text, checking him against the facsimile edition (C. E. Wright, *Bald's Leechbook*) and two editions in dissertation form: Deegan, *Critical Edition*, for the *Leechbook* books 1 and 2; and Olds, "Anglo-Saxon Leechbook III," for book 3. Though more recent, the Olds edition does not represent improvements over Cockayne for the recipes studied here. Cockayne's edition of book 3 also appears with a fresh translation in Pollington, *Leechcraft*, pp. 378–407.

7. Society-wide obsession with demonology leading to systematic torture of the mentally ill is not securely attested until after the Renaissance. Michel Foucault, in setting the stage for his account of the wide-scale institutionalization of the mentally ill in the seventeenth century, presented medieval treatment of the mentally ill as relatively tolerant. For Foucault, the mentally ill were haplessly drawn into the societal vacuum of "ritual exiles" left by the emptying of leprosaria (*Madness*, p. 10), and were drafted as counter symbols for reason, which was suddenly heralded as the defining characteristic of humanity. For criticism of Foucault's romanticized image of madness in the medieval West, see Scull, *Most Solitary*, pp. 5–7; Midelfort, "Madness," pp. 247–65. Of the various disciplinary responses to Foucault, Midelfort notes, "Happiest, perhaps have been the medievalists, for they have found in Foucault an unexpected defender. In his pages they can ignore the frequent cruelty of medieval society toward the mad, emphasizing instead its openness to folly and unreason" (251–52). Foucault does not treat of the early Middle Ages, but for the late medieval period, Foucault is certainly too facile in his poetic suggestion that madmen wandered at will with almost natural, romantic abandon, and he downplays the extent to which the insane posed a threat to medieval constructs of rationality, long before the age of reason.

8. Finucane, *Miracles*, p. 9. Elsewhere he notes, "Demoniacs were tied up and taken to medieval shrines and kept there for days or even weeks, until their rage subsided, though it was difficult to carry on the liturgy with much decorum during their screaming fits" (91). It should also be noted that Finucane's study focuses on a slightly later period than ours, mostly drawing from postconquest sources.

9. Richard Hunter and Macalpine, *Three Hundred Years*, p. 4. Bartholomaeus goes on to suggest that the mentally ill "shall be refreshed & comfortid—& withdrawen from cause and mater of drede and besy thoughtes" (4).

10. Sulpicius Severus, *Dialogi* 1.22 (Halm, *Sulpicii Severi*, p. 175).

11. Einhard, *Translatio et miracula sanctorum Marcellini et Petri* 3.20 (Waitz, *Translatio*, p. 255).

12. Colgrave, *Felix's Life*, pp. 126–28.

13. Thus Stanley Jackson: "In some instances these disorders [epilepsy, mania, phrenitis, melancholy, and uterine suffocation] were diagnosed as such but explained in terms of demonic possession; in other instances a 'diagnosis' of demonic possession was made *rather than* one in medical terms" ("Unusual Mental States," p. 292, and see p. 295).

14. In "On the Margins," as elsewhere, Jolly demonstrates the artificiality of many traditional generic categories that attempt to compartmentalize Anglo-Saxon devotional culture too strictly: "We need to change our view of what constitutes Christian prayer and ritual within the exegetical traditions of the early Middle Ages. The more medical *Lacnunga* and *Leechbooks* are semi-monastic or clerical ritual texts produced in a time when liturgical service books were themselves still developing and changing. What we find here in CCCC 41's margins is not much different in approach from that which we see in the Durham Ritual, the Leofric and Jumièges Missals, or the medicinal *Lacnunga* and *Leechbooks*. They all contain performative formulas rooted in similar assumptions about verbal rituals and the power of words" (pp. 173–74).

15. In hagiographic portrayals it is almost always the nuclear family which brings the sufferer to the saint or healing shrine. Considering the medical texts, Stanley Jackson adds, "the various therapeutic discussions all seem to imply that the patient was treated in the home" ("Unusual Mental States," p. 294). About half of the three thousand recorded miracles that Finucane examines from medieval England and France occur back in the patient's home, after they have returned from visiting the healing shrine (*Miracles*, pp. 69, 82). Sam Lucy, reviewing the respectful grave remains of several Anglo-Saxons with leprosy and paralysis, concludes: "Such cases throw interesting light on the caring nature of the communities in which these people lived, for care of the disabled and sick seems to have been prevalent" (*Anglo-Saxon Way*, p. 70).

16. Thus Sally Crawford: the "family" consisted of "a man, his wife and children rather than any more extended group, such as in-laws . . . the family perceived by the lawmakers as common to the average man seems to have been nuclear" (*Childhood*, p. 109). On the Anglo-Saxon family (which can mean either kin group or household, depending on context), see Stafford, *Unification*, pp. 162–79. The core of the household in this period remained the conjugal family of wife, husband, and children (164).

17. Orme and Webster mention that "hospitals in a free-standing independent sense remain elusive before 1066" (*English Hospital*, p. 20; see also p. 15). Rubin, however, refers to St. Peters at York, founded by King Athelstan ca. 937, and another house in Worcester, founded by Oswald before 992, both as "non-monastic houses which cared for the sick" ("Medical Practitioner," p. 69). For Anglo-Saxon hospitals, see Bonser, *Medical Background*, pp. 95–97. A twelfth-century record of St. Bartholomew's of London—England's first true hospital—records fifty-seven cases of "miraculous" cure, twenty-two of which are neurologic or psychiatric in nature (cases translated and discussed in Wilmer and Scammon, "Neuropsychiatric Patients," p. 2).

18. Bede, *HE* 4.24, 4.31, pp. 418, 446.

19. Orme and Webster, *English Hospital*, p. 17–20. Rubin notes, "Some of these places were certainly used as hospitals while others also shared this function with providing accommodation for travellers, pilgrims and others requiring hospitality" ("Medical Practitioner," p. 69). Talbot argues that throughout much of the Middle Ages what we now think of as "hospitals" also provided for the elderly, the homeless, and others needing to be cared

for, regardless of health (*Medicine*, p. 172). The *Regularis Concordia* encourages hospitality to poor travelers (chap. 10), and for ministrations to the sick in monastic houses see also chap. 12 (Symons, *Regularis Concordia*, pp. 62, 64–65). For the early evolution of healing in monastic contexts (specifically in late antique Egypt), see Crislip, *From Monastery to Hospital* (esp. pp. 78–81, for demons and demonic possession); and for Anglo-Saxon monastic infirmaries, see D'Aronco, "Benedictine Rule," pp. 235–51.

20. Bede, *HE* 4.19, p. 394; Asser, *De rebus gestis Ælfredi* 74 (Stevenson, *Assers's Life*, p. 54). See also the doctor in Bede, *HE* 5.6, p. 468.

21. Significant treatments of the Anglo-Saxon physician include Bonser, *Medical Background*; Cameron, *Anglo-Saxon Medicine*; Pollington, *Leechcraft*; and Rubin, "Anglo-Saxon Physician" (Rubin's arguments also appear in his monograph *Medieval English Medicine*). Also, still valuable are Grattan and Singer, *Anglo-Saxon Magic*; and Talbot, *Medicine*. Singer's patronizing assessment of Anglo-Saxon medicine (in his introduction to Grattan and Singer, *Anglo-Saxon Magic*) must be considered in light of more recent criticisms (e.g., Cameron, *Anglo-Saxon Medicine*, pp. 45, 117–29); and Rubin's curious conclusions that the Anglo-Saxon physician was "required to do no more than learn his material mechanically and uncritically, directly from his texts alone . . . from which no deviation was expected" ("Anglo-Saxon Physician," p. 8) are quite out of step with current critical consensus (see, for instance, responses to these arguments in Pollington, *Leechcraft*, pp. 44–45). For the transition to Anglo-Norman medicine and Gilbertus Anglicus (whom Getz calls "England's first major medical writer," 39), see Getz, *Medicine*.

22. Cockayne, *Leechdoms*, vol. 2, p. 350. For more on the joint participation of clerics and lay residents in such rites, see Jolly, "Tapping the Power," esp. pp. 61, 71–74.

23. Anon., *Vita Cuthberti* 4.17 (Colgrave, *Two Lives*, p. 136); Bede, *Vita Cuthberti* 32, 45 (pp. 258, 298), and Bede, *HE* 4.32, 5.2, pp. 448, 458.

24. We have three unequivocal names of Anglo-Saxon physicians: Bede's Cynefrith (*HE* 4.19, p. 394), and Oxa and Dun of Bald's *Leechbook* (Cockayne, *Leechdoms*, vol. 2, pp. 120 and 292). Bald, for whom the *Leechbook* was written, and Cild, who copied the book, may or may not have been doctors (Cameron, *Anglo-Saxon Medicine*, pp. 20–21; Rubin "Anglo-Saxon Physician," p. 8). We also know of a small handful of foreign physicians brought to England (such as Baldwin and Adelard), perhaps implying a relative dearth of native ones (see Kealey, *Medieval Medicus*, pp. 30–33). On women in Anglo-Saxon medicine, see Cameron, *Anglo-Saxon Medicine*, p. 22; Jolly, *Popular Religion*, p. 103; Meaney, "Women," pp. 21–23; Pollington, *Leechcraft*, pp. 45–57; Rubin, "Anglo-Saxon Physician," p. 11; Weston, "Women's Medicine," pp. 279–93.

25. Einhard, *Translatio et miracula sanctorum Marcellini et Petri* 3.16: "Hoc ubi mulierculis in eodem fundo habitantibus innotuit, adcurrunt herbisque et frivolis incantationibus malehabenti succurrere moliuntur" (When this [ailment] became known to some local women living on the same lands, they ran to assist the sick person with herbs and frivolous incantations; Waitz, *Translatio*, p. 254). See Pollington, *Leechcraft*, pp. 46–49.

26. Meaney, *Anglo-Saxon Amulets*, pp. 61–62, 65. The evidence from these few finds is admittedly slim, but continental Germanic analogues help provide a more complete picture (62–63).

27. Anne Van Arsdall defends the *Herbarium*, both in Latin and Old English translations, as an actively consulted text reflecting local practice in her recent translation of the Old English *Herbarium* (*Medieval Herbal Remedies*, pp. 80, 86). Earlier scholars believed that most of the medical texts extant from Anglo-Saxon England were scholarly artifacts even during the time of their production, and that since they were copied from classical

exemplars many times removed from the originals, they reveal little about contemporary Anglo-Saxon practices. The Old English *Herbarium Apuleii*, its companion treatise *Medicina de quadrupedibus*, and the *Peri Didaxaeon* are, demonstrably, translations of continental works. Linda E. Voigts, however, put to rest the older contention that Anglo-Saxon medical books were no more than scribal exercises in "Anglo-Saxon Plant Remedies," pp. 250–68. She argues that the *Leechbook* is "intelligently compiled for practical use" as a reference work (257), that the *Herbarium* deletes nonessential (magical) material in its vernacular translation while preserving details of plant habitat and preservation (266), and that the ingredients from warmer climates previously considered virtually inaccessible to Anglo-Saxon healers may have been more commonly available than once thought (259–66; see also Cameron, *Anglo-Saxon Medicine*, pp. 64, 100–106).

28. Jolly, "Magic," pp. 166–82; and passim in Jolly, *Popular Religion*, regarding the socio-religious context for all the charms; for *Lacnunga* in particular see *Popular Religion*, pp. 138–45.

29. Pollington calls the *Lacnunga Book* "a very humble work of non-specialist 'folk medicine'" (*Leechcraft*, p. 74), which is much less disparaging than the assessment by the manuscript's previous editor (Singer famously called it "a final pathological disintegration of the great system of Greek medical thought" [Grattan and Singer, *Anglo-Saxon Magic*, p. 94]). Jolly argues against such bifurcations of Anglo-Saxon healing and practice into professional versus folkloric (e.g., *Popular Religion*, pp. 101ff.). Contra Grattan and Singer, who believe the work was essentially a scribal exercise, Jolly considers that the *Lacnunga Book* may reflect actual practice specifically because of the unaffected, unselfconscious nature of its selection and presentation (107; and see Cameron, *Anglo-Saxon Medicine*, p. 47; and Pettit, *Anglo-Saxon Remedies*, 1:li–liv). Pettit believes the book may well have been intended for a wealthy tenth- or eleventh-century secular lord, or, "more likely," for his physician (1:liii). For broader discussion of early medieval manuscripts as organic, rather than lifelessly copied, see Riddle, "Theory," pp. 157–84; and Riddle, "Introduction," pp. 185–98.

30. Pettit, *Anglo-Saxon Remedies*, 1:xlvi, lii.

31. Cameron, *Anglo-Saxon Medicine*, p. 42.

32. Cameron provides an overview of which ones may have been known to the Anglo-Saxons in *Anglo-Saxon Medicine*, pp. 65–73.

33. Banham, "Millennium," pp. 234–36.

34. Jolly, *Popular Religion*, p. 172. She argues that liturgy, medicine, and folklore must be understood as an interconnected whole in order to understand the view of illness and healing presupposed in the charm collections: "In many ways in this early medieval period, the gap between liturgical books and medical books was so small that they belong together as a single, larger group of manuals for health and well-being, along with penitentials" (114).

35. Grattan and Singer, *Anglo-Saxon Magic*, p. 17.

36. Cameron, *Anglo-Saxon Medicine*, pp. 19–20; Rubin, "Anglo-Saxon Physician," p. 9.

37. Blair, *Church in Anglo-Saxon Society*, 484.

38. On insanity in the Middle Ages, see Doob, *Nebuchadnezzar's Children*. She points out the continuum in treatments of insanity from Caelius Aurelianus and Celsus through Bartholomeus Anglicus and Gilbertus Anglicus (38), adding that religious remedies such as prayers and exorcisms are also consonant with Greco-Roman practices. For mania, phrenitis, and melancholia, see Stanley Jackson, "Unusual Mental States," pp. 268–82; and for melancholia more specifically, see Stanley Jackson, *Melancholia and Depression*.

39. *Deofolseoc*: Gonser, *Das angelsächsische*, p. 152; translating *vexatus* (Felix, *Vita Guthlaci*

45 [Colgrave, *Felix's Life*, p. 138]). *Feondseocra monna*: Thomas Miller, *Old English Version*, vol. 1, p. 184; translating "obsessis . . . daemones" (Bede, *HE* 3.11, p. 246).

40. Catherine Lambert summarily reviews many of the terms in "Old English Medical Vocabulary," pp. 137–45; Bonser provides further detail in *Medical Background*, pp. 257–58.

41. *Herbarium* 132.4 (de Vriend, *Old English Herbarium*, p. 172).

42. *Herbarium* 96.2 (de Vriend, *Old English Herbarium*, p. 142).

43. Meaney, "Anglo-Saxon View," p. 25.

44. Clarke, *Mental Disorder*, p. 73.

45. Bede, *In Matthaei Evangelium Expositio* 1.4 (PL 92: col. 23C). References such as this to the moon's course may not literally represent a thirty-day cycle synchronized with the moon, but may simply imply a behavioral disorder that recurs periodically (Temkin, *Falling Sickness*, p. 93).

46. Zupitza, *Aelfrics Grammatik*, p. 305; Kindschi, "Latin-Old English Glossaries," p. 193.

47. Pheifer, *Old English Glosses*, p. lxxxix. The Épinal Glossary is Épinal, Bibliothèque municipal, MS 72 (2); Erfurt is Erfurt, Wissenschaftliche Allgemeinbibliothek, Codex Amplonianus f.42.

48. Pheifer, *Old English Glosses*, p. lxxxix.

49. Pheifer, *Old English Glosses*, p. lxii–lxiii, xc–xci.

50. Pheifer, *Old English Glosses*, pp. 21, 31. *Lymphaticus* is alternately glossed as *wæterseoc* in Brussels, Royal Library, MS 1650 (Goossens, *Old English Glosses*, p. 441), and as *gedwolan* in New Haven, Yale University, Beinecke Library MS 401 (Napier, *Old English Glosses*, p. 178; the manuscript is identified in Napier as Phillips [Cheltenham] 8071, but it was subsequently acquired by Yale in 1970).

51. Lindsay, *Corpus Glossary*, p. 92.

52. Leiden, Leiden University, MS Vossianus Lat. 69 (Hessels, *Late Eighth-Century*, pp. 9, 15). Pheifer dates the Leiden Glossary to the ninth century (*Old English Glosses*, p. xxxix).

53. *Lymphaticus* (Stryker, "Latin-Old English Glossary", p. 286), *freneticus* (214), *furias* (209), *inerguminum* (240), *insanum* (255), *frenesis* (21), *lunaticos* (277).

54. Aldhelm, *De virginitate* 50 (Gwara, *Aldhelmi Malmesbiriensis*, 2:671).

55. Source text: Aldhelm, *De virginitate* 52 (Gwara, *Aldhelmi Malmesbiriensis*, 2:697). Anatolia casts out the indwelling entity (*habitatore*) that keeps a consul's son, an energumen, in chains. See also Antwerp, Plantin-Moretus, MS 32 (Kindschi, "Latin-Old English Glossaries", p. 193).

56. The association of elves with the demonic is clear at least as early as the late eighth/early ninth century, when a prayer in the Royal Prayerbook (London, British Library, MS Royal 2 A.XX, fol. 45v)—to be used "ab omnibus insidiis inimici" (against all the tricks of the enemy)—places "elf" and "Satan" in apposition: "adiuro te satanae diabulus aelfae" (I adjure you, devil of Satan, of elf; Kuypers, *Prayer Book*, p. 221). For this passage, see Alaric Hall, *Elves*, pp. 71–72; Jolly, *Popular Religion*, pp. 144–45.

57. *Freneticus* (Oliphant, *Harley Latin-Old English Glossary*, p. 197), *frenesis* (197), *funeste* (203), *furor* (204), *furis* (204), *furia* (204), *furias* (204), *furalia* (204), *furiosus* (204).

58. Oliphant, *Harley Latin-Old English Glossary*, p. 123.

59. Oliphant, *Harley Latin-Old English Glossary*, p. 42.

60. The Roman *comitia* (plural of *comitium*, place of assembly) referred to the day of assembly when magistrates were elected. Since epileptic seizures occurring on this day were considered an ill omen, the assembly would adjourn; so epilepsy came to be called, among other things, *morbus comitialis*.

61. Oliphant, *Harley Latin-Old English Glossary*, p. 85.

62. Alaric Hall, *Elves*, pp. 149–51.

63. See Alaric Hall, *Elves*, p. 149.

64. Napier, *Old English Glosses*, p. 128: "limphaticum: þære gidigan"; cf. Brussels, Royal Library, MS 1650: "limphaticum: gy, uechordem, saul, þæne gidigan" (Goossens, *Old English Glosses*, p. 461).

65. *Middle English Dictionary*.

66. Alaric Hall, *Elves*, p. 149. For *dun-ælfa* and *land-ælfe*, see pp. 81–83; Stuart, "The Anglo-Saxon Elf," p. 317.

67. Peter Clemoes dates this work to around 992–1002 (*Chronology*, p. 34).

68. Healey, "Old English Glossaries."

69. Zupitza, *Aelfrics Grammatik*, p. 305.

70. Ælfric, *Dominica in Sexagesima* (*Catholic Homilies* 2.6; Godden, *Second Series*, p. 56).

71. Zupitza, *Aelfrics Grammatik*, p. 305.

72. Isidore, *Etymologiarum libri XX* 4.6.3 (PL 82: col. 185C).

73. *Ofsettan*: e.g., Ælfric, *Catholic Homilies* 1.4 (Clemoes, *Catholic Homilies*, p. 210); *gedrehtum*: e.g., Ælfric, *Life of Martin* (Skeat, *Lives of Saints*, vol. 2, p. 228).

74. Ælfric, *Passio Simonis et Iude* (*Catholic Homilies* 2.33; Godden, *Second Series*, p. 284); Ælfric, *Assumptio Iohannis Apostoli* (*Catholic Homilies* 1.4; Clemoes, *Catholic Homilies*, p. 210).

75. Brussels MS 1650: Goossens, *Old Engish Glosses*, pp. 341, 457; Bodl. Lib. Digby 146: Napier, *Old English Glosses*, pp. 82, 126; Plantin-Moretus MS 32: Kindschi, "Latin-Old English Glossaries," p. 193.

76. Goossens, *Old English Glosses*, p. 457.

77. Goossens, *Old English Glosses*, p. 457; Logeman, "New Aldhelm Glosses," p. 36 (fol. 71b); Thomas Wright *Anglo-Saxon*, 1:436, and 53. A gloss on Bede's *Vita Cuthberti* in Copenhagen, Det Kongelige Bibliotek Slotsholmen, MS Gl. kgl. samling 2034, explains *laruaribus* simply as *deoflicum gastum* (Meritt, *Old English Glosses*, p. 17).

78. Goossens, *Old English Glosses*, p. 7; following Ker, *Catalogue*, p. 7.

79. Goossens, *Old English Glosses*, p. 51.

80. Goossens, *Old English Glosses*; "freneticus: brægenseoc" (441), "freneticum: brægenseocne" (461).

81. Goossens, *Old English Glosses*, p. 441.

82. *Leechbook* 1.63, 1.66 (Cockayne, *Leechdoms*, vol. 2, pp. 136, 142). See Jolly, *Popular Religion*, pp. 132–68.

83. Jolly, *Popular Religion*, p. 146.

84. Chaps. 40, 41 (pt. 2), 64 (pt. 1), 67 (which may be two different recipes), and 68; Cockayne, *Leechdoms*, vol. 2, pp. 334, 334–336, 352, 354–356, 356.

85. Chap. 41 (pt. 1), 58, 62 (pt. 3), and 64 (pt. 2); Cockayne, *Leechdoms*, vol. 2, pp. 334, 342, 350, 352. See also chap. 1; Cockayne, *Leechdoms*, vol. 2, pp. 304–6. Meaney argues against translating *costunga* as "temptations" in this context: "the remedies suggested under this heading so resemble those for devil-sickness cited above that surely *costunga* must here mean something like 'afflictions, tribulations, torments'" ("Anglo-Saxon View," p. 17). She suggests epilepsy, madness, and Alzheimer's disease as candidates for such tribulations. Yet "temptations" (e.g., internal impulses and desires) may well be considered worthy of medical attention to the religiously minded. Meaney has nuanced her translation of "tribulations" more recently, however: see "The Devil Can Seriously Damage Your Health: Reflections on Anglo-Saxon Demonology" in Raiswell and Dendle, *Devil in Premodern Society*.

86. See Bonser, "Magical Practices"; Bonser, *Medical Background*, pp. 158–67; Clarke, *Mental Disorder*, pp. 47–48, 54; Jolly, *Popular Religion*, pp. 133–38, 144–68, Kieckhefer, *Magic*, pp. 73–74; Meaney, "Anglo-Saxon View," pp. 18–20, 24–25; Stuart, "Anglo-Saxon Elf"; Thun, "Malignant Elves." Meaney suggests cirrhosis of the liver for *ælf-sogoþa* ("Anglo-Saxon View," p. 30). For *ælf-sogoþa*, and for the idea of "elf-shot" in general, see Alaric Hall, "Calling the Shots." Hall argues that the literal conceptualization of elves firing missiles (such as invisible arrows) is perhaps a misunderstanding of terms such as *ofsceotan*, and that such terms probably suggested no more than "internal pains" to the people who used them.

The enigmatic *dweorg* (dwarf) of some medical texts has been interpreted as a reference to fits or seizures, especially those associated with fever: for instance, Peri Didaxeon: "hwile he riþaþ swylce he on dueorge sy" (sometimes he [an asthmatic or one who has trouble breathing] writhes as though he were "in," "on," or "at" a dwarf; Cockayne, *Leechdoms*, vol. 3, p. 118). It is hard to know what to make of the "dwarf" in such contexts. There may be some conceptual overlap between dwarves and possession, if dwarves were conceived as "riding" the victim (Stuart, "Anglo-Saxon Elf," p. 315), because demons are sometimes presented as riding an energumen. A demon sits on Avitianus's back in Sulpicius Serverus's *Dialogi* 3.8, depicted in the Hereford Troper (London, British Library, MS Cotton Caligula A.XIV, fol. 29r—see figure 1 in Dendle, *Satan Unbound*, also reproduced on the cover of that work). The *Middle English Dictionary* translates the phrase *on dweorge* as "possessed by a dwarf" (headword *dwergh*). For dwarves, see Grendon, "Anglo-Saxon Charms," p. 137; Motz, "Of Elves and Dwarfs," pp. 102–6; and Pettit, *Anglo-Saxon Remedies*, 1:xxxiii. The word may be etymologically related to Old Indian *drva-* (weakness, sickness), *dhvaras* (a demonic being), or Avestan *drva* (physical defect) (Pettit, *Anglo-Saxon Remedies*, 2:183). The Old English *Herbarium* translates the Latin *pollegion* (pennyroyal, *Mentha pulegium*) as *dweorge-dweosle*, and prescribes it against internal pains, nausea, and tertian fever (*Herbarium* 94; de Vriend, *Old English Herbarium*, p. 136). Pettit translates *dweorg* simply as "fever" in his edition of the *Lacnunga Book*, arguing that "it cannot be demonstrated that, for the Anglo-Saxons who composed, compiled and used these texts, the name of the putative dwarfish disease-demon had not come to denote the affliction itself" (*Anglo-Saxon Remedies*, 2:183). Pettit notes that, nonetheless, it still may be visualized as an independent "disease-demon." Cameron also tacitly accepts *dweorg* as "fever" (*Anglo-Saxon Medicine*, p. 10).

87. *Leechbook* 3.62 (Cockayne, *Leechdoms*, vol. 2, p. 350).

88. Bonser, "Magical Practices," p. 359; Thun, "Malignant Elves," p. 381. Stuart follows Cockayne in conceptualizing elves as physically possessing the body ("Anglo-Saxon Elf," pp. 314–16). She notes, "The ability to enter into a man and assume control of his mind and body can be viewed as an addition to the original elvish properties derived from the NT concept of penetrating demons" (314).

89. North, *Heathen Gods*, p. 52. He notes that *siden* in *ælf-siden* is cognate with *seiðr* (55), a claim supported by scholarly consensus (see Alaric Hall, *Elves*, p. 119). Whatever *siden* meant by the time of *Lacnunga*, however, analogues from Old Icelandic *seiðr* (North, *Heathen Gods*, pp. 55–56) are culturally remote from Anglo-Saxon England and do not themselves presuppose a strong Germanic tradition of recognizable demon possession (the unwilling usurpation of the will and personality by an alien being). *Seiðr* can imply a broad range of magical practices, and Hall translates *ælf-siden* rather as "the magic of *ælfe*" (Alaric Hall, *Elves*, p. 119).

90. Storms, *Anglo-Saxon Magic*, p. 249; see Alaric Hall, "Calling the Shots," p. 199.

91. Alaric Hall, "Calling the Shots," p. 205; see also n. 13 (pp. 205–6).

92. Grattan and Singer, *Anglo-Saxon Magic*, p. 56.

93. Aldred of Chester-le-Street's glosses to the Durham Collectar provide an instructive contrast; for instance: he glosses *spiritus inmundus* as *gast unclæne* (Lindelöf, *Rituale*, p. 120), *spiritalis nequitiae* as *gastlices woghful* (121), *demones* as *diovles* (121), and *creatura* (as in exorcisms of salt or water, e.g., *creatura salis*) as *giscæft* (120). In his glosses on the Lindisfarne Gospels, Aldred relies heavily on *diowl* and *diwles* when translating *daemonium* and *daemonia* (Boyd, *Aldred's Marginalia*, p. 18), and regularly glosses *creatura* as *gescæft* (Jolly, "Prayers," p. 106). Demons in the *Lorica of Gildas*: *tetri demones*, glossed there as *sweartan deoblu* (*Lacnunga* 65; Pettit, *Anglo-Saxon Remedies*, 1:355).

94. Thus Alaric Hall, "Elf and Elves," pp. 155–56, 174. Also, in "Calling the Shots" Hall ponders the fact that the *Leechbook* book 3 composer went to some lengths to preserve *ælfe*, as opposed to using *diaboli* or *demones* (205).

95. Liuzza, *Old Engish Version*, pp. 76–77. See also Luke 4:33 (Liuzza, *Old English Version*, p. 107), John 7:20 (172).

96. Liuzza, *Old English Version*, pp. 115, 97.

97. Liuzza, *Old English Version*, p. 96 (for Vulgate "eiecerat septem daemonia"). The demons are preserved, however, in the other account of Mary Magdalene's demons in Luke 8:2 ("awyrgdum gastum"; Liuzza, *Old English Version*, p. 116). Gospel glosses do not uniformly conform to the same pattern as the full Gospel translations: thus, while the Rushworth Gospels gloss *demonia* with an added *–seoc* suffix most of the time (e.g., *deofulseocne hæbbende* for *demonium habentem*), they also gloss without the suffix (*dioful hæfdun* for *demonia habebant*) (Skeat, *Holy Gospels*, pp. 81, 43). In the Lindisfarne Gospels Aldred never adds the *–seoc* element to gloss *demonia*.

98. It occurs in Matthew 4:24, 8:16, 8:28, 8:33 (Liuzza, *Old English Version*, pp. 8, 16, 17, 17); Mark 1:34, 1:39, 3:15, 3:22, 9:37 (pp. 64, 65, 67, 68, 81); Luke 8:27, 9:1, 9:49, 10:17, 11:14, 13:32 (pp. 117, 119, 122, 123, 125, 132).

99. Murdoch, "*Peri Hieres Nousou*," p. 149.

100. *Herbarium*, chaps. 10, 66 (de Vriend, *Old English Herbarium*, pp. 54, 108). *Monaþseoce* here translates the Latin *lunaticos*. Peony was for many centuries among the principal drugs for epilepsy (Temkin, *Falling Sickness*, p. 25).

101. *Medicina de quadrupedibus*, chap. 10 (de Vriend, *Old English Herbarium*, p. 263).

102. Clarke, *Mental Disorder*, p. 47.

103. *Herbarium* chaps. 11, 20, 132, and 179. In chap. 132, for example, mandrake is said to be good "wiþ gewitleaste, þæt is wiþ deofulseocnysse" (against witlessness, that is to say against devil-sickness; de Vriend, *Old English Herbarium*, p. 172).

104. *Elehtre* (x 6), *bisceopwyrt* (x 4), *beolone*, *cropleac* (x 2), *lybcorn*, *gyþrife* (x 4), *glæs*, *betonica* (x 3), *attorlaþe* (x 2), *cassuc*, *fane*, *finul* (x 2), *ciric-ragu*, *cristes mæles ragu*, *lufestice*, *cost*, *gotwoþe*, *hole-cerse*, *hofe*, *banwyrt*, *eofor-fearn*, *heahheoloþe*, *suþern finul*, *nefte*, *hindheoloþe*, *merce*, *cassia*, *alexandria*, *feldmore*.

105. *Leechbook* 1.63 (Cockayne, *Leechdoms*, vol. 2, p. 138).

106. In addition to the obvious magical associations of calling for lichen from a cross, Cameron explains that the identification of lichen is often facilitated by reference to its common substrates, as a sort of shorthand (*Anglo-Saxon Medicine*, p. 125).

107. Psalms 118, 67, and 68 (Vulgate).

108. Comprehensive sources include the "Anglo-Saxon Plant Name Survey," Institute for the Historical Study of Language (http://www.arts.gla.ac.uk/STELLA/ihsl/projects/plants.htm); Bierbaumer, *Der botanische Wortschatz*; and the ongoing *Dictionary of Old English*. See also D'Aronco, "Botanical Lexicon," pp. 15–33.

109. The recent tendency to valorize early medieval medicine as pharmacologically

efficacious should not be taken too far; see, for instance, Brennessel, Drout, and Gravel, "Reassessment," pp. 183–95.

110. *Herbarium* 132 (de Vriend, *Old English Herbarium*, p. 172).

111. *Lacnunga* 62 is a *slæpdrænc* recipe (a "sleeping drink"), which calls for radish, hemlock, wormwood, and henbane (Pettit, *Anglo-Saxon Remedies*, 1:30). On the alkaloids in henbane and other medieval psychotropic herbs, especially as surgical anesthetics, see Voigts and Hudson, "*A drynke*," esp. pp. 37–40.

112. Thun, "Malignant Elves," pp. 390–92. Cameron further discusses, and seems to support, Thun's identification in *Anglo-Saxon Medicine*, pp. 110–11. Aldhelm wrote a riddle articulating both respect and fear for the properties of woody nightshade (Enigma 98; Pitman, *Riddles*, p. 60; see also Cameron, *Anglo-Saxon Medicine*, pp. 111–12; von Erhardt-Siebold, "Hellebore," pp. 161–70).

113. *Leechbook* 3.61 (Cockayne, *Leechdoms*, vol. 2, p. 344).

114. There seems to be little basis for Bonser's claim that "[h]erbs, if used [against mental illness], are therefore of the unusual kind" (*Medical Background*, p. 261). The claim that hellebore "was largely used in cases of madness" is without support (262). Known as *tunsingwyrt*, white hellebore is prescribed for diarrhea in the *Herbarium* (140) and for internal worms of all sorts in the *Leechbook* 1.48. Though he cites the *Herbarium* entry for white hellebore, Bonser probably had in mind black hellebore or Christmas rose (*hamerwyrt*)—no doubt closer to what was meant by *wedeberge* ("madness-berries"). Black hellebore appears in the *Lacnunga* to combat headache, eye pain, and "flying venom and sudden eruption" (fleogendum attre ⁊ færspryngum; *Lacnunga* 18; Pettit, *Anglo-Saxon Remedies*, 1:10).

115. E.g., *Leechbook* 1.63 (for *feondseocum men* and *bræcseocum*); 1.66 (*ungemynde*); 3.61 (*ælfcynne*); and 3.64 (*ungemynde*). See Forster, Niklas, and Lutz, "Antispasmodic Effects," pp. 311–19.

116. *Leechbook* 3.41 (Cockayne, *Leechdoms*, vol. 2, p. 336). Jagiello-Wojtowicz, Jusiak, Szponar, and Kleinrok found sedative action and depressed motor activities in mice given chelidonine administration ("Preliminary Pharmacological Evaluation," pp. 125–31).

117. Akanmu, Honda, and Inoue, "Hypnotic Effects," pp. 309–10.

118. *Nefte*: *Leechbook* 3.64. Andreatini, Sartori, Seabra, and Leite find that valepotriates may reduce anxiety ("Effect of Valepotriates"), and the evidence for their sedative effects is reviewed in Houghton, "Scientific Basis"). Essential oils of *Nepeta caesarea* have been shown to have analgesic and sedative effects in mice (Aydin, Beis, Öztürk, Hüsnü, and Baser, "Nepetalactone").

119. Nucifora and Malone found a general depression of the central nervous system in rats after exposure to these alkaloids ("Comparative Psychopharmacologic Investigation"). More recently, a team of researchers found that lupinine, sparteine, and lupine seed extract had a sedative action on the central nervous system and delayed the onset of experimentally induced seizures in mice (Pothier et al., "Comparative Study").

120. See Dendle, "Lupines," pp. 96–97.

121. For a discussion of these conflicting interests in Merovingian Gaul, see Kitchen, "Saints," pp. 15–32.

122. Item 77 in Birch, *Cartularium Saxonicum*, vol. 1, p. 113. There is no consensus on the authenticity of the charter. Earlier commentators (e.g., Plummer, *Venerabilis Baedae*, 2:157) considered the charter spurious; Anton Scharer has recently reaffirmed that view, arguing that the charter bears all the hallmarks of a late eighth-century document (*Die angelsächsische*, pp. 150–51). B. Herbert Finberg notes that it is "thought to embody the substance of the original, but having some material, probably spurious, substituted or interpolated"

(*Early Charters*, p. 87 [item 199]). Eric John, however, defends the charter as essentially genuine: "There is nothing against a seventh century date for CS 77, and everything against supposing that it could be a late fabrication" (*Land Tenure*, p. 76).

123. By way of contrast, in an earlier period consider the seven exorcists who signed as witnesses to the Council of Arles in 314 (Gaudemet, *Conciles Gaulois*, pp. 58–62).

124. The early medieval *Epistula ad Leudefredum*, sometimes attributed to Isidore, reads, "It is for the exorcist to have exorcisms memorized, and to lay hands on those energumens and catechumens to be exorcized" (Ad exorcistam pertinet exorcismos memoriter retinere, manus super energumenos et catechumenos exorcizandos imponere; Ford, *Letters*, p. 10). Elsewhere (*De officiis* 2.13; PL 83: col. 792) Isidore implies that only exorcists can perform the exorcisms, citing 1 Corinthians 12:30 ("Do all possess gifts of healing?"). This section on the duties of exorcists is repeated by Hrabanus Maurus (*De institutione clericorum* 10; PL 107: cols. 304–5). On the authenticity of Isidorean and Pseudo-Isidorean tracts on the ecclesiastical ranks, see Roger Reynolds, *Ordinals*, pp. 118–21.

125. Article 62 (Munier, *Les Statuta*, p. 90). The *Excerptiones Ecgberti*, a collection of earlier canon law possibly by Ecgbert of York (eighth century), repeats the sentence verbatim (*Sancti Ecgberti Eboracensis Archiepiscopi excerptiones* 82 [PL 89: col. 389]). The *Excerptiones* does not, however, preserve the two following canons of the *Statuta*: (63) "Pavimenta domorum dei energumeni everrant" (energumens sweep the pavement of the houses of God); and (64) "Energumenis in domo dei assidentibus victus quotidianus per exorcistas opportuno tempore ministretur" (every day at the suitable time, exorcists give food to the energumens encamped in the house of God).

126. Canon 142 (Munier, *Concilia Africae*, p. 299), adapted from the *Concilio Laodicensi.*

127. Doble, *Pontificale Lanaletense*, p. 111; Vogel and Elze, *Le Pontifical*, vol. 2, p. 193. The lowest order I have found in early medieval sources performing solemn exorcism is the deacon, mentioned in an eleventh-century Spanish manuscript of a *Liber Ordinum* (Férotin, *Liber Ordinum*, pp. 74–80). Even so, this deacon—the lowest rank of the major orders—only performs the first half of the ceremony, while a priest recites the closing prayer (pp. 78–80). David Johnson detects the increased efficacy in using the sign of the cross to ward off the devil when employed by a bishop, as portrayed in Old English sources ("*Crux Usualis*," p. 92).

128. Bede, *HE* 3.11, p. 248; OE translation: Thomas Miller, *Old English Version*, vol. 1, p. 184.

129. The passage on the seven ecclesiastical ranks is referred to as D07G by Roger Reynolds in *Ordinals*, which provides an overview of its adaptive history, use, and contexts. Reynolds argues that, given its mixed Celtic and Gallican influences, the D07G may have originated in the British Isles (128). The formulation often found in Pontificals, in which Christ himself is seen as having exemplified the ranks, may also be a further Anglo-Saxon innovation (141). However, Anglo-Saxon Pontificals do not follow the traditional wording of D07G for the lower orders, substituting instead fragments from Isidore or from the *Liber de divinis officiis* (141, 149). Reynolds revisited and expanded his original study in "Christ as Cleric," pp. 1–50 (note that pagination of individual chapters [article reprints] are not continuous in this volume).

130. The explanation of *exorcista* as *adjurante* draws attention to the original sense of *exorcizo*, which is "to adjure" rather than "to cast out" or "expel" (thus, in its technical sense, *exorcizo* requires an object complement in the form of a verbal phrase: a priest cannot "exorcize a demon" but he can "exorcize a demon to leave"). The sense "to adjure" is preserved through most exorcisms of the Gelasian-Gregorian tradition: "Exorcizo te, inmunde spiritus

. . . ut exeas et recedas ab his famulis Dei" (I exorcize you, unclean spirit . . . to depart and withdraw from these servants of God; H. A. Wilson, *Gelasian*, p. 49).

131. London, British Library, MS Additional 57337, fol. 36v.

132. The passage, usually attributed to Isidore in most manuscripts of the tenth-century Romano-German Pontifical, also appears in Hrabanus Maurus (*De rerum naturis* 4.5) and others. In those places, and in a parallel section of the Corpus Canterbury Pontifical (CCCC 44, p. 201), the Latin equivalent is "adiurantes sive increpantes" (adjurers or accusers). See Fehr, *Die Hirtenbriefe*, pp. 256–58. There is further commentary on the "Ordinals of Christ" in Wulfstan's *Institutes of Polity*, chap. 24: "Exorciste beoð on getacnunge Cristes gespelian, syþðan hi, þone had underfoð, and þæt getacnað seo halsungboc, þe biscop heom on hand sylð, þonne he hi hadað. Þæt ealswa Crist wæs halsere, þa ðe he gehalsode, þæt ða deofla ut gewiten of ðam magdaleniscan wife, swa agen þa, þe ðone had underfoð, leafe ðurh Godes gyfe, þæt hi þurh gastlice hæse and halsunge magan and motan deofles costnunga oferswiðan and hine fram þam afyrsian, þe he to swiðlice dereð" ("Exorcists" stand as a symbol of Christ's utterances, when they accept the office, which is symbolized by the book of exorcisms that the bishop places into their hand when he ordains them. Christ was likewise an "adjurer," in that he adjured the devils to depart from the Magdalene woman; even so are "exorcists," when they accept the office, by permission and through the grace of God, that they through spiritual command and adjuration can and must conquer the devil's temptation [or affliction] and expel him from the people he hurts too severely; Jost, "*Institutes*," p. 231, and see Roger Reynolds, *Ordinals*, p. 87).

133. Pastoral Letter 2.103 (Fehr, *Die Hirtenbriefe*, p. 108). In the glosses *halsige* appears for *obsecro*, *adjuro*, *supplico*, *quaeso*, and *depreco*, as well as for *exorcizo*. *Halsigo* and *gihalsio* appear regularly for *exorcizo* in the Durham Ritual.

134. Pastoral Letter 1.32 (Fehr, *Die Hirtenbriefe*, p. 9). The reading cited here is from CCCC 190. A variant from Oxford, Bodleian Library, MS Junius 121 reads instead, following "wyllað menn dreccan," as follows: "him be-beodeð þurh þæs ælmihtigan naman" (commands them through the name of the Almighty; Fehr, *Die Hirtenbriefe*, p. 9). For Ælfric's pastoral letters, see Joyce Hill, "Monastic Reform," pp. 103–17.

135. This is the case, for instance, in Leiden, Rijksuniversiteit, MS Voss. Lat. Q 119, fol. 131r–v ("Exorcista oportet abicere demones et dicere populo qui non communicat de locum et aquam ministerii effudere"); Verona, Biblioteca capitolare, MS Lat XXXVII (35), fol. 59v; and Munich, Bayerische Staatsbibliothek, MS Clm. 19414, fol. 85v. Roger Reynolds discusses this text (*Ordinals*, pp. 135–37), and gives references to earlier medieval writers including Gregory the Great and Isidore who attribute this duty to the deacon (135–37).

136. The Sacramentary of Hildoard (Cambrai, Bibliothèque municipale, MS 164, fols. 35v–203r) is a first-generation copy of the Hadrianum.

137. Oxford, Bodleian Library, MS 579 (edited by Nicholas Orchard, *Leofric Missal*). The core text, called Leofric A, was probably written in the ninth or early tenth century.

138. Corrêa, *Durham Collectar*, p. 215.

139. These are sometimes called small exorcisms, as opposed to great exorcisms (another term for solemn exorcism; see Rodewyk, *Possessed*, pp. 58–59).

140. On judicial ordeal, see Bartlett, *Trial*; Hyams, "Trial," pp. 90–126; Keefer, "*Corsnæd* Ordeal"; Keefer, "Manuals," pp. 108–9; and Colin Morris, "*Judicium Dei*," pp. 95–111. The texts are collected in Liebermann, *Die Gesetze*, vol. 1, pp. 401–29. For the exorcists' role in ordeals, see Keefer, "*Corsnæd* Ordeal," pp. 240–41, 247.

141. H. A. Wilson, *Gelasian*, p. 115.

142. Jolly, "Prayers," p. 105.

143. Pettit, *Anglo-Saxon Remedies*, 1:108.

144. Bedingfield, *Dramatic Liturgy*, pp. 171ff.

145. The rites for infants and adults are somewhat blended in the lengthy series of prayers; sometimes the directions state that the subject is an infant ("super caput infantis," H. A. Wilson, *Jumièges*, p. 96), while elsewhere the catechumen is directed to speak. By Anglo-Saxon times infant baptism had long become the norm, and Wulfstan indicates that it is a sponsor who recites the appropriate phrases on behalf of the infant: "And ðeah þæt cild to ðam geong sy þæt hit specan ne mæge, þonne hit man fullað, his freonda forspæc forstent him eal þæt sylfe swylce hit sylf spæce" (and if the child is too young to speak when baptized, the sponsorship of his friends will stand for him as though he were speaking himself; *Sermo de baptismate* 3.c, Bethurum, *Homilies*, pp. 181–82). See also Ælfric, *In Aepiphania Domini* (*Catholic Homilies* 2.3; Godden, *Second Series*, p. 27). In modern Church parlance the term *infans* in its baptismal context has been reinterpreted to mean "initiate," without reference to the age of the individual.

146. The manuscript (Rouen, Bibliothèque Municipale, MS 274, Y.6) is from the late tenth or early eleventh century.

147. Bedingfield, *Dramatic Liturgy*, p. 175. He continues, "the series of passages from the Making of the Catechumen to the vesting has the feel of a single ceremony, closer to the quick ceremonies for the infirm that follow in each manuscript than to the structured, month-long process presented so carefully in the Gelasian" (176).

148. Bedingfield, *Dramatic Liturgy*, p. 184. Willis observes that as early as 787, the Council of Clovesho directs that baptism be ministered only at Easter and Pentecost, "which tends to show that even this was being neglected" (*Further Essays*, p. 234).

149. Cramer, *Baptism*, p. 139; J. D. C. Fisher, *Christian Initiation*, pp. 79, 82, 86–87.

150. Ine 2: "Cild binnan ðritegum nihta sie gefulwad; gif hit swa ne sie, XXX scill[inga] gebete" (A child should be baptized within thirty days; if it is not so, there is a fine of thirty shillings; Liebermann, *Die Gesetze*, vol. 1, p. 90). For further references in the *Canons of Edgar* and other places, see J. D. C. Fisher, *Christian Initiation*, pp. 82–86. The Council of Chelsea (787) tried to limit such irregular practices (p. 82).

151. *Norðhymbra preosta lagu* 10: "Æghwilc cild sy, we læreð, gefullod binnon nigon nihton, be wite VI or" (We instruct that each child must be baptized in nine days, on fine of six øre; Liebermann, *Die Gesetze*, vol. 1, p. 380).

152. H. A. Wilson, *Jumièges*, p. 93. The Leofric Missal, at the outset, alternately implores God to remove the demonic presence: "disrumpe omnes laqueos satane quibus fuerat conligatus" (break all the snares of Satan with which he had been bound; item 2480, Nicholas Orchard, *Leofric Missal*, 2:438).

153. H. A. Wilson, *Jumièges*, p. 95.

154. H. A. Wilson, *Jumièges*, p. 97.

155. H. A. Wilson, *Jumièges*, p. 97.

156. On the gradual separation of the rites of baptism and confirmation in the Middle Ages, see J. D. C. Fisher, *Christian Initiation*, chapter 6. Fisher believes that a driving consideration behind this trend was the propensity of infants and sick people to vomit back up the Eucharist, an unacceptable spectacle (pp. 102–3).

157. H. A. Wilson, *Jumièges*, pp. 100 and 101.

158. H. A. Wilson, *Jumièges*, p. 96; Leofric item 2497 (Nicholas Orchard, *Leofric Missal*, 2:443).

159. Ælfric, *Dominica iii in Quadragesima* (Pope, *Homilies*, vol. 1, p. 277). See also Lukken, *Original Sin*, esp. pp. 226–65.

160. Thus Kelly, "Struggle," pp. 9–10; Sorensen, *Possession*, p. 13.

161. H. A. Wilson, *Gelasian*, p. 111; H. A. Wilson, *Gregorian*, p. 229. This appears, for instance, in the Leofric Missal (item 2474; Nicholas Orchard, *Leofric Missal*, 2:434–45). Alternately, this could refer to someone subject to intermittent attacks (cf. Rodewyk, speaking of the need for demoniacs to confess as stipulated in the Roman Ritual: "it is obviously assumed, without particular emphasis, that the possessed has periods of being fully in command of himself"; *Possessed*, p. 46).

162. Kelly, *Devil at Baptism*, pp. 273–74; see also pp. 112–14.

163. Cramer, *Baptism*, pp. 14–15, 145–51.

164. For background tradition, see Barrett-Lennard, *Christian Healing*, pp. 262–64, 268, 270.

165. Augustine, *De beata vita* 18 (PL 32: col. 968C–D).

166. Cramer, *Baptism*, pp. 154–55; but see also Little, *Benedictine Maledictions*, pp. 82–83.

167. Cramer, *Baptism*, pp. 206–11; see also Plummer, *Venerabilis Baedae*, 1:lvi–lxii. See, more generally, Foot, "By Water," pp. 171–92.

168. Wulfstan, Homily 8a (Bethurum, *Homilies*, p. 169).

169. Wulfstan, Homily 8a (Bethurum, *Homilies*, p. 170). For possible influences of this liturgical action on Old English literature, see Thomas Hill, "When God," pp. 132–41. Daniel G. Van Slyke shows that there was inherently a difference between *insufflatio* and *exsufflatio* for Augustine and other patristic authors, though by the Middle Ages this distinction seems to have been lost and the two were used interchangeably in baptismal liturgies ("Emergence"; and "Augustine").

170. Wulfstan, Homily 8a (Bethurum, *Homilies*, p. 169).

171. Wulfstan, Homily 8b (Bethurum, *Homilies*, p. 172). The application of oil to the chest and shoulders protects the candidate from the devil's attacks: "se deofol ne mæg ænig his ættrenra wæpna on him afæstnian, naðer ne wiðforan ne wiðæftan, gif he þanonforð þurhwunað on rihtum geleafan" (the devil cannot then fasten any of his poisonous weapons in him, either from the front or from behind, if he thenceforth perseveres in the true faith; Homily 8b, Bethurum, *Homilies*, p. 173).

172. Wulfstan, Homily 8c (Bethurum, *Homilies*, p. 175; and see p. 181 for further development).

173. Ælfric, *Catholic Homilies* 1.21 (Godden, *Second Series*, p. 351).

174. There are references to "booklets in which exorcisms are written" (libellum in quo conscripti sunt exorcismi) as part of the ordination of exorcists as far back as the *Statuta ecclesiae antiqua*—books ceremonially handed to the exorcist during ordination, and apparently loaned to him since they come with the instruction that he should commit all the exorcisms to memory. It is not known, however, what these books were (Kelly, *Devil, Demonology, and Witchcraft*, p. 82; and see above, chapter 1). Probably they were earlier forms of the benedictionals and manuals that proliferated after the Carolingian reforms, in which the exorcisms only constituted but a small segment (contra the private communication by Professor Roger Reynolds cited in Gneuss, "Liturgical Books," p. 135). Thus the Samson Pontifical reads in the *Ordo* for exorcists that the candidate is given a *missalem* instead of the more usual phrase "libellum in quo conscripti sunt exorcismi" (CCCC 146, p. 111). London, British Library, MS Additional 28188 (an eleventh-century pontifical) and the Ramsey Pontifical both read "libellum, id est officialem, in quo scripti sunt exorcismi" (BL Add. 28188, fol. 65r; London, British Library, MS Cotton Vitellius A.VII, fol. 103v). It is unlikely the *libelli* that were the precursors of Sacramentaries were still in circulation; no such books for exorcisms are extant anyway (with the sole exception, possibly, of the Paris Supplement

to the Vatican Sacramentary, now bound with Paris, Bibliothèque nationale de France, MS lat. 7193). In referring to the ordination ceremony, Wulfstan's *Institutes of Polity* note that the bishop places a *halsungboc* into the exorcist's hand (chap. 24, *De ecclesiasticis gradibus*; Jost, "*Institutes*," p. 231); this word translates literally as "book of exorcisms" or "book of adjurations," but is otherwise unattested. The more general service books in which exorcisms are found may be what is meant by "libellum in quo conscripti sunt exorcismi." Exorcisms do not run more than a dozen pages or two, even in their most comprehensive clusters.

A marginal note in the tenth- to eleventh-century Sidney Sussex Pontifical (Cambridge, Sidney Sussex College, MS 100) glosses the phrase "libellum in quo conscripti sunt exorcismi" into Old English as "her þa onsong boc" (Banting, *Two Anglo-Saxon Pontificals*, p. 158; and see Gneuss, "Liturgical Books," p. 135). The meaning of *onsong* is unclear, but an eleventh-century reviser of Werferth's translation of Gregory's *Dialogues* (Oxford, Bodleian Library, MS Hatton 76) replaced *onsangum* with *galdrum* ("spells" or "incantations"; Banting, *Two Anglo-Saxon Pontificals*, p. xlii). The context in Werferth's text is the (ultimately unsuccessful) exorcism of a possessed woman by local sorcerers (*Dialogi* 1.10; Hecht, *Dialoge*, p. 73). This instance from Werferth's text is the only instance of *onsang* in the Old English corpus apart from the Sidney Sussex marginal note. It is possible that the later glossator felt that *onsong* was a proper and holy word—not one to be used in describing the ineffectual spells (*galdrum*) of these enchanters.

175. These are items 2471–73 and 2476–79 in Nicholas Orchard, *Leofric Missal*, 2:434–38.

176. Lanalet Pontifical: fols. 162r–167r; Anderson Ponifical: fols. 83v–86v. See also the Samson Pontifical, pp. 312–19.

177. Doble, *Pontificale Lanaletense*, p. 111. The Lanalet Pontifical (Rouen, Bibliothèque municipale, MS A.27, cat. 368) is a tenth-century book, with connections to Winchester, most likely from the monastery-bishopric of St. Germans in Cornwall (e.g., Winchester saints are included in the litany). See Doble, pp. xii–xiii.

178. Doble, *Pontificale Lanaletense*, p. 113.

179. Doble, *Pontificale Lanaletense*, p. 113.

180. Doble, *Pontificale Lanaletense*, p. 116.

181. Felix, *Vita Guthlaci* 41 (Colgrave, *Felix's Life*, p. 130).

182. This series of exorcisms from the Lanalet Pontifical also appears in the Anderson Pontifical and the Samson Pontifical, although unclear rubrics in those manuscripts make it less certain that the prayers are actually *contra demonum* (against demons), the way that they obviously are in Lanalet. In the Anderson Pontifical they still fall under the rubric "Oratio contra fulgora" (Prayer against lightning), and in the Samson Pontifical the last rubric prior to these rites refers to use in ordeals. The same series of exorcisms is also written in the Corpus Canterbury Pontifical (CCCC 44, pp. 389ff.), although there it is not a genuine medieval witness—this hand is a sixteenth-century imitation.

183. Leofric items 2471–73 (Nicholas Orchard, *Leofric Missal*, 2:434).

184. Leofric items 2474–76 (Nicholas Orchard, *Leofric Missal*, 2:434–35).

185. Leofric items 2480ff. (Nicholas Orchard, *Leofric Missal*, 2:438ff.).

186. H. A. Wilson, *Gregorian*, p. 136; H. A. Wilson, *Jumièges*, p. 100; CCCC 422, p. 392; Leofric item 2472 (Nicholas Orchard, *Leofric Missal*, 2:434).

187. H. A. Wilson, *Jumièges*, p. 100; Leofric item 2472 (Nicholas Orchard, *Leofric Missal*, 2:434). The Missal of Robert of Jumièges reading agrees with the Gregorian tradition (H. A. Wilson, *Gregorian*, p. 136).

188. "In cuius uirtute precipio tibi quicumque es, inmunde spiritus, ut exeas et recedas ab hoc famulo dei" (Leofric items 2497, 2472; Nicholas Orchard, *Leofric Missal*, 2:443, 434).

189. Nancy Caciola draws attention to exorcisms reshuffled for different uses, specifically in the tenth-century Vatican, Biblioteca Vaticana, MS Vat. Lat. 7701 and its (possibly) eleventh–century additions (*Discerning Spirits*, pp. 230–31).

190. Leofric items 2474 and 2478 (Nicholas Orchard, *Leofric Missal*, 2:434–45, 436–37), appearing in Lanalet Pontifical under the rubric "Exorcismus contra demonum" (Doble, *Pontificale Lanaletense*, pp. 115–16, 113–14). F. E. Warren similarly points out duplications, variations, and analogues to the exorcisms of the Stowe Missal in *The Liturgy*, pp. 207–15.

191. Anderson Pontifical, fols. 83v–86v.

192. Karen Jolly has shown similar adaptability in the prayer components for field blessings, demonstrating a "common strategy of modifying benedictional language and merging different sources to create a blessing specific to another context . . . such benedictions were regularly adapted to meet particular needs in the community, especially pragmatic ones involving sustenance" ("Prayers," pp. 115–16).

193. Missal of Robert of Jumièges, fols. 207r–11r (H. A. Wilson, *Jumièges*, pp. 286–94).

194. Item 634 in the Durham Collectar is in Old English (Corrêa, *Durham Collectar*, pp. 226–27), and rubrics are in the vernacular throughout this section (pp. 227–231). Old English judicial exorcisms also appear in BL Vitellius A.VII, the Samson Pontifical, and the Red Book of Darley (Keefer "Manuals," p. 108). These manuscripts have not been edited, but the texts of the Old English exorcisms are printed in Liebermann, *Die Gesetze*, vol. 1, pp. 409–15. See also Keefer "*Corsnæd* Ordeal," pp. 247–48 (n. 49).

195. Keefer touches briefly on a similar set of singular to plural form changes in certain ordeal texts ("*Corsnæd* Ordeal," p. 247), and the *ordines* for consecrations of the divine offices are changed from singular to plural in the Corpus Canterbury Pontifical (CCCC 44, pp. 210–11). The addition of plural grammatical endings above the singular ones are meant to provide two options, so that the ministrant can read one or the other as necessary (the same also frequently occurs for masculine and feminine forms). For this practice in the Sidney Sussex Pontifical, see Nelson and Pfaff, "Pontificals," p. 95.

196. Richard Kieckhefer posits a distinction between the formal exorcisms of the higher orders and the more popular exorcisms of the lower clergy (*Magic*, pp. 73–74).

197. The *Vita Romani,* chap. 15, states that Romanus and Lupicinus drive out the devil (along with "his minions and ministers" [satellitibus ac ministris suis]) so quickly that it is "sooner done than said" (dicto citius; Martine, *Vie*, p. 256). Of the possession cases from Anglo-Saxon England documented with any specifics, only two resemble the ritual exorcism implied by liturgical sources: Bede, *In Lucae evangelium expositio* 8.30 (PL 92: col. 438A); Felix, *Vita Guthlaci* 41 (Colgrave, *Felix's Life*, pp. 126–30). The rest are not technically exorcisms but distance or posthumous healings (Anon., *Vita Cuthberti* 2.8, 4.15; Bede, *HE* 3.11; Stephen of Ripon, *Vita Wilfridi* 39; Felix, *Vita Guthlaci* 42). See below, chapter 3.

198. Aldhelm, *De virginitate* 52 (Gwara, *Aldhelmi Malmesbiriensis*, 2:697).

199. Anon., *De SS. Anatholia*, p. 679.

200. Ælfric, *Natale Sancte Agnetis* (Skeat, *Lives of Saints*, vol. 1, p. 192); anon., *Vita Cuthberti* 4.18 (Colgrave, *Two Lives*, p. 138).

201. Logan, "Excommunication," p. 537.

202. See Little, *Benedictine Maledictions*, p. 117.

203. Treharne, "Unique Old English Formula," p. 189.

204. Treharne, "Unique Old English Formula," pp. 191, 202–203.

205. Treharne, "Unique Old English Formula," p. 209. Liebermann purports to present a number of Anglo-Saxon excommunication formulas (*Die Gesetze*, vol. 1, pp. 432–441), but Sarah Hamilton shows that Liebermann's collection relies on imprecise dating and

casts too wide a net ("Remedies," p. 95). She states: "it is perhaps surprising to realize that there is very little secure evidence for any Anglo-Saxon excommunication *formulae*" (94). Some localized exceptions include eleventh-century Worcester manuscripts and a charter anathema ("sit ipse alienus . . ."; pp. 99–101).

206. See Bartlett, *Trial*, pp. 63–64. In fact, one of the primary functions of the gruesome and somewhat arbitrary ordeals appears to have been the encouragement of private settlements among the disputants. Ordeals have numerous delays and "ways out" built into them. Stephen White argues that in eleventh-century France the very point of proposing an ordeal (or combat) was to initiate a different stage of conflict management, and thus redefine the stakes for all participants such that alternate means of resolution would be more aggressively pursued ("Proposing," pp. 89–123). The inherently unpredictable ordeal itself was of little use to either side: "the process of withdrawing from an ordeal, like the process of proposing one, was stylized, even ritualized" (107). Thus ordeals were proposed more often than they were completed (90).

207. On the limited resources—both material and textual—available to most rural priests in late Saxon England, see Jolly, *Popular Religion*, pp. 62–65.

208. Thus Jolly: "It is doubtful, then, that the priest would have used his liturgical training, however scanty, only in regular, perfunctory ways. Rather, it is likely he adapted his knowledge of Christian ideas, however inadequate, to meet local needs" (*Popular Religion*, p. 69).

209. See, for instance, instructions in *De exorcismis* on items 24–25 ("Deinde exorcista recitare potest, pro opportunitate, unum vel plures psalmos" [Then the exorcist may recite one or more psalms, as opportunity permits]), 34 ("si conveniens esse videatur" [if it seems to be appropriate]), 37, et al.

210. See, for instance, essays in Kiev, *Magic*. Colleen Ward reviews the evidence for the "success of indigenous therapies with emotionally based psychosomatic disorders, psychogenic organic malfunctions precipitated by emotional stress and conflict, and neuroses" ("Possession," p. 134). Michael Cuneo, skeptical himself of the existence of demons, notes that exorcism seems to offer at least temporary relief for many of the contemporary American believers who undergo it (*American Exorcism*, pp. 276–77).

211. E.g., Henderson, "Exorcism and Possession"; Ross, *Dissociative Identity Disorder*; and see Gardner, "Miracles," pp. 1927–33.

212. Schreiber, "Migration."

213. Ferracuti, Sacco, and Lazzari, "Dissociative Trance Disorder," pp. 528, 537.

214. Hale and Pinninti, "Exorcism-Resistant Ghost Possession," pp. 386–88.

215. See, for instance, Guthrie and Szanton, "Folk Diagnosis," p. 151; Prince, Leighton, and May, "Therapeutic Process," pp. 1171–83. Speaking specifically of Anglo-Saxon England, Clarke suggests, "the practical point about many of the direct cures, whether simple conversion cases or other conditions, seems to be that an authority-figure was able to intervene in a common-sense way before an inner conflict had turned a corner and become chronic" (*Mental Disorder*, p. 41).

216. Obeyesekere, "Idiom," p. 108.

217. Colleen Ward, "Possession," p. 135.

218. Brown, "Rise and Funtion," pp. 88–89; see also Brown, *Cult*, pp. 106–12.

219. Finucane, *Miracles*, p. 69. He adds, "if we expected to find as a daily occurrence cripples flinging away their crutches or mute pilgrims breaking out in a *Te Deum*, we would be disappointed" (75–76).

220. *Miracula Wulfstani* 11 (Darlington, *Vita Wulfstani*, p. 159).

221. Lapidge, *Cult*, pp. 312–14. The miracle is accepted as satisfactory because the man

had apparently prayed only to have his hearing restored (though the author acknowledges that the man is not at all guilty of the crime for which he was punished). For a reading of this partial cure, see O'Keeffe, "Body and Law," pp. 222–28. Ælfric dispenses with the problem somewhat when he relates the episode having only the man's eyes and ears mutilated in the first place (*Natale Sancti Swiðuni*; Skeat, *Lives of Saints*, vol. 1, p. 458). Finucane similarly refers to a crippled pilgrim miraculously "cured" by St. Simon to the extent that she only needed one crutch to walk (*Miracles*, p. 75). Einhard muses on the problem of partial cures, deciding that they serve to keep a person humble (*Translatio et miracula sanctorum Marcellini et Petri* 4.2; Waitz, *Translatio*, p. 257).

222. Finucane, *Miracles*, p. 101.

223. Major disorders are those which involve significant dysfunction and friction with family and community. Wen-Shing Tseng notes, "Major psychiatric disorders have prominent biological determinants and are less likely to be caused by psychological and sociocultural factors. The influence of cultural factors is secondary. . . . On the other hand, the origin of minor psychiatric disorders is more intimately tied to psychological and contextual factors, and therefore sociocultural factors are more critical in their etiology" (in Tseng and Streltzer, *Culture*, p. 8). See also Colleen Ward, "Possession," p. 136.

Chapter 3
Demon Possession in Narrative Portrayals

IT IS HARD TO IMAGINE Old English literature without demons. The loquacious demons of *Genesis B*, *Juliana*, and *Guthlac A* provide us with some of the more memorable flyting scenes in Old English poetry, while the hagiography of Cuthbert, Guthlac, and Dunstan emphasize dramatic physical confrontations with the demonic. However, all of these portray exterior battles. The great battles against demons in Anglo-Saxon literature are either the stylized Antonian conflicts of hermits contending with indigenous demons populating some desolate locale, or else the controlled debates of saint and demon while the saint enjoys divine protection. The demons in these scenes can be interpreted against the backdrop of popular folklore or against that of literary precedents, but in neither case is the saint out of control. Columba, Cuthbert, and Guthlac win their desired locations and drive away the autochthonous demons, but these are monsters roaming free rather than indwelling, medical demons.[1] Old English poetry knows nothing of demon possession, and Old English literature more generally shows little awareness of the idea apart from what it draws from continental source texts.

One of the major problems in interpreting Old English literature has always been situating it in the context of a particular readership or writing milieu. It is not easy to reconcile the erudite demonology of the literature, composed principally within monastic walls, with the presumed demonological beliefs of the average Anglo-Saxon. There is not much documentary support to help with imagining the relationship between early pastors in the Anglo-Saxon countryside, for instance, and the beliefs of their parishioners regarding possession. We are dependent on writers like Bede, who portrays the conversion in various regions as violent clashes of incompatible worldviews. Missionaries such as Augustine of Canterbury brought with them an inherited tradition that included the power of faith and discipleship, a belief in the justness of the church's authority on earth, and the conviction of unstoppable evangelical momentum. This tradition was passed down through specific role models and in fixed narrative paradigms. Missionaries understood their evangelizing in terms suggested by the Acts of the Apostles (both the canonical book and apocryphal accounts), and by the Gospel accounts of Christ's own ministry. They knew of such missions as St. Mark's among the Egyptians, and Bartholomew's and Thomas's among the Indians, from detailed apocryphal narratives that take up the story of Christianity's spread where scripture leaves off.[2] The Vercelli Book poem *Andreas* dramatizes that apostle's conversion of the Mermedonians in epic terms, and the poem immediately following it in the manuscript, Cynewulf's *Fates of the Apostles*, catalogs the missions and martyrdoms of all twelve apostles. Christ himself converted the Gerasenes, after spectacularly casting out a legion of demons (Mark 5:1–20). Perhaps none knew so well as Boniface—himself an Anglo-Saxon, gone to preach among continental heathens—the potential power of the rhetoric of bringing light to all the benighted corners of the earth, a rhetoric pervasive throughout his correspondence.

The fourth-century barbarians subsumed into the Roman Empire were converted, according to the fifth-century historian Sozomen, specifically because of the healing powers and the ascetic examples of the Christian missionaries.[3] Most striking is the account of Alaphion of Gaza, a man who was a friend of Sozomen's own grandfather.[4] Sozomen states that the man was possessed by a demon, and that the charms and spells of pagan and Jewish healers were ineffective. St. Hilarion cures the man by calling on Christ; Alaphion converts on the spot. This passage is especially valuable because it evidently records a healing miracle handed down in family lore—Sozomen perhaps heard it directly from his grandfather—rather than one gleaned from Jerome's *Vita Hilarionis* (no corresponding miracle is recorded there). The narrative shows the powerful role of exorcism specifically in times of cultural conflict, at the cusp of conversion—the very conditions under which possession seems to have made headway in seventh- and eighth-century Anglo-Saxon England.

Exorcism at the Intersection of Cultures

Brave medieval missionaries entering new, pagan lands may have expected to find people deliberately misled by the machinations of demons, and suffering under the yoke of ignorance, idolatry, and delusion. This is the way Bede and the documenters of the eighth-century English missionaries to the continent tell the story, following the literary and ideological precedents of Gregory of Tours, Sulpicius Severus, and other earlier narrators of conversion. Given their worldview and training, missionaries would naturally expect to find a population cringing under the tyranny of Satan's rule, in need of exorcism and healing as well as spiritual instruction. Such expectation, though, would not by itself produce widespread pathological behavior or muscle control disorders in the indigenous population. Minor behavioral conditions and anxieties could certainly be calmed, however, in a receptive community, while the more elaborate scripts of interactive exorcism would be slowly promulgated. It is possible that missionaries encountered people in trance states of various sorts among the native populations, and these they would have to begin slowly reinscribing as "demoniacs"; there would also be local seers, diviners, and wonder-workers, and these they would have to brand as "sorcerers" who draw their power from demons.[5]

Yet the saints' lives that record Anglo-Saxon missions to the continent are largely silent regarding native demoniacs among the unconverted. Just as Martin of Tours toppled pagan temples and revealed to the fourth-century inhabitants of northern Gaul that their pagan gods were demons, so Boniface, Sturm, and Willehad hewed down sacred trees and destroyed pagan idols in eighth-century Germany. According to Sulpicius Severus, Martin (though accustomed to energumens in and around Tours) did not encounter demoniacs in the countryside; there he converted the pagans through preaching alone.[6] Boniface likewise delivers the pagans of Hesse from "the captivity of demons" (a demoniorum captivitate)—by which he means the observation of pagan rites (*paganis ritibus*)—by preaching the gospel (*euangelica praedicando*); but the *Life of Boniface* does not indicate that he cured any possessed people.[7] In his correspondence Boniface continually decries paganism and its manifestations, but does not hint at possession among unconverted pagans. In his *Life of Sturm* Eigil of Fulda specifies that Sturm performs his exorcisms on those already converted: "quoties . . . immundorum spirituum habitationem a peccatoribus christianis expulit" (he often expelled evil spirits from sinning Christians).[8] Later Sturm preaches among the pagan Frisians and Saxons, but there is no mention of exorcisms among these unconverted peoples.[9] Willehad baptizes great multitudes in Saxony—as Anskar does in Denmark and Sweden, and Gall in Switzerland—but none of these saints encounters demoniacs.[10] In short, in these missionary accounts, exorcism is consistently associated with already converted populations. It is part of the relationship between Christian pastor and congregation, not the relationship between missionary and pagan.[11]

Recent missionary narratives can help elucidate the processes at work in acclimating a society to the expected norms of a new religion.[12] In order to assess the impact of newly introduced demonological beliefs, John Nevius, a nineteenth-century missionary to China, circulated a questionnaire among his fellow missionaries specifically asking about native possession behavior. The book he wrote based on the responses documents the well-established tradition of possession behaviors in native Chinese religions, and the easy transition from these to Christian demonological beliefs. As Nevius presents it, native possession resembled the Gospels' accounts in every particular, a common trope of missionary narratives.[13] Many natives are convinced to convert to Christianity after observing the efficacy of Christian prayer in healing demoniacs after their native remedies have failed.[14] The response from the Methodist minister W. J. Plumb to Nevius's circular could easily be mistaken for an excerpt from a medieval saint's life, in its almost parochial connection between conversion and demonology:

> In my native district, Chang-lo, there is a man who was formerly possessed by a demon. He believed in Christ, and entered the Christian religion, and was entirely relieved from the control of the demon. He afterwards turned aside from the truth, gave up his Christian profession, and the demon returned and tormented him until his death.[15]

Despite Nevius's conclusions, however, the examples he catalogs hint rather at the wide range of disparate manifestations of possession in various parts of East Asia and India. Unlike biblical demons, for instance, the demons possessing Chinese demoniacs claimed to be deceased relatives or to be "the fox" (a staple trickster of Chinese and Japanese mythology), chanted continuously in rhyme, demanded worship, and ordered that shrines be erected to them in people's houses.[16] The cultural distance between missionaries and the people they were attempting to understand seems even greater when the missionaries' accounts are compared with indigenous exorcism rites as described by the Chinese themselves.[17] In fact, the cases throughout this collection register the tense relationship between Christian pastor and local population, and—more importantly—the tense relationship between those members of the population already converted and those not yet converted.[18] A certain Mrs. Kwo, for example, is taken by her husband to the house of his newly Christianized brother-in-law, in the belief that a Christian household will offer more protection against evil spirits than their native one.[19] In this new house, while the family is preparing to attend the Christian services at a nearby town, Mrs. Kwo springs onto the table, throwing Bibles and hymnbooks to the floor. She is immediately joined in her raving by another woman, though the communal prayers of the Christian congregation soon calm them. The possession paradigm allows the women a model for expressing dissent at the rapid transition to Christianity in the family and community.[20]

Working among the nomadic Maasai people of Tanzania, Stanley Benson published a remarkable account of his experience with demon possession. He documents pathological trance states that (as with Nevius) seemed to him to resemble the demoniacs in the Gospel accounts, including violence, loud guttural sounds, seizures, and seemingly supernatural strength.[21] He attests, as a personal witness, that one woman spoke in Swahili, though she could not have known any, and she did so in a voice "not like hers in timbre or pitch."[22] It is the history of possession in the area, however, that is most curious. Benson reports that there were few accounts or memories of possession in the area before the late 1950s. The first cases reported were of people either living outside the area for a while who then moved back or of people having frequent contact with neighboring Swahili populations.[23] Benson charts the spread of possession among the Maasai in terms resembling the epidemiography of a flu or virus:

> [Demon possession] had its start among the Maasai speaking people whom they call the "WaLumbwa" (Wabariguyu). This tribe lives as semi-herding people in an area from near the coastal town of Bagamoyo westward into the Handeni district. They have been influenced greatly by their Swahili neighbors' customs and thoughts.
>
> From this tribe demon possession travelled into southeast Maasai district and moved slowly northward along the Ruvu River on the eastern boundary; westward following the southern border. There have been but a few isolated incidents reported in the western, central and northern areas of Maasailand even today. Most of the possession has taken place within the Kisongo section of the tribe in Tanzania. . . .
>
> Within Maasailand itself, there seems to be in the early history of the phenomenon, that it appeared closer to the market settlements and permanent water areas than away from these areas. In the more isolated areas, little was heard of this phenomenon.[24]

From this rare glimpse into possession behavior first taking root in a new population, it is clear that there must be contact with populations already having established possession behavior.[25] Nevius quotes a personal communication regarding exorcism in Christian missionary work in Japan from a Dr. Baelz of the Imperial University of Japan (presumably the influential German doctor Erwin Bälz, of whom there is still a statue at Tokyo University), who implies that possession is learned behavior: "Possession never occurs except in such subjects as have heard of it already and believe in the reality of its existence."[26] In the Benson case the neighboring Swahili-speaking population—one with a particularly "strong Islam and/or a strong mystical magical type of nativistic religion"[27]—provides the pattern for the behavioral anomalies then adopted by the Maasai. Since Maasai culture had no native curative responses to the phenomenon, they sought help from people outside the tribe.[28] The various tribal remedies employed were apparently useless, but starting in the late 1960s, as Benson reports it, Christian baptism was at last effective in preventing further attacks of possession among the population as a whole.

There is no indication of anything like demonic possession among the pre-Christian Anglo-Saxons.[29] Socially sanctioned trance states are sometimes evident in other pagan Germanic cultures, but there is little that resembles the particular dynamics of Gospel accounts. This is not to say that pre-Christian Anglo-Saxons did not have disease agents visualized as sentient, malicious entities attacking the patient from without: elves seem to have played such a role. By the time the *Leechbook* was compiled, elves had been largely assimilated with demons and other "nightmares" and "temptations," and had become associated especially with mental illness or behavioral disorders. There is no reference in Anglo-Saxon texts as a whole to a personality shift, though, such that an indwelling alien entity would be speaking through the patient's mouth, for instance. The closest we can get in native Germanic medicine are exorcisms intended to cast illness in general out of the patient.

The profile of possession that we encounter in Anglo-Saxon hagiography is manifestly Christian, derived ultimately from Near Eastern and Mediterranean traditions. Unlike exorcisms in other cultures, in the Judeo-Christian tradition the demon is purely an evil entity to be expelled and should never be bribed, entreated, flattered, or won over. The exorcism commonly begins with an overture by the demon, who often claims that the saint is a threat or that the demon is already in pain from the exorcist's mere presence. Then there is perhaps a dialogue in which the exorcist elicits the demon's name and extracts a confession concerning the demon's nature and past crimes. The two combatants threaten one another. The final adjuration from the exorcist directs the demon to depart, sometimes mentioning a specific place where the demon should go. Throughout this clash the demoniac adopts the persona of a fallen angel—now a demon and, as such, subject of the fallen archangel Lucifer. The source history of each of these elements is easily traceable, and in great detail, in early Judeo-Christian literature, but there is little trace of them in the Anglo-Saxon charms that presumably reflect echoes of pre-Christian belief systems. For the most part, the pagan Anglo-Saxons must have learned whatever possession behaviors they adopted through contact with Gallic, Irish, or Roman Christianity.

The seventh and eighth centuries were times of significant religious instability in Anglo-Saxon England. The king of a region was usually converted first, and then the population was expected to follow suit en masse. Backsliding into paganism was common from one monarch to the next, and even converted kings could turn apostate. Meanwhile, local populations reacted variously to the imposition of a new form of Christianity (in those few regions where British Christianity had remained current to some extent) or of an unfamiliar faith altogether (the vast majority of the populace, among whom Anglo-Saxon paganism had not appreciably assimilated British Christianity). St. Cuthbert, for one, was caught up in the dynamics of religious transition. His career ranged from the central Northumbrian monastery of Ripon to the isolated isle of Farne, covering areas that had generally been Christianized in the early to mid-seventh century. Bede notes that while prior of the monastery of Melrose, Cuthbert often had to contend with a populace ready to revert to the pagan gods of their ancestors (probably their grandparents or even parents) in times of duress:

> Aliqui etiam tempore mortalitatis, neglectis fidei sacramentis quibus erant inbuti, ad erratica idolatriae medicamina concurrebant, quasi missam a Deo Conditore plagam per incantationes uel fylacteria uel alia quaelibet daemonicae artis arcana cohibere ualerent.[30]
>
> [Some, in their mortal hour, turning from the sacraments of the faith in which they had been instructed, rushed to the fraudulent relief of

> idolatry, as though they could fend off a blow from God the Maker by means of incantations, amulets, or any other secrets of demonic craft.]

Even as late as 732 Bede complained that there were many rural areas in Northumbria that had no occasion to see a representative of the church for years at a time.[31] He remarked that King Aldwulf, who "lived into our own times," himself saw a shrine still standing that contained altars to both Christian and pagan gods.[32] The pagan Northumbrian site of Yeavering, the royal residence of King Eadwine, is an easy ride from Lindisfarne. Following his own conversion, at Yeavering, Eadwine, and King Oswald after him, allowed Paulinus to convert a large number of Bernicians.[33] In 747 the Council of Clovesho advised each bishop to travel throughout his diocese once a year to preach to those "qui raro audiunt verbum Dei" (who seldom hear the word of God).[34] Some areas of England were not converted at all until Bede's lifetime (Sussex in 681 and the Isle of Wight in 686, for instance). Therefore, in the period of our only detailed references to possession in Anglo-Saxon England, the country was still largely a religious frontier: paganism was fresh in the minds of many, backsliding was frequent, and the nascent church was struggling to establish authority and recondition a populace to the practices and conceptual categories of Latin Christianity. It is in this context that we find situated the small handful of statements that here or there an Anglo-Saxon was possessed. The anonymous hagiographer of Cuthbert asserts that in the saint's youth (probably around the 640s), Cuthbert "demones effugauit et insanientes uerbo orationis suae sanauit" (drove demons out and cured the insane with a word of his own prayer).[35] Such retrospective attributions of childhood miracles are common in saints' lives, and it is wise not to take them at face value. But the statement implies that, at the very least to the mind of the hagiographer, Northumbrians of Cuthbert's time—while not fully immersed in the Christian worldview, and while perhaps not fully conversant in the ritual drama of possession and exorcism—were actively accommodating local beliefs to the incoming Christian paradigm of possession.

Given the significant influence of Irish monastic spirituality in the conversion of the north of England in the seventh century, the question is worth asking whether that might be a possible source of possession behavior as well. Our knowledge of possession in seventh-century Ireland, however, must itself turn to only a small handful of sources that can be safely dated from this early period: Tirechan's *Life of Patrick* (or *Collection*, ca. 664–68), Cogitosus's *Life of Brigit* (ca. 680), Adomnan's *Life of Columba* (ca. 690s), and Muirchu's *Life of Patrick* (ca. 690s?).[36] These works do not indicate that exorcism contributed significantly toward the pastor-congregation relationship in seventh-century Ireland, however.[37] The Irish hagiographies of that time do not include any references to possession or exorcism, even though they provide catalogs of healings and other miracles.[38] In Jonas of Bobbio's sixth-century *Life of Columban*, Columban of Luxeuil is an Irish saint who cures demoniacs by the dozen, but these miracles occur on the continent. In any event, the vita is by a continental author, and surely reflects the mores of Gallic rather than Irish society.[39]

There is perhaps a more promising line of inquiry to account for why possession should apparently flourish in late seventh- and early eighth-century Northumbria and Anglia, as opposed to other times and places in Anglo-Saxon England: the religious context of northern England prior to and during the mid-seventh century. The Christianity of the Roman Britons in these areas was never of precisely the same character as Christianity in the south.[40] Christianity had taken most profound root (i.e., it more fully displaced Celtic polytheism and nature cults) in and around Romanized villa settlements, towns, and fortified centers—especially around the Thames and Severn estuaries—and perhaps on the militarized northern border. The lands north of Hadrian's Wall (including the area around Lindisfarne, Wearmouth-Jarrow, and Melrose) probably became Christianized relatively late (during the fifth and sixth centuries), at a time when the British church's infrastructure was already in collapse. John Blair writes, "the rituals of Romano-Celtic polytheistic cults can hardly have been eradicated totally, and syncretic fusions with Germanic paganism are not impossible."[41] In the south, Augustine of Canterbury was manifestly more interested in establishing Christianity afresh than in working closely with the surviving British clergy. His meeting with seven British bishops and a host of other learned men in 603 was, as Bede describes it, cold and antagonistic.[42] However, in the north and midlands there was greater scope for meaningful interaction between British priests and representatives of the new waves of conversion. In the early seventh century King Oswald and St. Aidan may have encouraged religious continuity in transitioning from the British church to reintroduced Catholicism.[43] Furthermore, the similarity between the Irish church and the British church probably facilitated a cooperative environment in the Irish sphere of evangelization.[44] Peter Hill claims that the early Northumbrian ecclesiastical incursions into Galloway "seem to show an unaccustomed regard for the sensibilities of the Britons."[45] Thus, for instance, the British saint Nynia was retained as patron of Whithorn, and British episcopal succession was preserved or else restored. Ecclesiastical sites in the north and midlands such as Carlisle, Abercorn, and Melrose even kept their British names.

Nonetheless, after the 660s any such situation of tolerance that may have existed had deteriorated: at the dedication of the Church of Ripon, Wilfrid read out the names of places which "clerus Bryttannus, aciem gladii hostilis manu gentis nostrae fugiens, deseruit" (the British clergy abandoned, fleeing before the sharpness of the sword in our people's hand).[46] Blair comments on the "more centralized and perhaps less tolerant religious-political world developing after the 660s," due in part to the establishment of endowed or royal minsters, which represented as much a political as a religious institution.[47] According to Bede, a devastating plague in May of 664 spread from the south to Northumbria: "corripiens atque acerua clade diutius longe lateque desaeuiens, magnam hominum multitudinem strauit" (it laid low a great multitude of people, attacking and raging furiously with bitter destruction, far and wide, for a long time).[48] This is known to have driven Christian converts back to paganism, including Sigehere of the East Saxons and his people.[49] By the 650s the foreign missionaries in Northumbria had been succeeded by the first generation of English-born bishops, and the church was becoming more localized in character. Also, it is probably around the 650s that many Anglo-Saxon kings who had adopted Christianity while (perhaps) continuing to permit pagan cults began to then suppress those cults. While there is no record of the specific time that pagan cults were suppressed in Northumbria or Mercia, Barbara Yorke calculates that

> [f]or those royal houses whose conversion Bede records in some detail, a hiatus can thus be recognised between the time of the first acceptance of Christianity and that of the formal abandonment of pagan worship which could be as long as forty to fifty years. No doubt there were others who followed Rædwald's practice of having altars to both christian and pagan gods. After all, to practitioners of a polytheistic religion there was no particular problem in extending worship to include another deity.[50]

King Eadwine of Northumbria converted in 627, so if Yorke is correct about a possible transitional period of tolerance for multiple religions, then the middle decades of the seventh century fall exactly into this timeframe. In short, the conversion of Northumbria and Mercia in the mid-seventh century involved an increasingly volatile progression over the course of the shift in local beliefs and practices. An initial period of assimilation with the native British clergy gave way around this time to instances of open hostility. Furthermore, the dual traditions of conversion—originating from Iona and Canterbury, respectively—produced further tensions as the Northumbrian church struggled to define itself.

These changes all took place about the time that possession first starts appearing in the Anglo-Saxon record, in the time of Cuthbert's youth (he would be in his twenties in the 650s).[51] The tensions have mostly resolved themselves, it would seem, by the time Bede writes his *Ecclesiastical History*, at the height of the Northumbrian golden age of learning and letters. As related in documents from throughout the first half of the eighth century, the last specific cases of possession mentioned are from the 710s (more on this below). It could be that possession and exorcism—so well suited to articulate and work through tensions in populations at the nexus of competing religious systems—were responding, in some way, to the particularly delicate and complicated circumstances of the evolving seventh-century church in the north of England.

Whatever the causes, in the seventh and early eighth centuries, possession as a behavioral paradigm was apparently adapting itself to the various personal and social needs of a recently converted population. The clergy might well tacitly encourage possession as an accepted means of channeling pain and frustration—it was, after all, something they knew how to deal with and something that reaffirmed the divine power of Christ and the earthly authority of the church. Possession at this time, however, probably exhibited an organic fluidity that made it more variable than the set patterns traditional church writings would indicate. Doubtlessly, not unlike the nineteenth-century missionaries to China in Nevius's account, the clergy interpreted what was actually a wide range of behaviors through the narrower lenses of biblical and hagiographical precedents. For example, a collection of canons included in what has come to be known as Theodore's Penitential (ca. 668–90) illustrates the disorganized nature of "demon possession" as a conceptual paradigm in the late seventh century.[52] The text provides a fascinating contrast to both hagiographic and liturgical models of possession:

> *X. De vexatis a diabolo*
> 1. Si homo vexatus est a diabolo et nescit aliquid nisi ubique discurrere et occidit semet ipsum quacumque causa potest ut oretur pro eo si ante religiosus erat.
> 2. Si pro desperatione aut pro timore aliquo aut pro causis incognitis Deo relinquimus hoc iudicium et non ausi sumus orare pro eo.
> 3. Qui se ipsum occiderit propria voluntate missas pro eo facere non licet, sed tantum orare et elemosinas largire.
> 4. Si quis Christianus subita temptatione mente sua exciderit, vel per insaniam se ipsum occiderit, quidam pro eo missas faciunt.
> 5. Demonium sustinenti licet petras vel holera habere sine incantatione.[53]
>
> [*10. Of Those Vexed by the Devil*
> 1. If a man is vexed by the devil and doesn't know anything except to run around all over the place, and he kills himself, there may somehow be cause to pray for him—if previously he had been pious.
> 2. If it was from desperation, from fear of something, or for unknown reasons, we leave its judgment to God and we do not dare pray for him.
> 3. It is not permitted to say masses for someone who kills himself willingly, but only to pray and dispense alms.
> 4. If a Christian loses his mind from a sudden attack or kills himself out of insanity, some people do say masses for such a person.
> 5. It is permitted to use stones or plants—but not incantation—for someone enduring a demon.]

Most obviously preoccupied with the taking of one's own life, this section implicitly equates demonic possession with suicide.[54] The penitential is uncomfortable allowing masses to be said for those whose suicides resulted from "unknown reasons," while "sudden seizure" and "insanity" receive softer treatment and permit tentative provisions for a mass. Here a desire is evident to strike a compromise between church orthodoxy and local custom. The last item—the only one to invoke demon possession rather than more general diabolic instigation—is only found in a minority of the extant manuscripts.[55] This challenging text serves, at the very least, to remind us of the wide range of social anxieties to which the demon possession idiom could be attached, and the imprecision with which the accepted ecclesiastical authorities responded to these anxieties.

Nine "Case Studies" from Anglo-Saxon England

I take as my starting point in this book a fresh premise: that we do not know whether widespread possession—not in the broader Anglo-Saxon sense of the term but in its modern sense implying personality displacement—ever existed significantly in Anglo-Saxon England. On the one hand, functional possession, in some form or other, has evolved as a sophisticated form of cultural expression in the majority of documented societies, both modern and premodern.[56] There would be nothing unusual in an Anglo-Saxon variant of such a practice. As a concept, possession would have been available to express a wide range of psychological states, from a simple need for individual attention or a way to display discontent with social pressures of various sorts to the expression of profoundly rooted emotional imbalances. Exorcism often performs positive social functions, such as the periodic articulation of cultural ideals and the public assertion of communal bonds.[57] Among the people potentially adopting possession behavior, some may have suffered from severe dissociation or functional psychosis. That is, some people with significant emotional damage (diagnosed as dissociation or "multiple personality" in secular spheres of the developed world) would act with a fractured sense of self, resembling possession in certain respects—this sometimes happens even in societies that have no beliefs regarding indwelling spirits or possession. Others with purely organic conditions such as neurological or muscle-control disorders would also sometimes have been considered possessed. Such organic conditions certainly existed, and the possession paradigm was a significant model for understanding such conditions in the early Middle Ages.

Yet there are only a small number of references to possession in Anglo-Saxon England, despite a relatively large documentary corpus. Furthermore, the accounts appear in notoriously stylized documents: the saints' lives produced within an ecclesiastical community whose inherited literary conventions—and whose perceptual categories and representational modes—were not necessarily representative of the Anglo-Saxon population as a whole. The highly symbolic and conservative nature of hagiography encourages the perpetuation of ancient tropes, and church writers of the period cast contemporary events into the narrative molds of earlier times and places as a matter of custom. Many of the accounts of demon possession bear suspicious resemblance (not just in detail but in actual wording) to earlier miracle healings from continental writings or from the Bible, leaving room for the genuine question of whether the accounts correspond to anything really happening in Anglo-Saxon society.

In the mid-sixth century Gregory of Tours initiated a project of systematically recording miracles at the shrine of St. Martin, with an eye toward preserving Martin's memory, demonstrating his holiness, and more generally promoting his cult.[58] Einhard compiled a similar collection of miracles in the ninth century for the relics of Marcellinus and Peter (ca. 834), which included his own catalog of miracles at Aachen and several other catalogs compiled at other locations.[59] This genre grew in the ninth and tenth centuries on the continent, following the pattern exemplified by Adrevald of Fleury's *History of the Translation of Benedict*.[60] By the twelfth century, popular shrines in England and France frequently employed registrars to verify and document miracles in extensive collections—such as Thomas of Monmouth's *Life of St. William* (completed around 1173, it contains miracle accounts compiled over twenty years of tending the shrine), and the two collections of Thomas Becket's miracles compiled by William of Canterbury and Benedict of Peterborough (together recording over seven hundred miracles occurring during their compilation in the 1170s).[61] There are some indications of a nascent miracle-recording program in Anglo-Saxon England, at least for St. Swithun: Lantfred of Winchester produced the *Translation and Miracles of St. Swithun* around 972–75, and this work was then versified, epitomized, and translated into Old English.[62] Aside from that miracle cycle, however, collections of *libri miraculorum* in Anglo-Saxon England are intermittent and poorly developed.[63] Even the prolific literary activity of the reign of Alfred and the monastic reforms of the tenth century never led to systematic collections of miracles. Thus Anglo-Saxon England presents us with far fewer contemporary accounts of possession than do Merovingian Gaul, Carolingian Germany, and Anglo-Norman England.

Anglo-Saxon hagiography is peppered with occasional references to demoniacs which state, for example, that "many were healed" at a given saint's tomb.[64] These are the stock-in-trade of a hagiographer's repertoire. It is much harder to find passages that tell us specifics about any particular possessed person—age, gender, social class, specific symptoms, etc. In fact, I know of only nine such passages from Anglo-Saxon England that provide any particulars at all. They are all from the seventh and early eighth centuries, and virtually all from northern England and Anglia. I include only stories about events purporting to take place in Anglo-Saxon England itself. Also, I have avoided miracle collections and other sources written or compiled in the postconquest period (such as the *Liber Eliensis*)—even when they retrospectively situate possession and exorcism in Anglo-Saxon England—because of the real possibility (demonstrable in some cases) of later contamination.[65] Also, I only include cases which seem to reflect actual medical, behavioral, or muscle-control conditions, not ideological differences of opinion or general moral censure. Demonic influence or diabolic instigation is sometimes attributed to someone with ill intent (as when Beccel apparently plots to murder Guthlac, in Felix's *Life of Guthlac*); while this can shed light on Anglo-Saxon rhetorical strategies and perhaps on contemporary psychology, it cannot safely be used to reconstruct actual disorders. I have only included such instances when they are explicitly accompanied by an additional statement of fits, pathological fury, or any other such identifiable dysfunction (such as Bede's account of King Eadbald or Boniface's account of King Ceolred).

Post-Roman Christianity first returned to the north of England through the small island of Iona, off the west coast of Scotland, where the Irish monk Columba had established a monastery by 565, some thirty years before Augustine's mission to southern England. In 635 the Irish bishop Aidan founded the island-monastery of Lindisfarne off the northeast coast of England. As early as 627 the missionary Paulinus had succeeded in converting King Eadwine of Northumbria (whose wife Æthelburh was already Christian). Eadwine insisted that his immediate entourage be baptized with him, and apparently convinced neighboring King Eorpwold of the East Saxons to convert also.[66] With the backing of powerful Northumbrian *bretwaldas* such as Oswald (r. 634–42) and Oswiu (r. 642–70), Christianity spread to other parts of the country. Even among the royalty, however, backsliding into paganism continued intermittently. By the late seventh century, Christianity had secured a more permanent foothold, allowing for a golden age of Northumbrian monastic culture. It is the literary production associated with the Northumbrian Renaissance that provides our only cases of Anglo-Saxon possession.

The anonymous *Life of Cuthbert* (ca. 699–705), one of the earliest extant literary productions of Anglo-Saxon England, gives us our earliest glimpse into demon possession, in seventh-century Northumbria. The author relates two specific cases and claims to have left many more unsaid:

> Nam etenim de hoc sileo quomodo in multis locis infirmantes demoniaci professi sunt, pro eo tantum futuro deseruisse demones, et numquam iterum possessuros, uel iterum quomodo praesens uerbo tantum alios sanauit.[67]
>
> [I will not say anything about how, in many places, demoniacs acknowledged that the demons left them because of Cuthbert, never to possess them again—nor about how, when present, he cured others with barely a word.]

The author writes further that Cuthbert cured various possessed persons later in his career, while at the monastery of Lindisfarne.[68] While such generalizations are commonplace in hagiography, it is hard not to sense a firsthand intimacy in the *Life of Cuthbert*; created shortly after the saint's death, the *Life* was written by a fellow monk of Lindisfarne who knew many of the people appearing in the work. A number of these are said to be still living,[69] and a paralytic is said to have been brought to Cuthbert's shrine "this very year."[70] The anonymous *Life* also gives explicit geographical information about the areas through which Cuthbert passed. There is little reason, then, to doubt the anonymous author's familiarity with his subject.

The first of the two specific possession cases detailed in the anonymous *Life of Cuthbert* occurs while Cuthbert is prior of Lindisfarne (probably in the 670s). The wife of Cuthbert's friend Hildmær is sorely possessed by the devil, but out of shame Hildmær is afraid to tell Cuthbert the nature of her illness:

> Fuit quidam uir religiosus specialiter carus homini Dei nomine Hildmaer, cuius uxor a demonio vexabatur nimis. Illa namque multum uastata et usque ad exitum mortis coangustata, frendens dentibus gemitum lacrimabilem emittebat. Supradictus uero uir de amara morte nihil dubitans ad monasterium nostrum proficiscens, uocauit ad se sanctum Cuðbertum, nam etenim illo tempore aecclesiae nostrae praepositus erat, indicans ei uxorem suam pene usque ad mortem infirmantem, non quae calamitas esset insaniae reuelauit. Iam enim erubescebat illam olim religiosam, tamen a demonio uexatam indicare. Nesciebat etiam nec intellegens, quod talis temptatio frequenter christianis accidere solet.[71]
>
> [There was a certain pious man named Hildmær, especially dear to the man of God, whose wife was greatly vexed by a demon. Indeed, she was severely devastated and oppressed to the point of death. Gnashing her teeth, she would let out tearful groans. Not doubting that she would die a bitter death, the aforementioned man, setting out for our monastery, called for the holy Cuthbert—because at that time he was in charge of our church—and informed him that his wife was sick almost to death. The man did not reveal that her misfortune was insanity (*insaniae*). In fact, he was ashamed to let on that she who had formerly been devout was now vexed to such an extent by a demon. He did not know or fully realize that such an attack frequently befalls Christians.]

While the author (writing twenty to thirty years after the incident) assures us that such possession is common, Hildmær himself considers his situation extraordinary. It is possible that possession had increased in frequency in the intervening period, and, living in the area in which the event occurred, the author knew of more reports. But it is equally possible that the monkish writer knows more about possession because he has read patristic commentary and continental hagiography, about which Hildmær of course knows nothing. In that case, we must equally watch out for literary embellishment.

Though Hildmær only wants to send for a physician, Cuthbert recognizes the true nature of the infirmity and volunteers to take care of it himself. They set out to ride back to Hildmær's house:

> Tunc uero preparauit se homo Dei, et omnes simul portati sunt equis, et uidens socium suum flentem et lacrimantem duobus causis, hoc est pro moriente uxore sibi deserto, et orbanis relictis, et maxime pro ignominiosa insaniae, in qua horribiliter redactam et inpudenter confractam et saliua pollutam, olim iam pudicam et castam, sciens homini Dei exspectanda erat, consolari eum cepit mitissimis uerbis, et omnem infirmitatem quam ei celauerat qualis esset reuelauit. Et postremo addit, prophetico ore dicens, Iam enim quando ueniemus ad habitacula uestra, uxor tua quam mortuam putas in obuiam mihi occurrens in acceptione habenarum istius equi quas nunc in manibus teneo per Dei adiutorium effugata demone saluata ministrabit nobis. Igitur peruenerunt sicut diximus, homo Dei ad uillam, et mulier quasi de somno surgens uenit in obuiam, et primo tacto freni plene pulsato demone sanitati pristine reddita.[72]
>
> [Then the man of God got ready and they all rode off together on horses. But he saw that his companion was crying and weeping, for two reasons: first because his wife was dying and he and his children would be left alone, but especially because of his wife's shameful madness, which he knew the man of God was about to witness. He would see her horribly reduced and shamefully broken, dirty with her own spittle—she who had once been modest and virtuous. Cuthbert began to console him with the calmest words, and he revealed the full nature of her condition though Hildmær had kept it hidden. At last, speaking prophetically, Cuthbert added: "When we arrive at your house, your wife—whom you think is just about dead—will run up to meet me and take the reins of this horse, which I now hold in my hands. She will attend to us healed, the demon having been driven away through the help of God." Sure enough, as we have said, they reached the villa, and the woman, as though just rising from sleep, came out to him. As soon as she touched the bridle, she was restored to her original health, the demon completely gone.]

This nonconfrontational exorcism is more obviously interested in the clairvoyance of the saint and in his ability to work miracles at a distance than in a dramatic conflict between demon and exorcist. In fact, this account studiously avoids any moment of verbal confrontation or violence between the demoniac and the saint. The demon is driven out "off stage." The wife's illness serves primarily as the backdrop for the conflict between Cuthbert and a man too ashamed to confide the full truth of his situation to the saint. The concern in this episode is to establish the authority of the holy man in the countryside, perhaps usurping some jurisdiction from physicians (Cuthbert is clear that this is a case for spiritual healing, not secular medicine) while still earning the trust of the local population at a personal level. The man should have confided in Cuthbert and confessed, as it were, his true situation. The only thing anyone has done wrong in the passage is to lie to a man of God.

The second case of possession related in detail in the anonymous *Life of Cuthbert* is a posthumous miracle, worked through a relic left over from the saint's burial. A man has to bring his possessed son to Lindisfarne in a wagon, so uncontrollable is the boy:

> Nam quidam pater familias filius suum a demonio fatigatum uociferantem et lacrimantem, lacerantemque corpus suum in plaustro ad insulam nostrum uehebat, et ad reliquias sanctorum apostolorum et martyrium Dei, ita ut occulte erat edoctus a presbitero sepe memorato nomine Tydi qui sanare filium eius, et fugare demonium non ualebat. Igitur sicut diximus clamante et uociferante demonioso, plurimorum aures horror inuasit. Multis namque disperantibus aliquod sanitatis remedium miserabili puero posse contulere, quidam tamen bone et integre fidei ad Deum spem ponens et deposcens sancti Cuthberti adiutorium, misericordia commotus, aquam benedixit, et partem humi de illa fossa in qua lauacrum corporis sancti episcopi nostri post obitum eius effusus est capiens aspersit in eam. Puer uero degustata aqua benedicta, a garrula uoce nocte illa desinit.[73]
>
> [A certain father conveyed his son, who was wearied by a demon—screaming out, weeping, and mutilating his own body—in a wagon to our island for the relics of the holy apostles and the martyrs of God. He had been advised to do this by the aforementioned priest Tydi, who was himself incapable of putting the demon to flight and curing the man's son. As we were saying, the demoniac, shouting and crying out, assaulted the ears of many with horror. Many people despaired of being able to secure any remedy for the miserable boy, but a certain man of good and pure faith who was moved to pity, placing his trust in God and entreating the help of St. Cuthbert, blessed some holy water and sprinkled in it some dirt from the ditch in which had been poured the bath water of the body of our holy bishop after his death. Once the boy tried the holy water, he desisted from his babbling that night.]

This boy's condition is more extreme than that of Hildmær's wife. In this account, which occurred sometime in the decade following Cuthbert's death (perhaps between 687 and ca. 700), the priest does seem to perform at least a skeletal rite by carefully preparing holy water for the patient to drink. Tydi's efforts signal a growing culture of exorcism: people apparently know to take such cases to priests, and priests have certain responses they are prepared to attempt. The anonymous priest whose response is at last successful performs only the most rudimentary "exorcism," without dramatic ritual or lengthy adjuration. Most of the procedural components of solemn exorcism are missing, both in this account and in the one involving Hildmær's wife. Neither Cuthbert nor the two priests mentioned in this chapter are explicitly said to lay on hands, sprinkle holy water, or recite prayers of adjuration over the possessed. The remedies we do see here are ad hoc charismatic and posthumous healings, not procedural liturgical rites.

Shortly after the appearance of the anonymous *Life of Cuthbert*, Bede wrote a brief verse account of the saint, and later a more expansive prose version (ca. 721). Finally, in 731 Bede provided an epitome of Cuthbert's career in his *Ecclesiastical History*. Though in the intervening years he collected what additional material he could find on Cuthbert's healing miracles, and spoke to those who knew Cuthbert or who witnessed miracles associated with him, Bede does not appear to have heard of any new cases of possession.[74] A great deal of modern work has begun to illuminate how Bede's hagiographic intentions differed from those of the anonymous writer before him.[75] Bede emphasizes didacticism, tightens the narrative by dwelling on moments of promotion and transition, and heightens the sense of continuity between Cuthbert and continental exemplars of holy men (such as those in Gregory the Great's *Dialogues*) while strengthening Cuthbert's profile as a Roman rather than an Ionan holy man.[76] There are some new details in Bede's retelling of the stories about Cuthbert, but it is perhaps safest to take these as representing Bede's understanding of exorcism, and not necessarily Cuthbert's.

Bede's version of the story of Hildmær's wife emphasizes both Hildmær's sense of shame at his wife's condition and Cuthbert's assurance that there is nothing to be ashamed about. In the anonymous version the man is ashamed because of his wife's "ignominious" (*ignominiosa*) insanity: she is "horribiliter redactam et inpudenter confractam et saliua pollutam" (horribly abased and shamelessly broken and polluted with spittle).[77] In Bede's version the man is more preoccupied by the moral implications, rather than the simple shame at her appearance and behavior: "timebat enim ne cum eam demoniosam inueniret, arbitrari inciperet, quia non integra Domino, sed ficta fide seruisset" (he was afraid that when Cuthbert found her possessed, he would begin to suspect that she had only served God with feigned rather than whole faith).[78] Cuthbert has to assure Hildmær that possession does not imply guilt, with a speech Bede now renders in direct discourse:

> Neque enim tali tormento soli subiciuntur mali, sed occulto Dei iudicio aliquotiens etiam innocentes in hoc saeculo non tantum corpore sed et mente captiuantur a diabolo.[79]
>
> [It is not only bad people who are subjected to such torments, but by the mysterious judgment of God, sometimes in this world the innocent are also taken captive by the devil not only in body but also in mind.]

What for the anonymous author was purely a healing anecdote—and thus for us, perhaps, a plausible glimpse into a real household whose insane mother and wife had become a source of shame—for Bede is an occasion for a brief meditation on illness and sin. It is the sincerity of the woman's religious convictions that most preoccupies Bede, rather than her public demeanor. Bede understands possession as a potential site of conflict between those of strong and those of wavering faith in the newly converted countryside.

Despite his prolific work in history and hagiography, to my knowledge, Bede only provides us with three detailed cases of demon possession in Anglo-Saxon England not found elsewhere.[80] The first is barely more than a mention: a moral indictment leveled against the pagan King Eadbald of Kent who refused to accept the newly-introduced Christian faith. Eadbald's reign, according to Bede, "magno tenellis ibi adhuc ecclesiae crementis detrimento fuit" (was a great detriment to the tender growth of the church).[81] In addition to refusing the new faith, Eadbald married his father's wife and so was *fornicatione pollutus* (polluted with fornication). Bede, perhaps bearing in mind Saul and his "unclean spirit" as a model, tells us that for his *scelere* (trespass), the king "crebra mentis uaesania et spiritus inmundi inuasione premebatur" (was overwhelmed by frequent mental insanity and possession by an unclean spirit).[82] Writing over a hundred years later, Bede is hardly in a position to have much insight into the specifics of Eadbald's condition. Of our nine cases, this account is both the least detailed and the furthest removed in time from the events it alleges to report. It is hard to know, in fact, whether Bede is reporting the king's final mental condition as it has been recorded elsewhere or otherwise handed down to him, or whether Bede himself has added the detail to ensure that the king comes across as having properly suffered for his apostasy.

The second case from Bede, again from his *Ecclesiastical History*, provides more of a detailed narrative. The drama occurs in late seventh- or early eighth-century Lincolnshire. Bede does not identify his informant for this story, though he mentions that Æthelhild, who obtained St. Oswald's relics from Queen Osthryth and who produced them at the appropriate moment, was still living at the time of writing.[83] It is intriguing to imagine Bede's having heard of the incident directly from somebody who was there, though he does not explicitly make that claim.[84] The story describes a team effort by those in possession of Oswald's relics to cure a visitor to Bardney Abbey:

> Transacto autem tempore aliquanto, cum [Æthilhild] esset in suo monasterio, uenit illic quidam hospes qui solebat nocturnis saepius horis repente ab inmundo spiritu grauissime uexari. Qui cum benigne susceptus post caenam in lecto membra posuisset, subito a diabolo arreptus clamare, dentibus frendere, spumare et diuersis motibus coepit membra torquere; cumque a nullo uel teneri uel ligari potuisset, cucurrit minister et pulsans ad ostium nuntiauit abbatissae. At illa aperiens ianuam monasterii exiuit ipsa cum una sanctimonialium feminarum ad locum uirorum, et euocans presbyterum rogauit secum uenire ad patientem. Vbi cum uenientes uiderent multos adfuisse, qui uexatum tenere et motus eius insanos conprimere conati nequaquam ualebant, dicebat presbyter exorcismos, et quaeque poterat pro sedando miseri furore agebat; sed nec ipse, quamuis multum laborans, proficere aliquid ualebat.

> Cumque nil salutis furenti superesse uideretur, repente uenit in mentem abbatissae puluis ille praefatus, statimque iussit ire ministram, et capsellam in qua erat adducere. Et cum illa adferens, quae iussa est, intraret atrium domus, in cuius interioribus daemonioses torquebatur, conticuit ille subito, et quasi in somnum laxatus deposuit caput, membra in quietem omnia conposuit. "Conticuere omnes intentique ora tenebant," quem res exitum haberet solliciti exspectantes. Et post aliquantum horae spatium resedit qui uexabatur, et grauiter suspirans "Modo" inquit "sanum sapio; recipi enim sensum animi mei."[85]
>
> [When Æthelhild was in her monastery (Bardney Abbey), it once happened that a certain visitor came who was used to being suddenly vexed very seriously by an unclean spirit, most often at night. After he was courteously taken in and after supper had gone to bed, he was suddenly seized by the devil and began to cry out, gnash his teeth, foam at the mouth, and fling his limbs about. Since no one could hold him down or bind him, an attendant ran and, knocking on the abbess's door, alerted her. She opened the monastery gate and went out, along with one of the nuns, to the men's quarters. She called for a priest and asked him to accompany her to the patient. When upon arriving they saw many people who were not strong enough to hold the demoniac or restrain his raging movements, the priest recited exorcisms and did everything he could to assuage the miserable man's ravings. However hard he tried, though, he was unable to make any headway.
>
> When nothing seemed to remain of the man's health for all the raving, the abbess suddenly remembered the aforementioned dust (from the washings of St. Oswald). She immediately had an attendant go and bring back the small box in which the soil was kept. The attendant brought it back as requested—and as soon as she passed into the entry hall of the house in which the demoniac was writhing, he suddenly became quiet and laid his head down as though in a deep sleep, and drew all his limbs back in peacefully. Everyone was quiet and held their breath, apprehensively waiting to see whether it would work. After an hour, the formerly troubled man sat up and, with a deep sigh, said, "Now I know sanity; I have recovered my mind."][86]

As with the exorcisms in the vitae of St. Cuthbert, a reader looking for a spectacular scene of conflict between saint and demoniac in the *Ecclesiastical History* will be disappointed. There apparently is such a scene—a failed exorcism, at least—but Bede passes over it quickly to focus instead on Oswald's sanctity, even at the most distant and deliberately capricious removes. Medievalists may be too used to such accounts of contact relics to appreciate the full impact of this episode: at his translation, Oswald's bones are washed before being placed in the casket. Some of the water spills onto the pavement, and some of the dust from this pavement is subsequently presented as a gift to Æthelhild. Some time later, faced with the raving demoniac, Æthelhild asks for the dust to be brought—and it does not even need to touch the demoniac or be in the same room. He is cured the very moment the servant bringing the dust nears the threshold of the building's entry hall. The man relates the moment in first-person speech:

> Mox ut uirgo haec cum capsella quam portabat adpropinquauit atrio domus huius, discessere omnes qui me premebant spiritus maligni, et me relicto nusquam conparuerunt.[87]
>
> [As soon as the maiden approached the entry hall with the small box she was carrying, all the evil spirits which were oppressing me departed, and having left me, were not apparent anywhere.]

Bede's interest here is more with spatial relations than with exorcistic confrontation—it is the distance of the healing saint that is stressed above all, through the precarious string of contact circumstances that nonetheless preserves intact the *potentia* of the saint (to use Peter Brown's term).[88] Contact relics, especially those efficacious at such removes, can be indicative of a society in which direct interaction with holy men is rare.

Bede's third report of possession is intriguing because it is much closer to home: it apparently happened in the environs of Wearmouth-Jarrow, though still related to Bede through second-hand report. In his commentary on Luke's version of the Gerasene demoniac episode (Luke 8:26–33), Bede mentions as an aside a local priest who was able to force a demon out of a nun through the power of confession, even when all else had failed:

> Sed et nostri temporis sacerdotes, qui per exorcismi gratiam daemones ejicere norunt, solent dicere patientes non aliter valere curari nisi quantum sapere possunt omne quod ab immundis spiritibus visu, auditu, gustu, tactu, et alio quolibet corporis vel animi sensu, vigilantes dormientesve pertulerint, confitendo patenter exponant. Et maxime, quando vel viris in specie feminea, vel in virili habitu feminis apparentes, quos daemones Galli Dusios vocant,[89] infando miraculo spiritus incorporei corporis humani concubitum petere se ac patrare confingunt. Et nomen daemonis, quo se censeri dixerit, et dejerandi modos, quibus amoris sui foedus alterutrum pepigerint, prodendos esse praecipiunt.
>
> Quae mendacio simillima res, sed adeo vera, et plurimorum est attestatione notissima, ut quidam vicinus mihi presbyter retulerit se quamdam sanctimonialem feminam a daemonio curare coepisse, sed quandiu res latebat, nihil apud eam proficere potuisse. Confesso autem quo molestabatur phantasmate, mox et ipsum orationibus caeterisque quae oportebat purificationum generibus effugasse, et ejusdem feminae corpus ab ulceribus, quae daemonis tactu contraxerat, medicinali studio adjuncto sale benedicto curasse.[90]
>
> [In our time the priests, who know how to cast out demons through the grace (or "gift") of exorcism, usually maintain that patients cannot be cured unless they openly reveal through confession everything they

> endured from the evil spirits in visions, sounds, tastes, tactile sensations, or through any senses whatsoever either physically or mentally. Especially when, appearing to men as women or to women dressed as men—which demons the Gauls call *Dusi*—they pretend to desire sexual intercourse with them and, an unspeakable marvel for an incorporeal spirit, to consummate with them in the flesh. And they advise that the demon's name—that by which he says he is known—and the ways in which they devised their mutual pact of passion by oaths, should be brought out.
>
> This may seem like a fable, but it is true insofar as there is the most notable testimony of many people that a certain priest in my vicinity related that he began to cure a certain holy woman from a demon, but as long as the matter lay concealed, there was nothing he could do for her. When she confessed what phantasm was troubling her, however, he quickly drove it out through prayers and other necessary kinds of purifications, and, applying consecrated salt with medical zeal, he cured the woman's body from the ulcers that had been brought about by the demon's influence.]

Bede's principal anxiety in this telling is to explain why an exorcism might not work. Even more clearly than in the episode of Hildmær, from the anonymous *Life of Cuthbert*, Bede focuses on the power of confession (though we should not yet imagine a fully developed tradition of auricular confession).[91] Patients must reveal to the priest all they have suffered before an exorcism can work. The local priest can have no success with the possessed nun until she herself acknowledges that she is troubled by an evil spirit. While downplaying sensationalistic elements of exorcism, Bede's approach does imply that the interrogation of the patient—the questioning of who is in the demoniac and why—is an essential feature of the process. It is only then that exorcism (which, in the particulars of "prayers and other necessary types of purifications," begins to sound increasingly like liturgical exorcism) can work.

Stephen of Ripon's *Life of Wilfrid* (ca. 710–20) reports a case of possession that can be fairly precisely dated to 680–81, during the nine months or so that King Ecgfrith of Northumbria had the controversial Wilfrid locked away in prison. Ecgfrith and his wife (this would be Ecgfrith's second wife, Eorminburh) had stopped at the Bernician royal monastery of Coldingham (a double house) while making the royal rounds through their kingdom. There, during the night, the queen is suddenly taken with a demon:

> Nam interim rex cum regina sua per civitates et castellas vicosque cotidie gaudentes et epulantes in pompa saeculari circumeuntes, tempore quodam ad coenobium, quod Colodaesburg dicitur, pervenerunt, cui praesidebat sanctissima materfamilias nomine Aebbae, soror Oswiu regis sapientissima. Illic enim regina illa nocte arrepta a daemone, sicut uxor Pilati multis flagellis fatigata, vix diem vivens expectavit.

Crastina die vero illucescente, mox sapientissima materfamilias veniens ad reginam, contractis membris simul in unum stricte alligatam et sine dubio morientem videns, regem adiit regique memorat lacrimabili voce, unde hoc miserabile malum secundum suam intelligentiam et ei evenisset, dicens audacter: "Ego scio et vere scio, quod Deo amabilem Wilfrithum episcopum sine alicuius sceleris piaculo de sede episcopatus abiecisti . . . in carcerem sanctum conclusisti. Et nunc, fili mi, secundum consilium matris tuae fac, disrumpe vincula eius et sanctas reliquias, quas regina de collo spoliati abstraxit et in perniciem sui, sicut arca Dei per civitates ducens, per fidelem nuntium emitte ei." . . . Iam enim rex oboediens matri castissimae factus est et sanctissimum sacerdotem nostrum resolutum cum suis reliquiis et cum suis sociis congregatis a se libere discedere concessit, et regina sanabatur.[92]

[While the king and his queen were going around the towns, forts, and villages, daily delighting and feasting along their worldly procession, they arrived on a certain occasion to the nunnery which is called Coldingham, which is presided over by the most holy and wise Abbess Æbbe, the sister of King Oswiu. There the queen was seized by a demon, and—wearied by numerous scourges just like the wife of Pilate—she hardly expected to live until daytime.

At break of dawn the next day, as soon as the most wise abbess came in to the queen—seeing that her limbs were closely constricted and drawn together as one and that she was undoubtedly dying—she went to the king and told him in a tearful voice why she thought this pitiable evil had befallen her, stating boldly: "I know and I know well that you threw out Bishop Wilfrid, dear to God and completely guiltless of any crime, from the episcopal see . . . you have shut the holy man up in prison. So now, my son, follow the advice of your mother: break his chains, and send forth to him by a loyal messenger the holy relics which the queen—to her own ruin—robbed by pulling them off his neck, carrying them through the towns like the ark of God." . . . Thus the king obeyed the holiest mother and allowed our most holy bishop to be released and to depart freely with his relics and with all his companions around him—and the queen was cured.]

Muscle-control disorders such as this are not mental disturbances in the modern sense, but they struck premodern observers in the same way that an alternate personality did: the subject is not in control of his or her own behaviors. Fully half the length of Stephen's chapter consists of Abbess Æbbe's speech of reprimand to the king (not quoted here in full); the queen's frightful condition is of secondary interest. Indeed, the entire episode is polemic in nature, and the final statement that the queen is cured ("et regina sanabatur") seems tagged on as a vindication of the abbess's position. Writing some thirty to forty years after the alleged incident, Stephen is not recording a medical case: in a transparently ideological passage he is employing possession as a sign of divine displeasure.

Further to the south, in East Anglia Felix's *Life of Guthlac* (ca. 730–40?)

records two cases of possession from the early eighth century. Felix follows the *Life of Cuthbert* in having his saint confronted by hordes of multiform demons when attempting to settle the wilderness, and he follows Athanasius's *Life of Anthony* in drawing these conflicts out into prolonged, detailed sequences.[93] However, Felix's accounts of actual healing miracles performed by Guthlac pale in comparison with these grand dramas. All but lost among a series of minor tricks of clairvoyance and prophecy are the two cases of demon possession. The first tells of a youth named Hwætred who is suddenly stricken by an evil spirit at home:

> [Q]uadam die domi sedens, subito illum nequam spiritus grassari coepit. In tantum autem inmensa dementia vexabatur ita ut membra sua propria ligno, ferro, unguibus dentibusque, prout potuit, laniaret; non solum enim se ipsum crudeli vesania decerpebat, quin etiam omnes, quoscumque tangere potuisset, inprobi oris morsibus lacerabat. Eo autem modo insanire coepit, ut eum prohiberi aut adligari nullius ausibus inpetraretur. Nam quodam tempore, congregata multitudine, cum alii illum ligare temtarent, arrepto limali bipenne tria virorum corpora letabundis ictibus humo sternens mori coegit. At cum bis binis annorum cursibus dira peste vesaniae vastaretur et exerti macilentia arido in corpore vires distaberent, tum demum a parentibus suis ad sacratas sedes sanctorum adductus est, ut a sacerdotibus episcopisque sacratis fontibus lavaretur. Cum ergo nullus eorum pestiferum funesti spiritus virus extinguere valuisset, tandem, exploratis reprobatisque omnium remediorum stigmatibus, domum reversi sunt.[94]
>
> [One day when he was sitting at home, a wretched spirit suddenly began to attack him. He was stricken with such intense madness that he lacerated his own limbs with wood, iron, and with his own nails and teeth as much as he could. Not only did he tear at himself cruelly and madly but he also tore at anyone he could reach with violent biting. He became so insane that he could not, by any hazard, be hindered or bound. Once when a large group had gathered around him and some of them tried to bind him, he grabbed a honed, double-edged battle-ax and sent three men to the ground with gleeful blows, killing them. When he had been devastated for four years with the awful plague of madness and his former strength had been drained from his emaciated body, at last his parents took him to the holy churches of the saints so he could be washed by the priests and bishops in the holy fonts. But since none of them could manage to extinguish the mortal pestilence of the hostile spirit, at length they returned home, every remedy for his scars having been tried and abandoned.]

Through word of mouth, Hwætred's parents learn of Guthlac's efficacy at healing and resolve to try their luck with him. Traveling an entire day, the parents bring their son with "limbs bound" (*ligatis membris*) to Guthlac's island. After hearing their troubles, Guthlac tries to console them and then begins to attempt a cure.

> Confestim enim, vexati manum arripiens [Guthlac], intra oratorium suum duxit, et illic continuis trium dierum ieiuniis, flexis genibus, orare coepit; tertia vero die, orto sole, sacrati fontis undis abluit, et, inflans in faciem eius spiritum salutis, omnem valitudinem maligni spiritus de illo reppulit. Ipse autem, velut qui de aestuantis gurgitis fluctibus ad portum deducitur, longa suspiria imo de pectore trahens, ad pristinae salutis valitudinem redditum se esse intellexit; ab illo enim tempore usque in diem exitus sui nullius molestiae inquietudinem ab inmundo spiritu pertulit.[95]
>
> [Straight away, seizing the hand of the distressed boy, he brought him into his oratory and there began to pray while kneeling and fasting continually for three days. Then on the third day, at first sunlight, Guthlac cleansed him in the waters of the holy font, and—blowing the breath of healing into his face—Guthlac repulsed from him all the force of the malign spirit. Just as one who is led to a harbor from the raging sea heaving with waves, the boy, letting out lengthy sighs from his innermost heart, understood that he had been brought back to his former state of health. And from that time until his dying day, he did not suffer anxiety from the vexations of that evil spirit again.]

Guthlac combats this spirit with the longest and most detailed procedural exorcism we have encountered so far in these case studies, and the one most resembling liturgical exorcism. Along with praying, fasting, and washing with holy water, Guthlac performs an act reminiscent of the *exsufflatio*—the ritual act of blowing in the candidate's face during baptism—indeed, this is the act that finally seems to drive out the demon.[96]

The symptoms relating to Hwætred in chapter 41 of the *Life of Guthlac* stress especially his violence, his self-mutilation, and the corporeal dimensions of his "madness" (*vesania*). In the subsequent chapter Felix recounts another healing miracle involving someone possessed by a demon, this time instead emphasizing the cognitive dimension:

> Alio quoque tempore, cum praefati exulis Æthelbaldi comes quidam, vocabulo Ecga, ab inmundi spiritus validissima vexatione miserabiliter grassaretur, ita ut quid esset vel quo sederet vel quid parabat facere nesciret. Corporis autem et membrorum vigor inlaesus permansit, facultas vero loquendi, disputandi intelligendique penitus defuit. Quadam die propinqui sui formidantes perpetuam vesaniam sibi venturam, ad praefati viri Guthlaci limina duxerunt; confestimque, ut se cingulo eius succinxit, omnem amentiam de se ablatam animumque sibi integre redditum persensit; se quoque illo cingulo semper praecingens, usque in ultimum diem vitae suae nullam a Satana molestiam perpessus est.[97]
>
> [And then another time, a certain retainer of that same Æthelbald named Ecga was attacked with the most severe disturbance of the unclean spirit, such that he did not know what he was or where he

> was or what he was going to do. His vigor of body and limbs remained unhurt, but his faculties of speaking, discussing, and understanding were utterly gone. One day, dreading that he would become permanently insane, his relatives brought him to the door of the aforementioned man, Guthlac. Immediately upon girding himself with Guthlac's belt, he clearly perceived that all his senselessness was lifted from him and his mind had become whole again. Always wearing that belt, up until the last day of his life he endured no further trouble from Satan.]

This entirely mental derangement complements the physical violence of the boy's derangement in the previous chapter, as though the two chapters collectively represent the totality of personhood. In this chapter it is Guthlac's belt (*cingula*) which cures the man, not anything that Guthlac says or does (other than presumably offering the man his belt).[98] In a sense Guthlac's belt now brings us full circle, recalling once again the horse's bridle that was the catalyst for a miracle cure in the first possession study (Hildmær's wife, in the anonymous *Life of Cuthbert* 2.8). Both of these symbols represent circularity, binding, and completion, and both attest to creative traditions of popular symbolism that stand apart from the known liturgical symbols of official exorcism rites.

Finally, our last case of possession in Anglo-Saxon England comes from the correspondence of Boniface, in a letter (ca. 746–47) to King Æthelbald of Mercia. In this letter Boniface mentions reports he has heard of the king revoking church privileges, and of the king's *prefecti* and *comites* (governors and companions) treating monks contemptuously.[99] Boniface implores the king to protect the church's estates and representatives, providing two negative role models to serve as cautionary examples. One is Osred, king of Bernicia and Deira, whom (according to Boniface) the "spiritus luxoriae . . . agitavit" (spirit of lust agitated), as seen in his "fornicantem et per monasteria nonnarum sacratas virgines stuprantem et furentem" (fornicating and defiling a convent of sacred virgins and raving in a fury).[100] Boniface notes that this dissolute monarch lost both his life and his soul, "contemptibili et despecta morte" (with a contemptible and despicable death).[101] The other cautionary example Boniface instructs Æthelbald to keep in mind is Æthelbald's own predecessor—Ceolred, king of Mercia. In fact, Æthelbald would need little convincing that his second cousin Ceolred was a disagreeable sort; Æthelbald had spent the reign of Ceolred (709–16) in exile (where he drew comfort from meeting with Guthlac in Crowland). Boniface alleges that Ceolred's *peccatis* (sins) included "stupratione et adulterio nonnarum et fractura monasteriorum" (ravishing and fornicating with nuns and destroying monasteries).[102] For his trespasses, Ceolred suffered an early and ignominious death, and now languishes in hell:

> Nam Ceolredum, precessorem venerande celsitudinis tuae, ut testati sunt qui presentes fuerant, apud comites suos splendide epulantem

> malignus spiritus, qui eum ad fiduciam dampnandae legis Dei suadendo pellexit, peccantem subito in insaniam mentis convertit, ut sine penitentia et confessione furibundus et amens et cum diabolis sermocinans et Dei sacerdotes abhominans de hac luce sine dubio ad tormenta inferni migravit.[103]
>
> [While Ceolred, the predecessor of your exalted reverence, as those who were there testified, feasted in splendor surrounded by his retinue, an evil spirit—which had seduced him to his own ruin through suggestion, away from the law of God—suddenly there in his sinning made him insane, such that without penance or confession, raving and senseless, and conversing with devils and cursing (or perhaps "repudiating") the priests of God, he traversed from this light, no doubt, to the torments of hell.]

This description paints a vivid and frightening portrait of a profligate monarch in the humiliating throes of helpless degeneration. Especially striking in this account is the image of Ceolred *cum diabolis sermocinans* ("conversing with devils"). We may be tempted by this wording to visualize Ceolred engaging in conversations with invisible beings—much like we perceive contemporary schizophrenics to be conducting half of a conversation, for instance. If this is what the wording does imply, then it is one of only a very few early medieval instances of "hearing voices," which is otherwise a predominantly modern phenomenon.[104] The accompanying phrase "sacerdotes abhominans" is ambiguous: Ceolred could be actively "cursing" the priests, or else simply "loathing" or "repudiating" them. In any event, though alleging to stem from firsthand accounts ("by those who were present"), Boniface's letter comes thirty years after the event, and it is probably unwise to try to pull too much out of his account as a literal description.

Patterns in the Nine Cases

Several conclusions can be drawn from these nine cases of Anglo-Saxon possession. First, we can sketch a rough profile of the range of conditions that were considered to be demon possession in these narrative accounts. In these few sources, demon possession refers perhaps most obviously to physical convulsions and uncontrollable seizures. Hildmær's wife gnashes her teeth, groans, and covers herself with her own spittle. She is said to be "horribly broken and shamefully reduced" as a result of her condition, and is apparently dying.[105] The visitor to Bardney Abbey suffers regularly from night attacks in which he cries out, gnashes his teeth, foams at the mouth, and flings his limbs about. When cured at last, he becomes peaceful and regains control of his limbs again.[106] Queen Eorminburh's sudden attack by a demon at Coldingham also manifests as a muscle-control disorder: her limbs are "constricted and drawn together as one" (contractis membris simul in unum).[107] The attack is severe enough that she is thought to be dying.

Insofar as these accounts can be trusted, these subjects apparently suffer from neurological conditions relating to the control of limbs, with no implication that their minds are deranged or that an alternate personality has taken over. If these are cases of functional possession, then the behaviors adopted very closely mimic neurological disorders.

The last six cases do in some way imply mental derangement or deliberative behavioral dysfunction. Of these six, two subjects exhibit violence and self-mutilation: this could range from isolated compulsions toward self-abuse to extreme psychotic episodes. A boy in the anonymous *Life of Cuthbert* is brought by his father to the saint in a wagon, screaming, weeping, and "mutilating his own body" (lacerantemque corpus suum).[108] More severe is the case of Hwætred in Felix's *Life of Guthlac*, who lacerates himself with wood, iron, and his own nails and teeth, and who tears and bites at anyone else who comes near.[109] He even kills someone with an ax, during an attempt to restrain him. Over its four-year course, the violent condition drains his energy, leaving him scarred and emaciated when he is at last brought to the saint.

The other four cases are rather harder to classify. There is very little to be learned from Bede's comment about King Eadbald of Kent (that he "was overwhelmed by frequent mental insanity and possession by an unclean spirit" [crebra mentis uaesania et spiritus inmundi inuasione premebatur]), other than that Bede disapproved of the apostate monarch.[110] Bede's mention of the holy woman in his vicinity who was possessed refers to some "phantasms" troubling her ("molestabatur phantasmate"), which at last go away once she confesses to a priest. Since the context of Bede's discussion is impure sexual thoughts, it is possible that this is what troubled the woman. In addition, however, the woman apparently has wounds or ulcers of some sort (*ulceribus*), which the priest also heals at the same time.[111] Boniface's moral indictment of King Ceolred describes him as raving and talking with devils, and implies that Ceolred dies in the course of this fit of madness.[112] Finally, Ecga, a retainer of King Æthelbald who lives with him in exile in the swamps of Crowland, is said to be possessed by a demon because he loses his mind completely—forgetting who or where he is, and losing his powers of speech and understanding. The man is perhaps driven to this state by the stresses of his exile in an unfamiliar place and in (no doubt) inhospitable circumstances. The comforting attentions of Guthlac and the gift of Guthlac's belt help restore him to soundness of mind.[113]

Other recurring themes in the narratives can help situate these Anglo-Saxon possession stories more broadly in their seventh-century context. To begin with, the accounts are concerned with establishing the Christian holy man as an authority to be trusted by rural Anglo-Saxons in their day-to-day lives, and by the royalty in their policy making. Hildmær unsuccessfully tries to hide the nature of his wife's condition from Cuthbert and learns that a saint can help him where a physician cannot. He should have confessed everything straight away (a theme also emphasized by Ælfric, much later). Bede's account of the holy woman in his vicinity likewise stresses that she continued to suffer from her demon until she "confessed" (*confesso*) truthfully to her priest what was troubling her. It is the secular rulers—King Ecgfrith and his wife—who mistrust the holy man Wilfrid, depriving him of his see at York and casting him into prison. The queen is stricken with an unclean spirit who only leaves once the royal couple admits that they are in the wrong and release the bishop. In the late seventh and early eighth centuries, then, exorcism was deployed as a sign of the intimate and immediate power of the holy man, in some ways bypassing conventional hierarchies of power and influence.

In addition to advocating trust in Christian holy men, these accounts also devote significant attention to the place of contact relics and to the "presence" (*praesentia*, again to borrow a term from Peter Brown) of the holy man even at a distance.[114] Thus, Oswald's relics serve to heal the visitor to Bardney Abbey even at many removes from the saint himself, and Guthlac's belt (though not technically a relic of the saint's body, it was nonetheless an item belonging to him) serves to restore sanity to Æthelbald's follower Ecga and to help keep him sane permanently. In this sense the possession accounts fall in line with the role of most healing and miracle stories of the time, which attempt to establish the cult of individual saints and to reinforce the importance of the church as a whole in shaping people's approaches to nature, their bodies, and themselves.

The narrative accounts of possession from this social context reveal an illuminating range of approaches on the part of the holy men. The priests, bishops, and hermits whose power is manifest in these healing miracles use a wide range of techniques in casting these demons out, techniques which are only loosely connected with "official" exorcisms of the liturgy—such as those found in the service books that Augustine of Canterbury might have had with him when he first came to England. These stories show the introduction and acclimation of native populations to the *materia magica* of the new religion: not the herbs, stones, pagan amulets, or other accoutrements that people's grandparents had perhaps used in healing rites, but the materials of the Christian liturgy—such as the water which is blessed by a priest and used to cure the boy brought to Lindisfarne in a wagon in the *Life of Cuthbert*, or the consecrated salt in Bede's commentary on Luke. Moreover, mixed in among holy oil and water are familiar domestic items, such as a bridle and a belt, that perhaps personalize the new church a little more to the local citizenry.

J. M. Wallace-Hadrill was struck by the failure of formal exorcism in the Bardney Abbey story in Bede's *Ecclesiastical History*, in which Oswald's dust at last enables the healing after a priest reciting exorcisms is unable to help.[115] Wallace-Hadrill comments, "it was possible for exorcism not to work, and this was a serious matter at a time when the church had to demonstrate the efficacy of its procedures to a semi-pagan population."[116] He argues that Bede's substitution of a local saint's relic for a solemn exorcism represents part of Bede's valorization of a particularly English and even Northumbrian Christian authority. Perhaps we should not make too much of what is a common hagiographic trope—the subject saint proving effective where some rival saint or other local churchman has proven useless—but Wallace-Hadrill is correct in drawing attention to a notable ambivalence toward procedural exorcism in these early Anglo-Saxon accounts. The competing interests of a regular church rite on the one hand (which emphasizes sacrament over the priest's character) and the independent authority of local holy men on the other (emphasizing immediate and spontaneous responses on the part of recognizable, familiar members of the community) play out in equal measure in these accounts, allowing us to witness the development of a regional church culture in organic response to local needs.

Really, of the nine accounts, two represent moral judgments rather than healing miracles. It is significant then that of the seven that relate "exorcisms," either official or otherwise, the failure of prior exorcisms is a prominent element in two. In addition to the Bardney Abbey account to which Wallace-Hadrill draws attention is the story in the *Life of Cuthbert* of the boy brought in a wagon to Cuthbert. Screaming and mutilating himself, the boy is advised to seek help from Cuthbert by a priest named Tydi, "who was himself incapable of putting the demon to flight and curing the man's son" (qui sanare filium eius, et fugare demonium non ualebat).[117] These are not anticlerical sentiments, of course; instead, they reveal the uncertain nature of exorcisms in these times. If possession and exorcism together represent a unified drama in which each participant plays a part, the recurrent anxiety of failed exorcism could represent a forge in which the proper roles are still being hammered out. Arguably, the exorcist and demoniac are not yet in synchronized agreement where there is a high rate of failed exorcism. The result is a miscellany of ad hoc responses in particular circumstances, a glimpse into a living tradition in a time before established Gelasian and Gregorian sacramentaries were commonplace, before the community and the church had negotiated a set of mutually acceptable roles in context.

Bede mentions in the commentary on Luke that priests expel demons specifically "through the grace of exorcism" (per exorcismi gratiam), but "exorcism" at that time may have represented a great diversity of practices. In the anonymous *Life of Cuthbert*, exorcisms are largely charismatic, completely unconnected with the directions for solemn exorcisms in the liturgy. Cuthbert's exorcism of Hildmær's wife amounts to little more than a prediction that she will be healed upon touching the horse's bridle. The *Life* simply states of Cuthbert's healing, "praesans et absens demoniacos sanauit, et alios uarios languores curauit" (he healed demoniacs both while present and absent, and cured various other weaknesses).[118] In revisiting the subject, however, Bede's *Life of Cuthbert* presents a more precise version of how these healings were performed:

> nonnullos ab immundorum spirituum uexatione non solum praesens orando, tangendo, imperando, exorcizando, sed et absens uel tantum orando, uel certe eorum sanationem praedicendo curauit.[119]
>
> [Some of those vexed by unclean spirits he cured not only while present, by praying, touching, commanding, and exorcising, but also while absent, either simply by praying or even just predicting they would be cured.]

Bede actively recasts the earlier anonymous account to bring it more in line with exorcism as a liturgical procedure rather than a charismatic gift. The four words Bede employs (*orando*, *tangendo*, *imperando*, and *exorcizando*) not only imply a longer and more systematic response but, more precisely, they reflect the specific language of the liturgy. The liturgy is of course principally composed of *orationes* (prayers), such as the series of prayers marked "Orationes super eos qui a daemonio vexantur" in the Leofric Missal.[120] The baptismal rites that include *ordines* direct the officiating priest to touch (*tangendo*) the candidate's nostrils, ears, chest, and sometimes shoulder blades ("Postea vero tangis ei pectus . . ."). *Imperando* is familiar from the *imperat tibi* refrain present in a number of solemn exorcisms, such as a rhetorically powerful series in the Leofric Missal:

> [I]mperat tibi dominus, imperat tibi filius et spiritus sanctus, imperat tibi apostolorum fides, sancti petri et pauli, et ceterorum apostolorum. Imperat tibi indulgentia confessorum. Imperat tibi martyrum sanguis, imperat tibi sacramentum crucis. Imperat tibi mysteriorum uirtus.[121]
>
> [The Lord commands you, the Son and the Holy Spirit command you, the faith of the apostles commands you—of Peter and Paul, and of all the other apostles. The mercy of the confessors commands you. The blood of the martyrs commands you, the mystery of the cross commands you. The power of the mysteries commands you.]

Finally, both solemn exorcism and prebaptismal exorcism require the cleansing of water and salt, usually employing the word *exorcizo* (e.g., "Exorcizo te, creatura salis"). Examples could be multiplied easily. Bede's commitment to valorizing the more liturgical approach comes out again in the commentary on Luke, where once the holy woman confesses, her priest casts out her demon, "orationibus caeterisque quae oportebat purificationum" (through prayers and other necessary [or "proper"] kinds of purifications).[122] The most involved exorcism in the narrative record is Felix's account of Guthlac healing the violent youth Hwætred: Guthlac brings him to the oratory and prays over him while kneeling and fasting for three days, at last washing him in the baptismal font. The final picture, then, is one of varied and creative responses to individual healing situations, on the part of priests and holy men in an age when the liturgical directions for solemn exorcism were part of the healing landscape but were not considered fixed or uniquely authoritative.

The late antique controversy over the Donatist heresy in North Africa was geographically and culturally quite removed from Anglo-Saxon England, but it can serve well enough as a model to help us understand the nature of what might have been at stake in the tensions between procedural and charismatic exorcisms. The Catholic position—the majority view in the Western church, as articulated forcefully by Augustine—maintained that the office of the priest, not his personal character, determined the validity of the sacraments. Upon reflection, it is obvious that this position is necessary for the basic functioning of the church and for social stability. Otherwise, if it is learned that a certain priest has been immoral in his conduct or heretical in his views, then all of a sudden the marriages, baptisms, last rites, etc., performed by him—perhaps over the course of many years—are revealed to have been illegitimate. The advantages in centralizing sacramental legitimacy in the ecclesiastical office, rather than in this or that individual, are evident for consolidating power and establishing stability. The Donatist position, on the other hand, emphasized greater scrutiny of the lives and character of individual priests, and in theory held church officials up to a higher standard of conduct. Donatism insists on an ideological vision in which the grace of God works through righteousness and the righteous, rather than bureaucratic offices and their appointed holders.

What we may be witnessing among these clerical writers of the Northumbrian Renaissance, then, is a local, largely internal church dialogue in which centralized control over "sanctity" was at some root level being worked out. To what extent English minsters would tolerate and even nurture cults of local holy men outside of their direct supervision was perhaps in the background of the way these healing cures are presented. The charismatic saints of this early golden age—Cuthbert, Oswald, Æthelthryth—would continue to be revered in the formal church liturgies throughout the Anglo-Saxon period, through generations which seemed to produce many fewer enduring saints. On the whole, in their insistence on the simple, immediate cure and their anxiety over the potential of procedural exorcism to fail, seventh- and early eighth-century narratives do not indicate a tradition in which protracted liturgical exorcism is being uniformly promoted as the most effective remedy for demon possession. In five out of the nine cases, a saint or holy man is not even present to perform the cure—the *praesentia* has already shifted to healing shrines and relics, rather than remaining vested in particular, living individuals. Once a saint is dead and safely buried in the sepulcher, the church as a body can then control what the saint "does" from that point on (e.g., authenticate visions or cures, interpret prophesies, etc.).

These nine cases, reported by five authors from the high period of Northumbrian letters, leave an initial impression of active epileptic and dissociative behavior, all of which is only poorly understood by the immediate family and community and is interpreted as demon possession by local clergy. The stories are restricted to a very specific time—they all occurred within a generation or two, from the 670s to the early 700s. All occurred in Northumbria and Anglia. All are distanced from the storyteller by at least one remove (or if the narrators were direct witnesses to these events, they do not specify that fact). Moreover, these cases stand as sole testimony in a time of thriving literary activity. There are numerous other sources in which we might expect to find mentions of possession, but in which there are none. Adomnan's early *Vita Columbae*, though filled with mythological demons inhabiting the wilderness, does not mention any demoniacs; nor are there any exorcisms in the anonymous eighth-century *Vita Ceolfridi* (sometimes called the *Historia abbatum*) by a monk of Wearmouth, the poetic *Miracula Ninie Episcopi*, Bede's *Historia abbatum*, or Alcuin's poetic narrative *De pontificibus et sanctis Ecclesiae Eboracensis*.[123] The authors of these latter sources lived in close proximity to the saints' tombs and therefore should have been well positioned to record directly whether healings occurred there, or to hear stories of any exorcisms performed during the saint's life. The nine cases of Anglo-Saxon possession all come from the same time and place, by and large, but we should also keep in perspective that they only form a very small part of the culture of healing and miracles even within that time and place. Perhaps in the context of Northumbrian and Anglian spirituality as a whole, the few possession narratives do not stand out as representative.

Tenth- and Eleventh-Century Sources

Looking beyond the narratives extant from seventh- and early eighth-century Northumbria and Anglia, the subsequent periods of Anglo-Saxon letters leave little with which to assess the existence or extent of possession in the ninth, tenth, or eleventh centuries. The early ninth-century poem *De abbatibus* by the Northumbrian poet Ædiluulf, while briefly documenting the lives and deaths of a half-dozen abbots, is very sparse on miraculous cures and is utterly devoid of demoniacs. The wide-reaching literary activity associated with the reign of Alfred in the later ninth century, though encouraging a range of genres and interests, does not leave us any insight into possession and exorcism in his time. Narrative sources such as Gregory the Great's *Dialogues* were translated into Old English, but original hagiographic composition was evidently not a priority for Alfred or his circle. Native demon possession is all but absent from the Anglo-Saxon literary records by this point.

The tenth-century monastic reform led to a resurgence of interest in native English saints and in hagiographic composition. In the mid 970s Lantfred of Winchester composed the influential *Translatio et miracula Swithuni*. A decade or so later, Abbo of Fleury wrote his *Passio Eadmundi* while living in England at Ramsey Abbey. In 996 Wulfstan of Winchester (also known as Wulfstan Cantor) wrote the *Narratio metrica de S. Swithuno*, based on Lantfred's prose work, and in the same year or shortly afterwards produced an original *Vita Aethelwoldi.*[124] Ælfric of Eynsham also wrote a Latin life of Æthelwold, based on Wulfstan's. Sometime between 984 and 998 a summary of Lantfred's *Translatio* now known as the *Epitome translationis et miraculorum S. Swithuni* was compiled, perhaps by Ælfric of Eynsham.[125] Also in the late tenth century (probably), a Winchester poet penned the metrical *Vita Iudoci*, based on an early tenth-century life of the Breton saint written in northeast France.[126] Two *vitae* commemorating the life of Dunstan, archbishop of Canterbury (d. 988), were written in the late tenth or early eleventh century by Adelard of Ghent and by an author known only by his first initial ("B").[127] Finally, Byrhtferth of Ramsey wrote a *Vita Oswaldi* and *Vita Ecgwini* in the early eleventh century.[128] It is in these saints' lives and miracle collections that we should most expect evidence of possession and exorcism activity in late Anglo-Saxon England. However, I am only aware of two brief mentions of it anywhere in these sources: one possible instance in the metrical *Vita Iudoci* notes that at the saint's tomb "nequam spirituum fugit infestatio mente" (wicked persecution of demons disappears from the mind); and the closing sentence of Byrhtferth's *Vita Oswaldi* states formulaically that "demons are driven out" (dæmonia effugantur) through appeal to Oswald's martyrdom.[129] The near absence of demon possession and exorcism in these documents of the tenth and eleventh centuries leaves us to wonder whether the cultural landscape had greatly changed in the two and a half centuries since the time of Bede.

Ælfric, the most prolific author of late Anglo-Saxon England, has almost nothing to say about possession and exorcism of his own period. In his compendious cycles of readings for the holy calendar (two complementary series of homilies) and in his *Lives of Saints*, however, Ælfric includes two- to three-dozen mentions of demoniacs and exorcisms—but these include references to Christ's own miracles and to miracles in early Christianity.[130] Since most of his subjects are foreign saints from earlier centuries, the vast majority of these are references borrowed from his sources. Even regarding English saints such as Oswald and Æthelthryth, he is necessarily dependent on Bede.[131] For more recent saints, Ælfric's explicit refusal to include the many popular stories he has heard, sticking instead to written sources, is frustrating for the modern student of popular religion: "Fela wundra we gehyrdon on folclicre spræce, be þam halgan eadmunde þe we her nellaþ on gewrite settan" (We have heard of many miracles, from popular hearsay, about the holy Edmund, which we will not set here into writing).[132] Thus Ælfric is virtually silent concerning demon possession in late Anglo-Saxon England. Even where miracles are present, demon possession is not emphasized. His treatment of St. Swithun, for instance, is largely a tissue of posthumous miracle stories—Ælfric laments that Swithun's own contemporaries did not leave more biographical material from which future hagiographers could draw.[133] The usual brigade of the lame and the blind are cured at his tomb, but nowhere are demoniacs mentioned.[134]

In a homily for the fourth Sunday after Pentecost, Ælfric states explicitly, "sind eac sume gecorene menn þe afligað þa awyriedan gastas fram ofsettum mannum" (also there are certain chosen people who drive unclean spirits from those afflicted).[135] In an intriguing and quite problematic section of his homily for Ascension Day, Ælfric tackles the problem of miracles directly, and it is interesting that he does so specifically in the context of demon possession and the casting out of devils. Following in the footsteps of Gregory the Great, Ælfric explains that miracles do not happen as often as they once did because now that Christianity has taken root people no longer require daily proofs. Malcolm Godden points out that Ælfric (following Haymo of Auxerre) departs from Gregory in asserting not just that miracles are less frequent but that they have ceased altogether: "syððan se geleafa sprang geond ealne middaneard, syððan geswicon þa wundra" (when belief spread throughout all the earth, then marvels abated).[136] Miracles were only necessary, apparently, at the beginning of the Christian era ("on anginne cristendomes").[137] Ælfric immediately clarifies this surprising position by explaining that miracles are in fact just as common as in the New Testament era, but that they are now "spiritual" rather than "bodily" miracles: "godes gelaðung wyrcð gyt dæghwomlice þa ylcan wundru gastlice þe ða apostoli ða worhton lichamlice" (every day the church of God still works the same marvels spiritually that the apostles worked bodily).[138] This digression is somewhat unfortunate for a homilist who will go on to include numerous bodily miracles of recent English saints in his *Lives of Saints*, and Godden has gone a long way toward making sense of it by explaining audience considerations and social context, and also by reminding us that Ælfric was a human being with various moods.[139]

The homily is especially interesting here, however, for its immediate context. Ælfric has been expounding on the "demonic" facet of sin in general. Someone who will not believe the truth of Christianity is, he explains, worse than a devil, because at least the devils recognized the divinity of Christ. Someone who believes but still sins is "like the devil" (se bið ðonne deoflum gelic).[140] After this, Ælfric restates Christ's promise to his disciples that those who follow him will see signs as proof: they will cast out devils, speak in new tongues, drive away serpents, enjoy immunity from poison, and heal the sick by laying on hands (Mark 16:17–18). Following the explanation that miracles are these days "spiritual" rather than "bodily," Ælfric points to the expulsion of the devil at baptism as an example. It is thus largely in a discussion of the demonic that Ælfric pauses to question why miracles are no longer evident. His position does not imply an audience for whom the literal casting out of demons is a frequent sight. Indeed, in a very curious passage, he pauses to gloss "having a devil" for his listeners, as though they won't necessarily know what it means:

> Twa bysmorlice word hi cwædon to criste. An is þæt he wære samaritanisc, oðer þæt he deofol on him hæfde, þæt we cweðað on englisc be wodum menn, "þu eart wod."[141]
>
> [They made two shameful accusations against Christ. The first is that he was a Samaritan, and the other that he "had a devil in him"—which in English is what we say about mad people when we say to them, "you are mad."]

This aside is not in Ælfric's source.[142] Even with a popular audience in mind, it is hard to imagine why possession should require such an explanation in late tenth-century England, save that the hermetically sealed world of monastic letters is perhaps by this point considerably out of step with common experience (or, at least, that Ælfric fears that is the case).[143]

In the postconquest period, possession stories and exorcisms quickly begin to appear in miracle collections. For example, an exorcism account appears in the *Miracula Swithuni*, a work compiled at the end of the eleventh century that adopts much from Wulfstan of Winchester's *Narratio metrica de S. Swithuno* but also adds new information.[144] The earlier healing miracles associated with St. Swithun made no mention of the insane or possessed. Folcard's *Vita S. Johannis* (the life of John of Beverley) has that saint curing a demoniac and states that at his tomb, "dæmones effugantur" (demons are put to flight).[145] Sometime between 1095 and 1113 a monk named Coleman wrote the *Vita Wulfstani*, a life of Wulfstan of Worcester (not to be confused with either Wulfstan of Winchester, or the famous homilist Wulfstan of York). Though originally written in Old English, the work only survives in the Latin translation of William of Malmesbury. Mary Lynn Rampolla finds it significant that six of the thirteen miracles in the *Vita Wulfstani* involve curing the insane (four of whom are explicitly described as demon possessed).[146] She interprets this high proportion of mental disturbances as a symptom of a disordered society: "the stories of madmen, who so clearly disrupt the social order, parallel the condition of England."[147] Whether or not the preconquest period was an "ordered" society, that era exhibits a notable resurgence in awareness of and interest in the mentally ill and the possessed. This revitalization of possession narratives casts into sharper contrast the previous three centuries, in which possession and exorcism activity is very poorly attested in England.

Overview

Possession beliefs and behaviors can be fragile and extremely context dependent. The ritual of possession and exorcism, taken together as a dyad, is especially reliant on all the actors (demoniac, healer, and community) internalizing their roles and continuing, presumably, to benefit from the convention. The widespread increase in possession and exorcism in late twentieth-century America—sparked in large part, as is now well documented, by the 1973 movie *The Exorcist*—should remind us how subject such practices are to influence and example, and how quickly even deeply held beliefs and attitudes toward the demonic can radically shift in a very short period of time.[148] The picture that emerges from Anglo-Saxon letters is one of a brief period of possession behavior in the recently converted rural areas of Northumbria and Anglia, within the scope of a single generation. The stories from this time are energetic, personal, and exhibit significant diversity. The sources that come after are largely silent. This may reflect the abatement of possession behaviors, but it may also reflect shifts in literary interest: after the Northumbrian Renaissance, hagiography (our primary genre for possession stories) recedes from the literary landscape for over two hundred years. It returns, however, under the auspices of the broader reform agenda of the tenth-century Anglo-Saxon church, but that may have discouraged some of the dynamic, creative impulses fueling the earlier accounts. Indeed, Christian hagiography itself was, as a genre, two hundred years more mature when it reappeared in England in the late 900s. The extensive writings of Carolingian authors had left an indelible stamp on the genre by the time of Æthelwold and the Anglo-Saxon church reformation.

The narrative sources from which our nine case studies are taken operate according to literary conventions (largely influenced by hagiography) that make them subject to at least a healthy skepticism. Bede may have, as he states, known a local priest who performed an exorcism on a nun or it may have been something more like a "friend of a friend." The aims of hagiography make it conducive to employ realism as a literary device, in the sense of creating an air of verisimilitude—but not necessarily conducive to record historical or factual material. It is perhaps safest to take the early stories not as events which necessarily happened but as events which the (primarily) monastic audiences such as those at Wearmouth-Jarrow, Ripon, and Crowland would have recognized as typical or at least plausible, either from personal experience or from their other readings in hagiography.

NOTES

1. Adomnan, *Life of Columba* 1.1, 3.8 (Anderson and Anderson, *Adomnan's Life*, pp. 194 and 480); Bede, *Vita Cuthberti* 17 (Colgrave, *Two Lives*, pp. 214–15); Felix, *Vita Guthlaci* 29–36 (Colgrave, *Felix's Life*, pp. 94–116). The Old English poem *Guthlac A* is exclusively a rendering of Guthlac's fight with the demons of the island he wishes to inhabit. There is no fight against indwelling demons—no exorcism—related in any Old English poem.

2. Mark: Ælfric, *Passio S. Marci* (Skeat, *Lives of Saints*, vol. 1, pp. 320–26); Bartholomew: Ælfric, *Passio S. Bartholomei* (*Catholic Homilies* 1.31; Clemoes, *Catholic Homilies*, pp. 439–

50); Thomas: Ælfric, *Passio S. Thomæ* (Skeat, *Lives of Saints*, vol. 2, pp. 398–424). See also O'Leary, "Apostolic *Passiones*."

3. Sozomen, *Ecclesiastical History* 2.6: "many priests of Christ who had been taken captive, dwelt among these tribes; and during their residence among them, healed the sick, and cleansed those who were possessed of demons, by the name of Christ only, and by calling on the Son of God; moreover they led a blameless life, and excited envy by their virtues. The barbarians, amazed at the conduct and wonderful works of these men, thought that it would be prudent on their part . . . if they should imitate [them] . . . the people were taught and baptized, and subsequently were gathered into churches" (trans. in Hartranft, *Ecclesiastical History*, pp. 262–63).

4. Sozomen, *Ecclesiastical History*, 5.15 (Hartranft, *Ecclesiastical History*, p. 337).

5. On this process, see Boureau, *Satan*, p. 146; Waegeman, "Medieval Sibyl"; and the refreshingly direct presentation in Wiśniewski, "La consultation." Erik Sorensen's monograph *Possession and Exorcism in the New Testament and Early Christianity* argues that Christianity owed much of its conversion successes to the gradual reinscription of Greco-Roman conceptions of ecstatic, divine possession as demon possession (pp. 222–25).

6. Sulpicius Severus, *Vita Martini* 12–15. He converts pagans exclusively by preaching (*praedicatione*: chap. 15; Halm, *Sulpicii Severi*, p. 125). For exorcism miracles back among his Christian fold, see chapters 17–18.

7. Willibald, *Vita Bonifatii* 6 (Levison, *Vitae Sancti*, pp. 27, 31–32). It is not until after his death that demoniacs are cured at his shrine in Fulda (*Vita Bonifatii* 8; Levison, *Vitae Sancti*, pp. 54–55).

8. Eigil, *Vita Sturmi* 3 (Pertz, *Eigilis*, p. 366).

9. Eigil, *Vita Sturmi* 15 and 22 (Pertz, *Eigilis*, pp. 372–73, 376).

10. *Vita Willehadi* 3–5, 8, pp. 843–44, 845; Rimbert, *Vita Anskarii* 7, 11–12, et al. (Waitz, *Vita Anskarii*, pp. 26–29, 32–34); Strabo, *Vita Galli* 1.4–1.8 (Krusch, *Passiones* [MGH, SRM 4], pp. 287–91). Demoniacs are eventually cured at Gall's tomb after his death (*Vita Galli* 2.5, 2.23; Krusch, *Passiones*, pp. 316, 328).

11. Note also the wording of the ordination rite for exorcists in the liturgy: "Accipe et commenda, et habeto potestatem imponendi manum super energumenum, sive baptizatum sive catechumenum" (Accept and commit these exorcisms [to memory], and receive the power of laying hands on an energumen, whether already baptized or whether a catechumen; H. A. Wilson, *Gelasian*, p. 145). In envisioning only those already baptized or those currently in the catechumenate, the rite does not acknowledge jurisdiction over anyone completely outside of the Christian fold.

12. See, for instance, Kilger, "Devil," pp. 213–22; Oesterreich, *Possession*, pp. 131–46; and Verdun, *Le Diable*.

13. Nevius, *Demon Possession*, pp. 108–9. Hugh White, a Southern Presbyterian missionary in China, writes, "Demonism as seen today is the same as in the time of Christ. The terminology is so identical as to make one feel that he is walking the streets of Nazareth or Capernaum" (quoted in Mooneyham, "Demonism," pp. 209–19, 211).

14. Nevius, *Demon Possession*, p. 76.

15. Quoted in Nevius, *Demon Possession*, p. 52; see also pp. 81–82.

16. Deceased relatives: Nevius, *Demon Possession*, pp. 76, 274; fox (104–5); chant in rhyme (37, 31); demand worship (65–67, 402). The "fox" is said to enter the human either through the breast or underneath the finger nails (105). Guo stresses the importance in Chinese traditions of the evil or vengeful ghost as the primary entity in need of exorcism, and the

exorcist's correlative assumption of a ghost identity to be an effective opponent (*Exorcism*, p. 130).

17. See, for instance, the account in an 1870 Yixian County gazetteer (itself critical of the "superstitious" rites): "In the Seventh District, there are the procession for the sun and the subduing of the [spirit-possessed] children, which are particularly absurd. . . . On the days of the procession for the sun, the *xiangtong* [spirit-possessed children] are enacted by children from bondservant households, which produce hereditary sorcerers. The *shiwu*, or the master of the *xiangtong*, performs witchcraft to have the children possessed by spirits, making them jump and leap wildly. [He] then uses a sharp knife and cuts the forehead [of each *xiangtong*], so that their blood floods down to the breast. This is called 'breaking the heavenly gate.' In addition, a huge cauldron is set up to heat cooking oil; when it is hot, the bean curd is thrown in. [The xiangtong children] then use their bare hands to take the bean curd out [from the cauldron of still burning oil]; they do so several times and distribute the burned bean curd to the audience. After all of the bean curd has been taken out, their hands are not burned" (Guo, *Exorcism*, p. 107).

18. For a nuanced study of the often intense conflicts Christians faced in China during this period, see Sweeten, *Christianity*.

19. Nevius, *Demon Possession*, pp. 30–35.

20. Further accounts in Kenneth Taylor, *Demon Experiences*, support the idea that accounts of possession appear especially at moments of cultural transition, forming a bridge between pagan and Christian. In that collection, N. Daniel states that demons in India have power over "those who are only nominal Christians" (21), and David Ekstrom notes that a common element in all the possession cases he knows about in Guatemala involve Christians "in a backslidden condition" (108). See also Verdun, *Le diable*, vol. 1, pp. 254–55 and 259–60.

21. Stanley Benson, "Conquering Sacrament," pp. 54–55.

22. Stanley Benson, "Conquering Sacrament," p. 55.

23. Stanley Benson, "Conquering Sacrament," p. 52.

24. Stanley Benson, "Conquering Sacrament," pp. 52–53.

25. Thus Bourguignon: "It is as if the exorcists had raised this issue in the minds of the people, and had thereby stimulated the development of the evil they were out to fight" (*Possession*, p. 53). Lewis traces the migration patterns of other possession behaviors in east Africa—for instance the *zar* possession that began with Ethiopian women and moved into neighboring Somaliland, Sudan, and Egypt ("Spirit Possession," p. 315). For *zar*, see especially Boddy, *Wombs*; and Sengers, *Women*.

26. Nevius, *Demon Possession*, p. 105.

27. Stanley Benson, "Conquering Sacrament," p. 52.

28. Stanley Benson, "Conquering Sacrament," p. 56. Donald Jacobs reports occurrences of Maasai exorcists in the late 1960s who are unable to cast out a certain "strange and highly malevolent demon" by traditional means. Noting that those already baptized by Christian missionaries were immune to this particular demon, many in the community were converted to Christianity "as a sort of immunization against attack" ("Possession," p. 183).

29. See above, chapter 2.

30. Bede, *HE* 4.27, p. 432.

31. Bede, *Epistola ad Ecgbertum Episcopum* 7: "Audiuimus enim, et fama est, quia multae uillae ac uiculi nostrae gentis in montibus sint inaccessis ac saltibus dumosis positi, ubi nunquam multis transeuntibus annis sit uisus antistes" (Indeed, we have heard—and it is well known—that many of the farms and villas of our people in the hills are inaccessible and

situated in wooded areas thick with thorny overgrowth, where the priest might not travel at all for a number of years; Plummer, *Venerabilis Baedae*, 1:140).

32. Bede, *HE* 2.15, p. 190.

33. Bede, *HE* 2.14, pp. 186–88.

34. *Council of Clofesho* 3 (Haddan and Stubbs, *Councils*, pp. 363–64).

35. *Vita Cuthberti* 1.7 (Colgrave, *Two Lives*, p. 72).

36. Tirechan, *Collectanea*: Bieler, *Patrician Texts*, pp. 122–66; Cogitosus, *Vita Brigidae*: PL 72: cols. 775–790D. Adomnan, *Vita Columbae*: Alan Orr Anderson and Marjorie Ogilvie Anderson, *Adomnan's Life*. Muirchu, *Vita Patricii*: Bieler, *Patrician Texts*, pp. 66–122. Other works which sometimes depict possession in Ireland (e.g., the *Vita Samsonis* 1.38 [Flobert, *La Vie Ancienne*, pp. 200–202]) are very difficult to date. For context and dating of early Irish hagiography, see Sharpe, *Medieval Irish Saints' Lives*.

37. The exorcizing of indwelling demons does not feature prominently in, for instance, the lives printed in Plummer, *Vitae Sanctorum Hiberniae*. Plummer cites only two examples specifically (clxxv, clxxx); one is the later text *Vita Fursei* 2.3, in which Fursey exorcizes a woman named Ermeneflad in the northern Gallic town of Arras (edited in Smedt and de Backer, *Acta Sanctorum Hiberniae*, p. 103). I have not found any possession references in seventh-century Irish materials which would be relevant for a background study of Anglo-Saxon spirituality in the late seventh and early eighth century.

38. There are references to St. Patrick performing exorcisms in fifth-century Ireland—for instance, in the *Annals of the Four Masters* (under the year 493; see O'Donovan, *Annals*, pp. 156–57)—but the *Annals* was compiled in the early seventeenth century, from sources now mostly lost. The earliest lives of Patrick—those from the seventh century, by Tirechan and Muirchu—do not make reference to exorcisms.

39. Jonas of Bobbio, *Vita Columbani* 39–41, 46, 49 (PL 87: cols. 1034A–1035D, 1037C, 1038D–1039A).

40. Blair, *Church*, pp. 26–27; Higham, *Rome*, pp. 97–98.

41. Blair, *Church*, p. 13.

42. Bede, *HE* 2.2, pp. 136–40; but see Stancliffe, "British Church," pp. 121–31.

43. Blair suggests tentatively these two may have "allowed more continuity of religious personnel and structures, when absorbing British territory in the 630s, than King Ecgfrith and St Wilfrid would do in the 670s" (*Church*, p. 30); see also p. 187.

44. Stancliffe, "British Church," p. 110.

45. Peter Hill, *Whithorn*, p. 18.

46. Stephen of Ripon, *Vita Wilfridi* 17 (Colgrave, *Wilfrid*, p. 36).

47. Blair, *Church*, p. 30.

48. Bede, *HE* 3.27, p. 312. On this plague and its effects throughout England, see Maddicott, "Plague," pp. 7–54.

49. Bede, *HE* 3.30, p. 322.

50. Yorke, "Reception," p. 164. The first suppression of pagan cults according to Bede was by Eorcenberht of Kent (r. 640–64; Bede, *HE* 3.8, p. 240–44).

51. There is only scant and imperfect evidence of possession being known to the Christianized Britons prior to the arrival of the Anglo-Saxons. The *Vita Samsonis* describes two cases of possession in southern Wales (chaps. 1.18–19 and 2.8 [Flobert, *La Vie Ancienne*, pp. 174–78, 250–54]), but this work was written in northern France perhaps several centuries later. Traditional composition dates range either in the early seventh century or the ninth century, but the most recent editor prefers the mid-eighth century (Flobert, *La Vie Ancienne*, p. 111).

52. None of the penitentials associated with Theodore of Tarsus are thought to be his own work. For the text cited here (by the *Discipulus Umbrensium* or "Disciple of the Northumbrians"; Finsterwalder's U in *Die Canones*), see Charles-Edwards, "Penitential," pp. 141–74. Charles-Edwards notes that by the late eighth century this text was "perhaps the most authoritative penitential even in Ireland" (162). Book 2 of this collection—not a penitential at all but a collection of canons—often traveled independently of book 1.

53. Theodore's Penitential, book 2 (Finsterwalder, *Die Canones*, p. 324).

54. For demonic instigation in suicide, see Nie, *Views*, pp. 233–34. Very little is known about suicide or the lack of it in Anglo-Saxon England; see, for instance, Toso, "And Then There Was Silence," pp. 237–42.

55. The item appears in only three of the ten manuscripts containing book 2 of the Penitential (Haddan and Stubbs, *Councils*, p. 198).

56. Surveying the literature for 488 societies from across the globe, Bourguignon found "possession beliefs" (in which spirits are thought to cause illness, without implying displacement of personality) in 360, or 74 percent (*Possession*, p. 31). "Possession trance" (displacement of personality) appeared in 251 societies, or 52 percent. Possession trance is lowest in Native American societies, and is associated more with societies that are sedentary, agricultural, more populous, and more hierarchically organized beyond the local level than societies without possession trance (*Possession*, pp. 42–45). For further breakdown of societies into trance and possession types, see Bourguignon, *Religion*, pp. 3–35, 321–39.

57. See Waxler, "Mental Illness," pp. 233–53.

58. Gregory of Tours, *Libri de virtutibus sancti Martini episcopi* (Krusch, *Miracula et opera*, pp. 134–211); and see above (chapter 1).

59. Einhard, *Translatio et miracula sanctorum Marcellini et Petri* (Waitz, *Translatio*, pp. 238–64). Possession stories appear sporadically at this point, and include three possession healings associated with St. Denis (ca. 835), nine associated with St. Philibert (ca. 837–38), and eventually twelve associated with St. Wandrille (ca. 886). For these tabulations, see figs. 5 and 6 in Lysaght, "Fleury," pp. 100–102.

60. Lapidge, *Cult*, p. 233. Adrevald's *Historia translationis Benedicti* is edited in PL 124: cols. 901A–909B, and in Lysaght, "Fleury."

61. Thomas of Monmouth, *Vita et passione S. Willelmi*: Jessopp and James, *Life*. William of Canterbury, *Miraculorum Gloriosi Martyris Thomae*: James Robertson, *Materials*, pp. 137–546. Benedict of Peterborough, *Miracula S. Thomae*: James Robertson, *Materials*, pp. 21–281. Ronald Finucane discusses these collections (*Miracles*, pp. 118–26), and more generally, the practice of miracle documentation at healing shrines throughout the later Middle Ages (*Miracles*).

62. *Translatio et miracula S. Swithuni*: Lapidge, *Cult*, pp. 252–332.

63. An invaluable overview of hagiographic activity and sources in Anglo-Saxon England is Lapidge and Love, "Latin Hagiography," pp. 203–325.

64. General mentions that demoniacs are healed: Felix, *Vita Guthlaci* 45 (Colgrave, *Felix's Life*, p. 138); *Vita Cuthberti* 1.7, 3.1, 4.18 (Colgrave, *Two Lives*, pp. 72, 94, 138); Bede, *HE* 1.17, 3.11, 4.19, pp. 56, 246, 396; Byrhtferth, *Vita Oswaldi* (Raine, *Historians*, p. 475).

65. The almost immediate attachment of exorcism miracles to the cult of Wulfstan after the conquest (see below) demonstrates the need for caution. Similarly, the *Miracula Ninie Episcopi*, a hexameter work from late eighth-century Whithorn, does not refer to any demoniac encounters associated with that saint; but by the twelfth century, the *Vita Niniani* (perhaps by Aelred of Rievaulx) states that in converting the Picts, Nynia set free those oppressed by demons ("oppressi a demone liberantur"; *Vita Niniani* 6 [Forbes, *Historians*, p. 147]). In addition to miracles retrospectively attributed to preconquest saints, fresh

possession accounts also begin to appear at this time, such as the demoniac Edwin during the reign of William I in *Liber Eliensis* 2.129 (Blake, *Liber Eliensis*, pp. 208–9).

66. Bede, *HE* 2.15, p. 188.

67. *Vita Cuthberti* 4.18 (Colgrave, *Two Lives*, p. 138).

68. *Vita Cuthberti* 3.1: "praesans et absens demoniacos sanauit, et alios uarios languores curauit" (he healed demoniacs both while present and absent, and cured various other weaknesses; Colgrave, *Two Lives*, p. 94).

69. E.g., the widow Kenswith (*Vita Cuthberti* 2.7), the priest Beta (4.3), and the monk Walhstod (4.12; and see also more general references in 2.2, 4.8).

70. *Vita Cuthberti* 4.17: "in praesenti anno factum est" (Colgrave, *Two Lives*, p. 136).

71. *Vita Cuthberti* 2.8 (Colgrave, *Two Lives*, pp. 90–92).

72. *Vita Cuthberti* 2.8 (Colgrave, *Two Lives*, p. 92).

73. *Vita Cuthberti* 4.15 (Colgrave, *Two Lives*, pp. 132–34).

74. Bede's prose *Vita* does include eight miracles not found in the anonymous *Vita*; two additional ones appear in the *Historia ecclesiastica* (4.31–32, pp. 444–48).

75. See, for instance, Berschin, "*Opus deliberatum ac perfectum*," pp. 95–102; Cavill, "Some Dynamics," pp. 1–20; and Stancliffe, "Cuthbert," pp. 21–44.

76. Thacker, "Bede's Ideal," pp. 130–53, 136–42.

77. *Vita Cuthberti* 2.8 (Colgrave, *Two Lives*, p. 92).

78. Bede, *Vita Cuthberti* 15 (Colgrave, *Two Lives*, p. 204).

79. Bede, *Vita Cuthberti* 15 (Colgrave, *Two Lives*, p. 206).

80. There are numerous references in the *HE* to saints or their relics healing a variety of ailments (e.g., 2.16, 3.2, 3.9, 3.17, 5.18), but only a few references to the healing of the possessed: 1.17, 3.11, 4.19.

81. Bede, *HE* 2.5, p. 150.

82. Bede, *HE* 2.5, p. 150; 1 Samuel 16:14 (*spiritus nequam*).

83. Bede, *HE* 3.11: "quae usque hodie superset" (who is still living at the present time; p. 246).

84. A meeting between Queen Osthryth and Abbess Æthelhild would probably have occurred around the turn of the eighth century, give or take ten years. Nothing is known of Æthelhild, but Osthryth, King Oswiu's third child with Eanflæd of Whitby, would have been born around 645, and presumably would not have lived much longer than her younger sister Ælfflæd, who died in 713.

85. Bede, *HE* 3.11, p. 248.

86. When Alcuin retells this episode in his *Versus de patribus regibus et Sanctis Euboricensis ecclesiae* some fifty years later, he adds the detail that the "restless demon" (uagus hostis) flees "into the empty air" (uacuas . . . in auras; Godman, *Alcuin*, p. 36).

87. Bede, *HE* 3.11, p. 248. The importance of the threshold is well established in magic and demonology, and is a tradition surviving in the Anglo-Saxon literary record. Pagan Anglo-Saxons buried animals at the doorways to timber buildings, and a human with a goat's skull and horns at his feet was found at the threshold of a Bernician timber hall from the early seventh century. Animal deposits at doorways continue to be attested into the twelfth and fourteenth centuries, perhaps (originally) as foundation sacrifices. The human skeleton at the east gate of the Bernician hall is aligned with the central axis of the hall. See Merrifield, *Archaeology*, pp. 116–18. A demon in Jerome's *Vita Hilarionis* enjoys power over an innocent virgin and makes her insane only so long as a tablet (*bred*, as translated in the *OE Martyrology*) engraved with spells remains secretly buried under the threshold of her house (*OE Martyrology*, October 21 [Kotzor, *Das altenglische*, 2:236–38]; Jerome, *Vita*

Hilarionis 21 [PL 23: col. 38A–39A]). An Old English charm from the *Leechbook* book 3 instructs a person afflicted by the "devil's temptation" (*feondes costunge*) to hang a certain herb over the door to the house and place it under the pillow (*Leechbook* 3.58: "Rudniolin hatte wyrt weaxeþ be yrnendum wætre. Gif þu þa on þe hafast, and under þinum heafodbolstre and ofer þines huses durum, ne mæg ðe deofol sceþþan, inne ne ute" ["Red stalk" (or "water pepper") is the name of an herb that grows near running water. If you keep it on you, and under your pillow and over the doors of your house, the devil cannot harm you, inside or out]; Cockayne, *Leechdoms*, vol. 2, p. 342). See also *Medicina de quadrupedibus* 1.7 (de Vriend, *Old English Herbarium, p.* 236).

88. Brown, *Cult*, pp. 106–27.

89. Bede could have obtained this detail from Augustine, *De civitate Dei* 15.23 (Dombart and Kalb, *Sancti Aurelii*, 2:108), or Isidore, *Etymologiarum libri XX* 8.103 (PL 82: col. 326B).

90. Bede, *In Lucae Evangelium expositio*, for Luke 8:30 (PL 92: col. 438B).

91. On the development of confession, see Lea, *History*; C. M. Roberts, *Treatise*, esp. pp. 88–89 for Bede.

92. Stephen of Ripon, *Vita Wilfridi* 39 (Colgrave, *Wilfrid*, p. 78). The traditional attribution of this text to Eddius Stephanus is no longer maintained.

93. Kurtz lines up thematic and verbal parallels between the *Vita Guthlaci* and Evagrius's *Vita Antonii* ("From St. Anthony," pp. 104–16), arguing that while Felix very obviously walks in Evagrius's footsteps, Felix is one of the few early medieval hagiographers to preserve the "psychological realism" of the demonic encounters of the *Vita Antonii* (111–12).

94. Felix, *Vita Guthlaci* 41 (Colgrave, *Felix's Life*, pp. 126–28).

95. Felix, *Vita Guthlaci* 41 (Colgrave, *Felix's Life*, p. 130).

96. See above, chapter 3.

97. Felix, *Vita Guthlaci* 42 (Colgrave, *Felix's Life*, pp. 130–32).

98. Felix is sometimes cited as a case study in uncritical hagiography (thus Kurtz, "From St. Anthony," and see especially Charles Jones, *Saints' Lives*, pp. 54–55). Jones believes that Felix stitched the story of Hwætred together from the anonymous *Vita Cuthberti* 4.15 and from Bede's *Vita Cutherberti* 41 ("the same stories appear in different guise," *Saints' Lives*, p. 74); but the stories are only roughly analogous and I cannot find verbal similarities of any note. For instance, the initial description of the demoniac in each of the three accounts in question runs as follows: Anonymous—"filium suum a demonio fatigatum uociferantem et lacrimantem, lacerantemque corpus suum" (Colgrave, *Two Lives*, p. 132); Bede—"puerum . . . atrocissimo demone uexari, ita ut sensu rationis funditus amisso clamaret, eiularet, et uel sua membra uel quicquid attingere posset, morsibus dilaniare niteretur" (Colgrave, *Two Lives*, p. 288); Felix—"quidam iuvenis . . . in tantum autem inmensa dementia vexabatur ita ut membra sua propria ligno, ferro, unguibus dentibusque, prout potuit, laniaret" (Colgrave, *Felix's Life*, pp. 126–28). Perhaps there is a verbal echo of Bede's *dilaniare* in Felix's *laniaret*, but this sort of parallel hardly seems to warrant Jones's charge. Felix's youth is a violent, ax-wielding killer, unlike the boy Cuthbert heals. Colgrave states that Felix's story of the possessed man Ecga being cured by Guthlac's belt is "reminiscent of, and perhaps based on" an episode in the *Vita Cuthberti* (*Felix's Life*, p. 189). In the episode he cites, Ælfflæd is stricken with a sort of paralysis, which is cured by a belt that Cuthbert sends her. The presence of a belt that heals and protects is the only similarity in the two stories. For further meditation on Felix's *Vita Guthlaci* and the range of its dependence on earlier authors, see Meaney, "Felix's Life," pp. 29–48.

99. Boniface, Letter 73 (Tangl, *Die Briefe*, p. 152).

100. Boniface, Letter 73 (Tangl, *Die Briefe*, p. 153).
101. Boniface, Letter 73 (Tangl, *Die Briefe*, p. 153).
102. Boniface, Letter 73 (Tangl, *Die Briefe*, p. 152).
103. Boniface, Letter 73 (Tangl, *Die Briefe*, p. 153).
104. See below, chapter 4.
105. *Vita Cuthberti* 2.8 (Colgrave, *Two Lives*, pp. 90–92).
106. Bede, *HE* 3.11, pp. 246–50.
107. Stephen of Ripon, *Vita Wilfridi* 39 (Colgrave, *Wilfrid*, p. 78).
108. *Vita Cuthberti* 4.15 (Colgrave, *Two Lives*, pp. 132–34).
109. Felix, *Vita Guthlaci* 41 (Colgrave, *Felix's Life*, pp. 126–30).
110. Bede, *HE* 2.5, p. 150.
111. Bede, *In Lucae Evangelium expositio* (PL 92: col. 438B).
112. Boniface, Letter 73 (Tangl, *Die Briefe*, p. 153).
113. Felix, *Vita Guthlaci*, p. 42 (Colgrave, *Felix's Life*, pp. 130–32).
114. Brown, *Cult*, pp. 86–105.
115. Bede, *HE* 3.11, p. 248.
116. Wallace-Hadrill, *Bede's Ecclesiastical History*, p. xxx, and see also p. 104.
117. *Vita Cuthberti* 4.15 (Colgrave, *Two Lives*, p. 132).
118. *Vita Cuthberti* 3.1 (Colgrave, *Two Lives*, p. 94).
119. Bede, *Vita Cuthberti* 16 (Colgrave, *Two Lives*, pp. 208–10).
120. Leofric item 2471 (Nicholas Orchard, *Leofric Missal*, 2:434).
121. Leofric item 2478 (Nicholas Orchard, *Leofric Missal*, 2:437).
122. Bede, *In Lucae Evangelium expositio*, for Luke 8:30 (PL 92: col. 438B).
123. Charles Jones believes that since Bede does not mention any miracle in his personal letters, miracles may largely be a convention of hagiography rather than a feature of Bede's perceived quotidian world (*Saints' Lives*, p. 54).
124. *Narratio* edited in Lapidge, *Cult*, pp. 372–550; *Vita Aethelwoldi* edited in Lapidge and Winterbottom, *Wulfstan*. On dating and authorship see Lapidge, *Cult*, pp. 336–41.
125. Lapidge argues for Ælfric as author (*Cult*, pp. 553–61).
126. Edited in Lapidge, "Metrical *Vita*." The date and provenance of the poem are both matters of conjecture (the manuscript is from the late eleventh century), but Lapidge makes a coherent case for the possible circumstances of its composition.
127. Edited in Stubbs, *Memorials*, pp. 3–52.
128. The *Vita Oswaldi* is edited in Raine, *Historians*; the *Vita Ecgwini* (or *Vita quorundum Anglo-Saxonum*) is edited in Giles, *Vita quorundum*, pp. 349–96. Byrhtferth may also be the author of the life of Alfred traditionally ascribed to Asser.
129. *Vita Iudoci* 1.401 (Lapidge, "Metrical *Vita*," p. 294); Byrhtferth, *Vita Oswaldi* (Raine, *Historians*, p. 475). The mention of miracles at the saint's tomb in the *Vita Iudoci* is a novel addition to the source text (the first prose *Vita Iudoci*), probably devised to assert the authenticity and potency of the relics of Iudoc at Winchester. Lapidge explains that in 977—probably shortly before the writing of this metrical vita—the monks of Saint-Josse claimed to have rediscovered the relics of Iudoc in northern France, relics which had otherwise resided at Winchester since 901 (pp. 267–68). If these suppositions are correct, then there is obvious political motive in embellishing the miracles at the saint's tomb. The prose *Vita Iudoci* is edited in Le Bourdellès, "Vie de St Josse," pp. 915–28.
130. For Gospel accounts, see Ælfric's Passion of Mark (Skeat, *Lives of Saints*, vol. 1, p. 320), his homily on "Memory of the Saints" (vol. 1, p. 346), *De auguriis* (vol. 1, p. 376–78), *Dominica ii in Quadragesima* (*Catholic Homilies* 2.8; Godden, *Second Series*, p. 68), and his

account of Abdon and Sennes (Skeat, *Lives of Saints*, vol. 2, p. 60). For early Christian sources, see his accounts of Apollinaris (vol. 1, pp. 476–78), Eugenia (vol. 1, p. 32), Sebastian (vol. 1, p. 140), Maur (vol. 1, pp. 158–60), Agnes (vol. 1, pp. 192 and 194), and Martin (vol. 2, pp. 252, 254, 256, 292–94), the *Depositio* of Martin (*Catholic Homilies* 2.34; Godden, *Second Series*, p. 293–94), Bartholomew (*Catholic Homilies* 1.31; Clemoes, *Catholic Homilies*, pp. 441 and 447), Thomas (Skeat, *Lives of Saints*, vol. 2, p. 414), Stephen the Protomartyr (*Catholic Homilies* 2.2; Godden, *Second Series*, p. 12), and Benedict (*Catholic Homilies* 2.11; Godden, *Second Series*, pp. 100 and 104–105).

131. In his *Lives of Saints*, Ælfric includes four English figures: Æthelthryth (Skeat, *Lives of Saints*, vol. 1, pp. 432–40), Swithun (vol. 1, pp. 440–70; and now Lapidge, *Cult*, pp. 590–608), Oswald (Skeat, *Lives of Saints*, vol. 2, pp. 124–42), and Edmund (vol. 2, pp. 314–34). Ælfric addresses the issue directly at one point in his life of Edmund: "Nis angelcynn bedæled drihtnes halgena. . . . Synd eac fela oðre on angel-cynne halgan þe fela wundra wyrcað" (Nor is England deprived of the saints of God. . . . There are also many other English saints who work many miracles; vol. 2, pp. 332–34).

132. Ælfric, *Passio Eadmundi* (Skeat, *Lives of Saints*, vol. 2, p. 332).

133. Ælfric, *Natale Sancti Swyðuni Episcopi*: "Þæt wæs þæra gymeleast (þe on life hine cuþon) þæt hi noldon awritan his weorc and drohtnunge þam toweardum mannum ðe his mihte ne cuðon . . . nu næs us his lif cuð" (it was careless for those who knew him in life not to write down his works and way of life for future generations who would not know of his power . . . now his life is unknown to us; Lapidge, *Cult*, p. 590).

134. Posthumous miracles: Swithun (Lapidge, *Cult*, pp. 590–608), Æthelthryth (Skeat, *Lives of Saints*, vol. 1, pp. 438–40), Oswald (vol. 2, pp. 136–42), Edmund (vol. 2, pp. 326–34).

135. Ælfric, *Dominica iiii post Pentecosten* (*Catholic Homilies* 1.24; Clemoes, *Catholic Homilies*, p. 375).

136. Ælfric, *In Ascensione Domini* (*Catholic Homilies* 1.21; Clemoes, *Catholic Homilies*, p. 351). See Godden's comments in *Introduction* (p. 172). The immediate source in Gregory is *Homily* 29 (PL 76: cols. 1215 B–C; see McCready, *Signs*, pp. 19, 30–32), but this is a recurring anxiety for Gregory: the apparent absence of contemporary miracles is the frame pretext of the entire *Dialogi* (Prologue 7–8; *Dialogues*, vol. 2, pp. 14–15). See also Augustine, *De civitate Dei* 22.8, for discussion of the fact that, to many of his contemporaries, miracles do not seem to occur anymore as they are said to in scripture (Dombart and Kalb, *Sancti Aurelii*, vol. 2, p. 566).

137. Ælfric, *Catholic Homilies* 1.21 (Clemoes, *Catholic Homilies*, p. 350).

138. Ælfric, *Catholic Homilies* 1.21 (Clemoes, *Catholic Homilies*, p. 351).

139. Godden, "Ælfric's Saints' Lives," pp. 83–100.

140. Ælfric, *Catholic Homilies* 1.21 (Clemoes, *Catholic Homilies*, p. 350). For Ælfric on the devil in general, see Locherbie-Cameron, "Ælfric's Devils," pp. 286–87; Jeffrey Burton Russell, *Lucifer*, pp. 151–54.

141. Ælfric, *Catholic Homilies* 2.13 (Godden, *Second Series*, 130).

142. Augustine, *In Iohannis Evangelium Tractatus* 43 (Willems, *In Iohannis Evangelium*, pp. 373–74); cf. Haymo, *Homily* 56 (PL 118: col. 329C). Ælfric frequently seems to provide a gloss or explanation when he mentions exorcists: see Pastoral Letters 1 and 2 (above, chapter 2), and his account of St. Martin in *Lives of Saints*: "exorcista, þæt we hatað halsigend þe ðe bebyt deoflum þæt hi of gedrehtum mannum faran" (*exorcista*, which we call "adjurer," because he commands devils to leave troubled people; Skeat, *Lives of Saints*, vol. 2, p. 228). The Old English translation of the *Rule of Chrodegang* likewise feels the need to gloss *exorcista* as well as *accolitus* (chap. 83): "Ne sceal nan accolitus, þæt is husolþen,

forsecgan nanne subdiacon, ne nan exorcista, þæt is halsere, forsecgan nanne accolitum, ne nan rædere forsecgan nanne halsere, ne nan duruweard nanne rædere mid nanre wrohte" (An acolyte—that is, the Eucharist attendant—must not speak before a subdeacon, nor must an exorcist—that is, adjurer—speak before an acolyte, nor a lector speak before an adjurer, nor a doorkeeper [speak before] a lector with reproach; Napier, *Old English Version*, p. 97).

143. For this homily, Godden notes, "Ælfric seems in his opening remarks to have the monks and clergy as much in mind as the laity" (*Introduction*, p. 466).

144. *Miracula Swithuni* 41 (Lapidge, *Cult*, p. 676).

145. Folcard, *Vita S. Johannis* 13 (Raine, *Historians*, p. 260); and see also chap. 12 ("dæmonem ab homine expulit").

146. Rampolla, "Mirror," pp. 99–102.

147. Rampolla, "Mirror," p. 109.

148. Thus Cuneo, *American Exorcism*, pp. 11–13, 270–81 (and for a different point of view, from a Catholic priest—for the unleashing of genuine demons on a pandemic scale following Vatican II—see p. 39). Cuneo concludes, "the practice of exorcism in contemporary America has also been deeply influenced by the popular entertainment industry. . . . During the mid-seventies, after decades of neglect, decades of near-invisibility, exorcism suddenly became a raging concern. Almost overnight, untold numbers of people were complaining of being afflicted by demons, and new exorcism ministries couldn't spring up fast enough to meet the soaring demand" (271). Alongside William Peter Blatty's novel *The Exorcist* (1971) and William Friedkin's film adaptation by the same name (late 1973), Malachi Martin's *Hostage to the Devil* (1976) was an important catalyst of this surge in possession beliefs. In 1975 an English translation quickly appeared (under the name *Possessed by Satan*) of Adolf Rodewyk's 1963 book *Die dämonische besessenheit* (Aschaffenburg: Paul Pattloch Verlag) explaining and defending, in popular terms, the Catholic Church's official position on possession and exorcism. For an Anglican counterpart, produced shortly before the outset of this rise in popular demonological beliefs and behaviors, see Petitpierre, *Exorcism*.

Chapter 4
Neurological and Behavioral Pathologies in the Early Middle Ages

"Now a certain contemplative man—an excellent person—has remarked that this phenomenon is due to the passion of vainglory and also to the influence of a demon who stimulates a specific site of the brain and thus agitates the cerebral circulation..."—Evagrius Ponticus, *Chapters on Prayer*[1]

NOT ALL DISSOCIATIVE STATES are pathological. Possession by divine forces is valorized as an important spiritual experience in many religious traditions, and appears in the Christian tradition through such phenomena as ecstatic communion, prophecy, and speaking in tongues. Pathological ("demonic") possession is distinguishable from a positive trance state by the presence of undue distress placed on either the subject or the surrounding community. The diagnosis can come either from the subject or—in case the subject does not acknowledge possession or demonic influence—from the community. Although in the late Middle Ages the problem of distinguishing demonic from divine possession had become acute, this was not yet a problem in the early Middle Ages. "Discernment" was by and large the private gift or practice within an individual of distinguishing good impulses from evil ones, not the public evaluation of prophetic or ecstatic claims on behalf of a member of the community. Certain core behaviors considered pathological and thus in need of treatment are shared by the early Middle Ages and the contemporary world (e.g., violent outbursts, excessive withdrawal, inability to perform social roles), and these can provide a point of potential contrast. This chapter focuses on some of the nonfunctional pathologies that likely formed the physiological core of possession behaviors in Anglo-Saxon and numerous other premodern societies. Though the behaviors are described here through the prism of secular medicine and psychiatry, within a number of religious communities many of these continue to be considered the work of demons.

Medieval energumens and their indwelling demons insist that they are distinct identities. Fragmentation of the self is the core of possession as it is currently understood, and is implicit in premodern models which visualize a separate entity to have taken over part or whole of an individual's personality or functioning. Where dissociation (the manifesting of distinct personalities or compartments of consciousness) is prevalent, fugue states can sometimes hide disparate elements of the personality from one another. The subject claims to be someone or something else and acts accordingly, and then has limited or no recollection of the event once the normal personality retakes control. Such dissociation (with or without loss of memory) must underlie any exorcism scene in which there is a dialogue between the exorcist and the indwelling demon.

Alongside dissociative behavior, muscle-control disorders regularly struck premoderns as cases of spirit possession. A demonic explanation for such disorders as epilepsy was not required, however—sometimes the evaluation remained purely physiological:

> Quedam in uicino quodam uico matrona morabatur, quam dira ualitudo que grece paralisis latine dissolutio membrorum dicitur inuaserat, inuasam miserabiliter detinebat, detentam intolerabiliter detorquebat. Hec nec manus ad os ducere, nec fronti crucem pingere, neque de loco cui assedisset per se ualebat exsurgere, sed eius ori seruientium manibus inferebatur edulium, ab eis erigebatur, ab eis deportabatur. Nam acerbissime huius passionis ex humorum frigiditate semper aut in toto corpore aut in parte accidentis cruciante seuitia, marcuerant membrorum compagines, totaque natura corrupta, inutile corpus manebat.[2]
>
> [There was a certain wife living in the vicinity, whom a fearful condition that is called "paralysis" in Greek and "loosening of the limbs" in Latin had taken over. Having been miserably seized thus, she was twisted intolerably. She could neither bring her hand to her mouth, nor trace the sign of the cross on her forehead, nor even get up from the place she was sitting by her own strength, but food was put in her mouth by the hands of servants, and by them she was lifted up, by them moved around. In this most bitter affliction, arising from the coldness of the humors—the torturous savagery always either befalling the whole body or just a part—the limbs atrophied together, the body remained useless, and its whole nature have been corrupted.]

Similarly, the anonymous *Life of Cuthbert* relates an account of a paralyzed boy (who is cured through Cuthbert's shoes), an account which fails to mention any presence of the demonic either before or after the cure.[3] When Bede retells the same story of the paralyzed boy, though he draws out the episode significantly, he continues to emphasize a medical interpretation rather than a spiritual one: he adds that the Greeks call the illness "paralysis" ("ea quam Greci paralisin vocant infirmitate").[4] Such scenes could have been read alternately as instances of demonic attack or as natural bodily dysfunction, without perceived contradiction. Paralysis could perhaps appear symptomatic of alternate agency (such as indwelling demons) because the inability to use limbs or muscles properly is not connected with externally visible trauma. Uncontrolled motions, jerking, and convulsions were even more understandably attributed to a foreign will or agent. An epileptic is presumed to be possessed in Bede's account of a visitor to Bardney Abbey.[5] In the anonymous Frankish *Life of Genovefa* (perhaps sixth century), a psalm singer "lanians proprius artus, quos mente captus esse alienus credebat" (tore his own limbs, which, because of his seized mind, he believed to be alien objects) during mass.[6] On other occasions an author is content with the medical diagnosis of "epilepsy," as in Gregory of Tours's *Life of the Fathers*:

> Phronimi igitur Agatensis episcopi famulus epilentici morbi accentu fatigabatur, ita ut plerumque cadens ac spumans, linguam suam propriis dentibus laceraret.[7]
>
> [The servant of Phronimus, bishop of Agde, had been plagued by a stroke of epileptic sickness, such that he would often fall to the ground, foaming at the mouth, and he would lacerate his tongue with his own teeth.]

In the twelfth-century *Book of the Foundation of St. Bartholomew's Church in London*, epilepsy (*fallynge evill*) is, according to physicians, a "syknes that compressith the ventriclis and the weys of the brayne" in one passage, while in the very next chapter a case of epilepsy is considered to be directly caused by the devil ("malignyng enemy, spirite of malice").[8] Both spiritual and medical models were available throughout the Middle Ages, and were not necessarily exclusive. Though our early medieval sources predominately prefer demonic to physiological explanations, this may reflect the clerical nature of the written record. We should be cautious about presuming that all of society attributed as much pathology to demons as ecclesiastical authors did.

It would be impossible to enumerate all the possible conditions that could have struck the medieval observer as demonic (in a religious worldview this might include any state or condition—medical or otherwise—perceived as undesirable).[9] Despite the theoretical difficulties in mapping current pathology categories onto medieval possession accounts, it is nonetheless a necessary step in visualizing and understanding what was happening that so captivated the attention of witnesses. Barring the religious explanation itself—that invisible demons exist and controlled people's behavior—the secular medical explanation (though imperfect and under continuous revision) is a powerful interpretive tool and has the greatest claim to cross-cultural objectivity. It is equally important to tread with caution, of course, and to determine as thoroughly as possible whether or not a given category is applicable to other cultures, modern or ancient. Borderline personality disorder, for instance, may seem to reflect the volatile spontaneity of possession, culminating at times in violence; but the condition as currently understood is too rooted in the stresses of the modern world to be safely applied to past eras.[10] For some disorders (for example, epilepsy), a determination is easy enough, while for psychiatric disorders such as dissociative identity disorder and post-traumatic stress disorder, modern clinical and experimental findings can only be a starting point in potentially understanding early medieval accounts, and behaviors must be interpreted in light of differing cultural contexts.

On the whole there is little evidence for a flourishing culture of possession and exorcism in Anglo-Saxon England, in the sense of dissociating subjects assuming the persona of a demon. There is no question, however, that some people from time to time suffered from the sorts of neurological conditions that could have been perceived by the community as demon possession. It may be useful to ascertain what some of these conditions were and what they may have looked like, in trying to reconstruct the broader social landscape, outside the monastery walls in which Old English literature was promulgated. My final chapter thus presents a redescription of demon possession in modern clinical terms, geared especially toward the descriptions of demoniacs in early medieval sources. I will focus especially on those organic conditions that form the bedrock of possession behaviors, disorders rooted most securely in neuropathology. In fact, these provide us with the majority of symptoms described in the early Middle Ages as demon possession. While some modern diagnoses such as borderline personality disorder and schizophrenia that we might be tempted to read back into the Middle Ages turn out to have problematic cross-cultural profiles, epilepsy, Tourette's Syndrome (and related disorders), and post-traumatic stress disorder prove more fruitful lines of inquiry. My hope is that by applying what we know now about these conditions' symptoms and how they can affect functioning, we can construct a more nuanced understanding of early medieval possession, as experienced both by the subject and the community.

Together these conditions provide us with a rough yet plausible overview, in varying proportions, of the range of behaviors that confronted the saint and exorcist. I make every attempt to determine cross-cultural applicability for these neurological conditions. This overview is meant to be neither exhaustive nor definitive: it is a work in progress, necessarily "trapped" by seeing through the lens of the current generation of medical understanding. This exercise can, however, help us focus on some of the conditions that explain more unusual behaviors and that raise some of the more interesting questions about identity and community.

Epilepsy

Epilepsy refers not to a specific disease (i.e., a particular pathogen), but to a complex of neurochemical events that can vary greatly among individuals. The condition is marked by recurring cerebral seizures, general or localized, arising from a number of possible causes (an isolated seizure, from whatever cause, is by definition not epileptic).[11] A seizure is a brief, paroxysmal neuronal discharge in the brain, whose outward manifestation(s) depend on which part(s) of the brain are affected. The excessive, simultaneous discharge of neurons usually begins in the cerebral cortex (including the hippocampus) or the amygdala, but can then spread to any structure in the central nervous system. The term "epilepsy" is reserved for those recurring seizures not directly caused by an identifiable proximate insult or metabolic disorder. Despite unparalleled advances in the twentieth and twenty-first centuries, the electrical and chemical mechanisms of epilepsy are not well understood. Most anticonvulsants currently in use were discovered by accident, and researchers are not always in agreement on exactly how they work.

Epilepsy has a fascinating and unusually well-documented history. It was believed at various times and places to be divine as well as demonic, hence its popular Greek designation, "the sacred disease."[12] It is possible epilepsy was among the conditions treated in prehistory by trepanation, a practice still attested in Anglo-Saxon England.[13] There are treatises or chapters of treatises from very early times devoted entirely to epilepsy. The Babylonian medical treatise *Sakikku* attributes epilepsy to a "demon or departed spirit."[14] The Greeks did not necessarily share such a belief in demons as intrusive disease agents, though they did believe that someone subject to seizures was inspired by a *daimon* in some sense and was thus imbued with a prophetic spirit. The earliest Greek treatment of the subject (the Hippocratic treatise *On the Sacred Disease*, ca. 400 BCE) is the work of a professional physician who attacks this popular belief, arguing that epilepsy is simply a natural disease like any other.[15] Connections have often been observed (or invented) between epilepsy and personalities with exceptional artistic or spiritual acumen. As a result, epilepsy has been ascribed quite loosely to historical figures of genius or note, including Alfred the Great.[16]

Gregory of Tours offers a provocative description of epilepsy from Merovingian Gaul, including a difference in terminology used by professional physicians and rustics:

> Quidam ex Viennensi terreturio Landulfus nomine graviter a lunatici daemonii infestatione vexabatur, ita ut plerumque ab hoste se vallari putans in terram corrueret, cruentasque ex ore spumas emittens, tamquam mortuus habebatur. Quod genus morbi ephilenticum peritorum medicorum vocitavit auctoritas; rustici vero cadivum dixere, pro eo quod caderet.[17]
>
> [A certain man named Landulf from the province of Vienne was greatly troubled by an indwelling "lunatic" demon. He would often fall to the ground as though defending himself against an enemy, emitting bloody spittle from his mouth. He was thought to be a dead man. The authority of expert doctors called this type of illness "epilepsy;" but the country people said it was "falling sickness," because he would fall down.]

("Lunacy" refers here to periodicity, and is not necessarily linked with lunar cycles.) The observers perceived the subject to be "defending himself against an enemy," which raises interesting questions about the interiority/exteriority of the putative demon assaulting the man. It is probably the essence of the "demon" as a construct that occupies an ambivalent, liminal position at the cusp of interior and exterior.

There is significant evidence for epilepsy and seizure disorders in Anglo-Saxon England. The Antwerp-London Glossary associates two vernacular terms with *epilepsia*: *fylle-seoc* and *bræc-coðu*.[18] Bede's account of the man at Bardney Abbey cured by Oswald's relics is very likely a case: "subito a diabolo arreptus clamare, dentibus frendere, spumare et diuersis motibus coepit membra torquere" (suddenly he was seized by the devil and began to cry out, gnash his teeth, foam at the mouth, and fling his limbs about).[19] Fits of some sort that include gnashing teeth (*frendens dentibus*) also afflict Hildmær's wife in the anonymous *Life of Cuthbert*.[20] Items in the medical recipes—found in, for example, the *Lacnunga Book* or the *Leechbook*—are sometimes translated as being against "seizures" in modern translations, though these interpretations are not certain.[21] Wilfrid Bonser cites as "obviously a case of epilepsy" a miraculous cure appearing in the *Life of Wilfrid* in which a reeve's wife becomes rigid and cold, closes her eyes, and foams at the mouth.[22] Beyond these symptomatic similarities, however, it is important to bear in mind that although we now think of epilepsy as a specific cluster of symptoms, medieval references to *epilepticos* or the *fellseoc* included a wide range of nervous disorders causing convulsions, trembling, or seizure (in the same way that *leprosus* referred to much more than the specific disease caused by *Mycobacterium leprae*). Thus the Northumbrian missionary Willibrord, who converted the Frisians and founded the monastery of Echternach, went on to become one of the patron saints of epilepsy (along with St. Valentine), after Echternach became associated with deliverance from a "dancing mania" of the later Middle Ages.[23]

The word "epilepsy" itself means "seized upon," referring to the patient's loss of motor control. "Generalized" seizures affect the entire brain, while "partial" seizures are restricted to a localized region. Seizures can be so mild that even the subject is unaware of the event, or so extreme that the subject loses consciousness and suffers extensive cerebral and/or motor dysfunction. Aside from well-known motor convulsions such as jerking or twitching, seizures can manifest themselves in a variety of behaviors—for example, blank stares, cessation of bodily motion, sweating, tingling sensations, or hearing buzzing sounds. Tonic-clonic seizures (generalized seizures formerly known as grand mal) provide a more dramatic scenario: the patient typically loses consciousness, falls to the ground, lies rigid for a minute, and then convulses for two to three minutes. The patient may discharge the bladder or bowels, or bite the tongue or lips, and after the episode may have no recollection of the attack. The lack of voluntary motor function combined with a lack of recollection could lend support to the belief that another will has taken over the body. Most impressively, not all seizure-induced automatisms (unwilled motor actions) are random jerkings: seizures can occasionally result in semi-purposive activity, such as undressing, searching for something, wandering, or beginning to cook a meal. These automatisms usually last under five minutes, and the patient usually has complete amnesia of the episode.[24] To onlookers in the Middle Ages, such an episode would have appeared uncanny and inexplicable, and an indwelling, intelligent agent such as a demon would no doubt have provided a natural and satisfying explanation.

There are experiential facets of seizures which may also have caused the appearance of an alternate entity inhabiting a person, such as dysphasia (impairment in speaking or understanding speech), déjà vu, and jamais vu (the impression that a familiar sensation is novel). When seizures occur in the temporal lobe (limbic system seizures), visual, auditory, and olfactory hallucinations can result. For example, the sufferer may perceive people or objects drawn from past experience, in hallucinations of varying complexity from flashing lights to structured scenes.[25] In temporal lobe seizures the patient may furthermore experience acute but intense fear, causing the patient to run in fright spontaneously or cower under the bed.[26] Thus a medieval epileptic may on occasion have acted as though an invisible person or object were present.

Seizure-induced hallucinations can sometimes assume a formidable array of demonic appearances. Caelius Aurelianus (the fifth-century Latin translator of Soranus) mentions visions "araneorum cassibus aut nubibus tenuissimis similia, aut parvulis volantum animalibus ut sunt culices" (like spider webs or very thin clouds, or small winged animals like gnats) as possible hallucinations from epilepsy.[27] Though that physician treats the condition as a purely medical phenomenon (in true Hippocratic tradition) and does not entertain the possibility of demon possession, his description is certainly reminiscent of the tiny winged demons sometimes surrounding a sufferer in medieval manuscript illustrations.[28] The *Charaka Samhita*, a principal text of the Ayurvedic tradition, characterizes the hallucinations of epilepsy (*Apasmāra*) as the condition "in which the patient believes that he is pursued by a black or red complexioned creature and becomes insensible as soon as the creature touches him."[29] Olfactory hallucinations in partial seizures are usually unpleasant; patients describe the smells as resembling burnt onions, excreta, or simply as "indescribable but horrible."[30] Gustatory hallucinations may be pleasant, but are often described as "metallic."[31]

Most epileptic attacks are not nearly as severe or dramatic as those I have described. I have only drawn attention to some of the possible behavioral and physiological manifestations of epilepsy that may have occasionally given the appearance of a conscious, foreign, indwelling entity. From its unmistakable characteristics, epilepsy is easily recognizable as a condition that has consistently afflicted humankind throughout the period of written records, and one that has both awed and frightened observers. It has also proven among the most intractable of disorders to treat medically, until the accidental discovery of bromide (the first anticonvulsant) in 1857. Modern commentators often criticize former ages for branding epileptics as demoniacs, but the condition is highly irregular in its manifestations and extremely unresponsive to traditional therapeutic and pharmacological cures.

Given its perceived association with an indwelling spirit, epilepsy has long been treated in premodern cultures with exorcism and other ritual responses. An especially wide range of charms and amulets are associated with such convulsive disorders in medieval Europe and, indeed, throughout the world. Medieval attempts to counter seizures with amulets or prayer would have done little to regulate brain chemistry, but, as Brian Murdoch argues, "the unconscious, possibly foaming patient would be back to normal within the time that it takes to repeat a charm and some prayers perhaps three times."[32] Additionally, the most common herbal responses in Anglo-Saxon England (lupine) and medieval Europe more generally (peony) may have lowered seizure threshold or provided a buffer against the full extent of potential neurologic effects, although it is hard to imagine this could be counted upon to regularly offer relief.[33] The seizures would have played themselves out naturally in any event, and this would give the impression of effective treatment.

Personality Disorders

Personality disorders are sensitive to cultural factors, perhaps more than any other medical condition.[34] Modern categories implicit in diagnoses of bipolar disorder, dissociative identity disorder, or post-traumatic stress disorder arguably rely on a Western, post-Enlightenment concept of the "self." Each culture evolves a construct of the self differently, and an internal negotiation of one individual's integration of moods, beliefs, and personality states may not be perceived as such by observers from another time and place.[35] Only an immediate circle of friends and family, in concert with communal traditions as a whole, can ultimately decide when a person is no longer acting like him- or herself. Laurence Kirmayer writes, "Cultures differ in their tolerance for gaps in narratives, unmotivated events, happenings attributed to extrinsic agencies, and the radical shifts in perspective that accompany shifts in states of mind."[36] A strong insistence on the individual as monadic entity, for instance, may be a fairly recent, Euro-American trend, and other cultures may more readily allow a fluidity in the boundaries of the self. In that sense, the theoretical problems inherent in interpreting historical societies are similar in many ways to those inherent in interpreting any foreign culture.

The shifting categories of contemporary psychiatry are clumsy, controversial, and in a state of continual revision—but they are not arbitrary. Joel Paris observes that there is growing evidence for a stable core of "reaction patterns" to distress, and that culture mediates primarily its expression.[37] Underlying biological processes are undeniable, though, however important the role of culture is in their interpretation: "biological correlates of personality disorders may provide an empirical basis to the notion of biological predispositions to psychological functions."[38] Recent successes in pharmacological treatment and predictive epidemiology support a cross-cultural interpretation for many of the more pronounced of these conditions: "Many professionals would argue that normal personality traits and personality disorder symptoms ultimately have a biological, mostly genetic basis."[39]

Modern psychiatry has identified a range of personality and mood disorders, but for the most part these bear only a superficial resemblance to medieval portrayals of demon possession.[40] Though it is easy to recognize isolated elements of paranoid, antisocial, narcissistic, schizoid, and histrionic personalities in the behaviors appearing in early narratives, people in the Middle Ages did not attribute most behavioral and emotional excesses that arose naturally in everyday life to supernatural intrusion. Wild mood swings, maladjusted social relationships, contrarian impulses, and introverted phases are surely part of the human condition, and have been present to varying degrees in every society, in any age. The taxonomy of psychiatric disorders is in a perpetual state of revision, especially as the international community strives to standardize terminology and diagnostic guidelines. Various psychiatric manuals such as the *Diagnostic and Statistical Manual of Mental Disorders* (DSM) in the US and the *International Classification of Diseases* (ICD) in the UK and elsewhere variously subdivide overlapping disorders. Even within a single society, various communities recognize and tolerate varying degrees of eccentric behavior, only the extremes of which warrant such diagnostic labels as "possessed" (in religious parlance) or "psychotic" (in a secular perspective). Nonetheless, the labels of contemporary psychiatry are helpful because they are our labels: they form a necessary facet of the prism through which the past is refracted to us.

Depression

Clinical depression has captivated the popular imagination over the past several decades, in parallel with significant advances in therapeutic options for treatment. Depressed individuals suffer prolonged periods of either sadness or emptiness (lack of any emotion), with diminished pleasure in the normal activities of life. They may also lose weight or suffer sleep disorders. They might report feelings of worthlessness, excessive guilt, or an inability to concentrate. Finally, they may dwell excessively on death or on thoughts of suicide.[41] Depression is more prominent in women than men; a study by the APA estimated lifetime risk for major depressive disorder at 5–12% for men and 10–25% for women.[42] The risk may increase with childhood adversity, such as sexual abuse, severe physical abuse, or neglect.[43] A cross-cultural study found that rates of depression were on the rise globally: earlier age of onset and increased severity of depressive symptoms were found over time in cohorts from North America, Puerto Rico, Western Europe, the Middle East, Asia, and the Pacific Rim.[44] Such rapid fluctuations should alert us to the sensitivity of this condition to social and cultural factors.[45] Genetic factors seem to play some role in predisposing an individual to major depression, but the manifestation is heavily reliant on neurochemical and psychosocial variables. Decreased levels of cerebrospinal fluid 5-HIAA, the principal metabolite of serotonin, has been consistently found in depressed individuals who have committed suicide.[46] A problem with serotonin regulation is thus strongly implicated in depressive systems, and the most commonly prescribed antidepressants in the United States (such as Paxil, Prozac, and Zoloft) are selective serotinin reuptake inhibitors. Successful advents in the pharmacological treatment of depression have renewed attention to the potentially neurochemical basis of the condition. When depression is combined simultaneously or alternating with extended periods of mania (inflated self-esteem, grandiose thoughts, decreased need for sleep, racing thoughts, dangerous excesses in pleasurable but risky behavior), the person is instead diagnosed as bipolar (formerly "manic-depressive").[47] John Cassian offers an intriguing analogue for contemplation, drawn from a monastic setting:

> Hic igitur beatus Danihel inquirentibus nobis, cur interdum residentes in cellula tanta alacritate cordis cum ineffabili quodam gaudio et exuberantia sacratissimorum sensuum repleremur . . . oratio quoque pura emitteretur ac prompta et mens plena spiritalibus fructibus preces suas efficaces ac leues etiam per soporem supplicans ad deum peruenire sentiret, ac rursum nullis exsistentibus causis tanto subito repleremur angore et inrationabili quadam maestitia premeremur, ut non solum nosmet ipsos huiusmodi sensibus arescere sentiremus, uerum etiam horreret cella, sorderet lectio, ipsa quoque instabilis ac nutabunda et quodammodo ebria emitteretur oratio. . . .[48]
>
> [Then we enquired of the holy Daniel, why sometimes, residing in our cells, we are filled with great cheerfulness of heart along with a certain indescribable joy and overflowing of the holiest feelings . . . and pure prayer comes forth unhesitatingly and with a mind filled with spiritual enjoyment, and even the one praying in sleep senses that his prayers reach God readily and lightly; but then on the other hand, we might suddenly and powerfully be filled with anguish and overwhelmed by a certain irrational sorrow, for no reason at all, such that we would feel that not only we ourselves were languishing under these feelings, but even the cell itself became dreadful, our readings were despicable, and our praying itself—as though we were intoxicated—would come forth unsteadily and with doubt. . . .]

This could well represent an insight into the strictures of monasticism, though, rather than a chemical imbalance. The spectrum of moods which in many occupations and forms of life are readily accepted as normal become exaggerated in a rigorous discipline of "prayer without ceasing," and in which many ascetics are known to have asked impossible things of themselves. Anglo-Saxon men of the cloth—just as their Mediterranean antecedents—struggled continuously with deciding when the extremes of asceticism became "pathological" (articulated in the Middle Ages as inspirations coming from the devil rather than from God).[49]

Melancholy served an important place in classical, late medieval, and Renaissance medicine as one of the four humors in the Hippocratic model of human physiology. In early medieval northern Europe, though, the humoral theory was greatly atrophied, and indeed throughout Latin Christendom it survived in largely simplified forms prior to the rise of Salernitan and then scholastic medicine. Some Mediterranean and Byzantine authors continued to actively employ and build on humoral theory, such as Alexander of Tralles in the sixth century and Paul of Aegina in the seventh. A Latin translation of Alexander of Tralles's twelve books on medicine became an important staple of European medicine for several centuries. Stanley Jackson summarizes the wide range of emotional states implicit in Alexander's understanding of melancholy:

> the euphoric, the rageful, the sluggish and withdrawn, the fearful, the suicidal, and the homicidal . . . it is clear that he included under the rubric of melancholia a much more extensive group of types of madness than did most medical writers on this subject.[50]

Although the humoral theory of medicine was never thoroughly understood or integrated into Anglo-Saxon medicine, some awareness of "black bile" does appear in the glosses and in Byrhtferth's *Enchiridion*, and it also receives some discussion in the late *Ramsey Scientific Compendium*.[51] In glosses (from Aldhelm's *De virginitate*) found in BL Cleopatra A.III *melancholia* is translated as *ðæs sweartan galgan* in one place and a little later as *gealla*.[52] In both places the term glosses a passage from Aldhelm's account of Athanasius, when a prostitute hired to bear false testimony against him instead finds herself vomiting up "fetidam melancholiae nauseam" (the fetid retch of black bile).[53] In such occurrences melancholy is hardly more than a poison or ichor—there is little awareness of its role as a natural and necessary fluid within the body's humoral balance.

Depression was by and large demonized only in a very specific context in the early Middle Ages: the sin of *acedia* (glossed as *biternes* in BL Cleopatra A.III).[54] Evagrius Ponticus and John Cassian brought wide attention to this mood or affliction of the soul as being a particular danger for monks and hermits. In the beginning *acedia* was a form of "spiritual sloth" particular to ascetics—it represented a wavering or uncertainty in the commitment to leave friends, family, commerce, and the world to go pray unceasingly to God in the desert. It could also manifest in particular moments of boredom during offices or prayer, or in moments of distaste for work. Accoring to Cassian's *Institutes*, *acedia* is

> taedium siue anxietatem cordis . . . adfinis haec tristitiae . . . denique nonnulli senum hunc esse pronuntiant meridianum daemonem, qui in psalmo nonagensimo nuncupatur. . . . Qui cum miserabilem obsederit mentem, horrorem loci, cellae fastidium, fratrum quoque, qui cum eo uel eminus commorantur, tamquam neglegentium ac minus spiritalium aspernationem gignit atque contemptum. Ad omne quoque opus, quod intra saepta sui cubilis est, facit desidem et inertem.[55]
>
> [weariness or anxiety of heart . . . not far from dejection . . . some of the fathers speak of this as the "mid-day demon," which is mentioned in the ninetieth Psalm. . . . When it takes control of a pitiable mind, it gives rise to dread of the place, a loathing of the cell, and also disdain and contempt of the brothers who live either close to him or distant, as though they were careless and without spirituality. For whatever kind of work there is to do within the walls of his cell, it makes him idle and lethargic.]

Evagrius is among those who explicitly demonize *acedia* as the "midday demon" (*daemonio meridiano*) from Psalm 90. The state makes the sun seem to crawl in the sky or stand still, and makes the day seem 50 hours long.[56] The demons, of course, would like nothing better than for the ascetic to give up and return to secular life. *Acedia* was also linked with *desperatio* (despair); again, this might conceivably rise to the level of perceived demonic influence if it results in suicide.

Acedia was less familiar in Anglo-Saxon England than in earlier monastic sources, because Gregory the Great dropped it from his list of seven sins (by subsuming it under *tristitia*)—but it still worked itself into lists of sins on occasion.[57] Homily 3 in the Vercelli Book lists both *tristitia* and *acedia*, in Old English as *unrotnes* and *sleacmodnes*, while counting them together as a single sin.[58] Ælfric includes some discussion of both *tristitia* (*unrotnys*) and *acedia* (*asolcennys* or *æmelnys*) in his homily for the middle Sunday in Lent:

> Se fifta leahtor is unrotnys ðissere worulde, þæt se man geunrotsige ongean god for ungelimpum ðises andwerdan lifes. Of ðam bið acenned yfelnys and wacmodnys, heortan biternys and his sylfes orwennys. Twa unrotnyssa sind: an is ðeos derigendlice, oðer is halwendlic, þæt gehwa for his synnum unrotsyge mid soðre dædbote. Se sixta heafod-leahtor is asolcennys oððe æmelnys. Se leahtor deð þæt ðam men ne lyst nan ðing to gode gedon, ac gæð him asolcen fram ælcere dugeðe. Nis se leahter pleolic geðuht, ac he gebrincð swa ðeah ðone mann to micclum yfele. He acenð idelnysse and slapolnysse, gemagnysse and wordlunge, worunge and fyrwitnysse.[59]
>
> [The fifth sin is unhappiness with this world, when a man is unhappy with God for the misfortunes of this present life. From this is born wickedness and faintheartedness, bitterness of heart and despair for himself. There are two types of sadness: one is this noxious sort, the other is salutary, when someone is unhappy with his sins in sincere

> repentance. The sixth deadly sin is sloth or slackness. This sin makes it so that a person has no pleasure in doing anything good, but he turns idly from everything seemly. This sin is not thought dangerous, but it does nevertheless bring a person to great wickedness. It gives rise to idleness and sleepiness, impudence and gossip, wandering and curiosity.]

It is hard to know how clinically to read such homiletic treatments of behavioral patterns.[60] The detail that "men ne lyst nan ðing to gode gedon" (a person has no pleasure in doing anything good) is strikingly reminiscent of the common claim among people with depression that they can find no joy in the normal pleasures of life.[61] Nonetheless, by the end of the passage Ælfric seems to have in mind restless students or monks pursuing normal signs of boredom, more than depressed people on verge of suicide.[62] The classical construct "melancholy" is of limited application to understanding the Anglo-Saxons' own perception of their disease states.

Our modern understanding of "depression" (a term which came into wide use in the eighteenth century) is also of limited application to Anglo-Saxon pathologies, not because we can be sure that it didn't exist in some form or other but because introverted and withdrawn behavior was not by itself demonized. Lethargy, inattention, apathy, and sadness do not appear as symptoms in those recipes linked with demonic influence in the medical books, and the behaviors are not indicated as symptoms in the narrative accounts of demoniacs brought forth for healing. On the contrary: it is the excesses of rage and violence that stand out as requiring a demonic explanation (perhaps corresponding, in some instances, to the "manic" phase of bipolar disorder). In the survey of glosses and medical literature above (chapter 2), demonic illness was associated primarily with anger and violence (*wuhunga*, "rage, fury, madness"; *repnes*, "cruelty, harshness"; *hatheortnessa*, "rage, anger, passion") and remained clustered around Latin concepts of excess energy or passion (*bacharis*, *furia*, *freneticus*, *lymphaticus*). One imagines that only when depression reached the level of self-violence or suicide would demonic forces be implicated (suicide and demon possession are linked in the Anglo-Saxon penitential tradition—see above, chapter 2)—though this is not necessarily the case even for later medieval England.[63] Levels of depression in the modern West were on the rise in the twentieth century, and we may have a disproportionate sense of its historical prevalence or profile. Stressors such as the breakdown of social and religious support structures and changes in eating, sleeping, and work habits may contribute to contemporary depression. There are demographic differences that also present problems: records from twelfth- to fourteenth-century England (none are available for Anglo-Saxon England directly) indicate men were committing suicide almost twice as often as women, a metric that does not strongly support comparisons with depression as it is currently known.[64] Doubtlessly, cultural factors (such as cultural attitudes toward suicide and violence, the relationship of martial prowess to ideas of masculinity, etc.) affected manifestations of depression as well as levels of suicide. On the whole, however, if depression (or early analogues of it) afflicted individuals to the point of social dysfunction and ongoing personal unhappiness in Anglo-Saxon England, this was not strongly equated with the demonic, and was never explicitly equated with "demon possession." In their brooding internal meditations, the implied narrators of *The Wanderer*, *The Wife's Lament*, *The Seafarer*, and other elegies seek consolation through further meditation on God's broader promise of salvation, or through (one imagines) the cathartic act of poetic expression itself, and are not portrayed as needing exorcism.

Impulse Control Disorders and Inhibition Breakdown

Various obsessive-compulsive, phobic, panic, and anxiety disorders (formerly known collectively as "neuroses") can produce behaviors reminiscent of possession symptoms, but all of these are subject to degrees of severity. The *Vita Gildae* (ca. perhaps the eighth century), by an anonymous monk of Ruys, Brittany, portrays a robber who has lost his mind after killing a man and who goes about naked after rending his own clothes. Rending clothes and going about naked is something of a literary motif (the medieval "wild man" is a well-known trope), but the subsequent detail is quite particular:

> Huic si quis pro misericordia aliquod indumentum porrexisset, ille, si forte sub arbore sedisset vel in quolibet loco, non discedebat, donec ipsum indumentum omnino discidisset. Et si quidem laneum vel lineum fuisset, in ipso loco diffilabat eum, si vero pelliceum, et ipsum ad nihilum redigebat.[65]
>
> [If, out of pity, someone offered him some garment—whether he happened to be sitting under a tree, or wherever—he would not leave until he had completely cut that garment into pieces. If it was woolen or linen, he would unthread it in that very place; if it was made of hide, just the same, he would reduce it to nothing.]

Not being able to leave the spot until a garment is completely cut into pieces is a novel image of compulsive fixation. This, along with other evident self-destructive impulses, apparently impel the author to attribute this behavior to demonic possession—"correptus a daemonio" (seized by a demon).[66]

While obsessive-compulsive behavior by itself should rarely escalate to such dysfunctional levels as to invite a diagnosis of possession, it forms part of a spectrum which can certainly exhibit extremes. Perhaps the compulsive behavior most reminiscent of demoniac behavior is Tourette's Syndrome (TS).[67] The inexplicable muscle movements and sudden, loud vocalizations (collectively known as tics), especially in swearing and in articulating socially or politically subversive thoughts, can help illuminate some of the most opaque facets of demon possession in the Middle Ages. Even without the swearing, TS would present a disturbing challenge to populations unaware of the workings of the central nervous system, and the indwelling of a foreign spirit would adequately account for the observed symptoms. Given the cross-cultural universality of TS, it is chilling to read such an account as the following, retrospectively imagining something similar occurring in a small early medieval village:

> At age 17, Abe's parents brought him for evaluation tied to a chair to prevent his horrible, self-injurious behavior. He lurched forward, banged his head, threw whatever came to reach, yelled and cursed. At his worst, he was tied to a bed or allowed to simply thrash about for hours. His mind and body were trapped by rituals of touching one part of the body and then another, repeating, jerking, calling out. His eyes would be magnetically attracted to particular patterns, especially intersecting lines and squares, from which he could not disengage. For an hour or two, he would sit in frozen concentration, moving his eyes from one corner to another of the pattern, unable to detach. He would become drenched with sweat and finally would be able to pull himself back by a force of great will when he felt, for some reason, that he had done the pattern "just right" and "correctly." He had "crazy" ideas that he had to hold himself back from. Between paroxysms of tics and compulsions, he begged for help.[68]

John Berecz explains that TS subjects "often appear behaviorally 'possessed,' and if demonology were a currently popular paradigm . . . people with compulsive disorders would be prime candidates for dunking stools, trephinations, and a variety of 'cures' designed to drive out the demons within."[69]

In the early twentieth century the outbursts of swearing commonly associated with TS lent fuel to psychoanalytic schools of thought that considered TS the expression of suppressed primal rage, or the reverberations of childhood traumas. The school of Freudian psychoanalysis prevalent in the first half of the century distracted attention from the organic features of TS, focusing instead on family dynamics and developmental emotional instability. Unfortunately, this often led to accusations of bad parenting and counterproductive therapies attempting to decondition patients. The same breakthrough in neuroleptics that redefined professional opinions of schizophrenia also revived the organic view of TS, since dopamine blockers were proven effective for treating both disorders. These behavioral abnormalities were increasingly seen as neurochemical. The controversy has still not fully subsided,[70] but as in many other dimensions of contemporary psychology, the breakthroughs in effective pharmacological treatment currently support the biochemical explanation: "The uniformity of response to medication suggests a common biologic basis to TD [Tourette's Disorder] independent of culture or geography."[71] Psychosocial factors still play a part in behavioral expression, but to the extent that TS results from dopamine and serotonin levels—rather than from parenting practices or cultural factors—it is likely to have existed in the early Middle Ages.[72]

TS is equally prevalent across ethnic and racial boundaries.[73] Robertson and Baron-Cohen state that "Tourette Syndrome occurs in all cultures where it has been looked for."[74] Specifically, it has shown consistent patterns across thirty-five hundred patients in twenty-two countries, including China, Japan, Argentina, Brazil, Turkey, South Africa, and Norway.[75] It occurs across all social classes.[76] Furthermore, there is no reason to think TS is a recent medical phenomenon. Shapiro et al. review possible cases of TS in history, starting with a priest described in the fifteenth-century *Malleus Malleficarum.*[77] It is likely that Anglo-Saxon communities were on (rare) occasion confronted with an exceptionally severe case of this condition, and this must have posed a unique range of challenges to family and local clergy alike.

In this genetic behavioral disorder, subjects exhibit recurrent, involuntary tics starting at an early age, which can include anything from grimacing, lip smacking, and eye blinking, to clothes tugging, teeth grinding, and kicking. The average age of onset is around seven years old for motor tics, and eleven for vocal tics. Eye blinking and shoulder shrugging are common early tics, and complex tics involving several muscles in coordination can eventually develop (compulsively hitting or biting one's self, smelling fingers or objects, popping knuckles, etc.). Combinations of motor movements can recur in ritualized and repetitive patterns, such as turning around three times and squatting down, or taking two steps forward and one step back. Subjects may feel the need to touch a certain object in a certain way, or to complete a series of actions in a certain order, and will be increasingly consumed by the thought until they do. Failing to reach out and touch a tree when the urge strikes, for instance, may result in the person coming back many hours later and performing the seemingly trivial act, having been unable to think about anything else in the meantime. Vocal tics include producing animal noises, barking, belching, grunting, screaming, sniffing, snorting, or spitting. Some subjects are apparently quite good impersonators of animal noises, so good in fact that "people think the animal is just around the corner."[78]

Vocal tics are various, and include echolalia—the repeating of the last word or phrase someone else present has just said—and, more famously (but not more commonly), coprolalia, or uncontrollably inappropriate language.[79] Swearing is a common form, but any religiously, politically, or socially unacceptable articulations are possible. An oft-cited case is that of an eleven-year-old girl with TS in Communist China, who repeatedly expressed reactionary political sentiments such as "down with Chou En-lai" (a revered veteran of the Communist revolution).[80] The age of onset, usually around twelve to fourteen years, is somewhat later for this symptom than for more basic motor tics. This can be the most devastating symptom for people with TS, rendering normal social functioning difficult if not impossible. Sometimes the very awareness that a particular time and place is highly inappropriate for certain speech is the very thing the sufferer fixates upon—thus increasing the urge that much more. Much to the patient's embarrassment, racial and sexist slurs and a wide range of devastating personal observations about others can easily come out, precisely because they happen to have flitted through the patient's mind for whatever reason and the patient is intensely afraid of saying them aloud. It is a compulsion toward the forbidden.[81] A married patient may repeatedly call out the name of a previous spouse.[82] One boy asked his mother to tape his mouth shut before he boarded an airplane, to prevent him from yelling out "hijack" once in the air.[83] Those with TS do not feel the desire to swear around speakers of a foreign language who will not understand. It is clearly a communicative act—though an unwilled one—and not just a random, explosive outburst.[84] Throughout even the most shocking of these displays, the person is still alert and rational. The patient struggles to suppress the urge or to cover tics by integrating them somehow into more acceptable routines, and so it is easy to see where onlookers may be given the impression of an indwelling entity in cases of severe TS—of there being two competing wills within the single body.

John Berecz describes coprolalia as a form of social brinkmanship, in which the subject compulsively releases carefully gauged utterances whose psychological effect on the listeners is, if not controllable, intimately appreciated.[85] Clearly, crowded public spaces can represent stressful and potentially humiliating milieus for those with TS. In the early Middle Ages mass would have been one of the few organized, public occasions in rural communities, other than market days or seasonal festivals, and unlike festivals or market days, mass was an occasion requiring solemnity if not silence (though it is uncertain precisely how quiet or boisterous church services in early medieval England were).[86] One modern patient reported avoiding church altogether, as well as the movies, for fear of inappropriate outbursts.[87] Not just stress but enjoyable excitement (such as going to the circus) can also exacerbate coprolalic symptoms, as can the presence of authority figures. Medieval possession cases are reminiscent of such compulsions, although of course the nature of the available evidence makes such comparisons suggestive at best. For instance, a girl brought to the monastery of St. Gall in Walafrid Strabo's *Life of Gall* is stricken with a demon as soon as she enters: "horrendo clamore spurcissima verba coepit effundere" (she began to pour out most foul language in a dreadful cry).[88] An Anglo-Saxon analogue is perhaps King Ceolred of Mercia (who "talked with devils and deprecated the priests of God" [cum diabolis sermocinans et Dei sacerdotes abhominans])—though I am entirely skeptical that we should take this report from Boniface's letters literally, as opposed to reading it simply as Boniface's disapproval of Ceolred's attitude toward the church in general.[89]

The uniquely difficult circumstances of TS can lead to adaptive and behavioral difficulties, especially in an environment in which family and peers do not understand the nature of the condition.[90] Those with TS can become withdrawn and unresponsive. There can be delusions of persecution or of grandeur (e.g., the sense of having extrasensory perception and/or powers). Symptoms may come on suddenly, or disappear suddenly. Self-destructive behaviors may manifest, such as cutting oneself with a knife, and sufferers may be obsessed with sexual or scatological topics far beyond the normal childhood and adolescent curiosity for those subjects.[91] Rage attacks are not uncommon, and can continue into adulthood. The striking incongruence between violent outbursts and the subject's normal character is often described as a "Jekyll and Hyde" phenomenon.

There is substantial overlap in some of the more dramatic symptoms of TS (and related compulsive disorders) and medieval descriptions of demon possession. Tics in TS often manifest in hissing, growling, barking, or other seemingly nonhuman vocalizations that often suggest animal noises to those present. Beyond vocalizations, medieval demoniacs are also often said to be continuously tearing or biting at themselves. A woman in Cyprian of Carthage's *On the Lapsed* (mid-third century) shreds her own tongue by biting; a young man with a demon in Sulpicius Severus's *Dialogues* tears at himself with his teeth; an adolescent girl is brought to Austreberta of Pavilly crying and "tearing herself to pieces" (vociferans atque se discerpens).[92] In Anglo-Saxon England, the boy brought to Cuthbert's tomb lacerates his own body ("lacerantemque corpus suum"), and the young man Hwætred "tears [or "plucks"] at himself cruelly and madly" (se ipsum crudeli vesania decerpebat).[93] Demoniacs, like people with TS, can speak out ostensibly against their own will—for instance, directing a tirade against the attendant saint or healer, or disrupting public services.[94] While Bishop Ambrose of Milan is preaching, according to Paulinus a man in the crowd begins to cry out that he is being tortured by the bishop.[95] Ironically, the point of this story is not that Ambrose heals the man, but simply that the saint makes him shut up so that the service can continue. In Arles Bishop Caesarius is interrupted by a woman who terrifies the entire congregation with her wailing and crying out ("eiulans et proclamans").[96] The comments made to saints by demoniacs are often abusive: a cripple tended by St. Eulogius for many years turns against him ("multisque eum probris coepit insequi, adeo ut eum etiam appeteret maledictis" [he began to reproach him with many accusations, indeed, even attacking him with insults]); and in Gregory of Tours's *Passion and Miracles of Julian*, a group of energumens "plerumque evoment in sanctum Dei convitia" (spewed forth many insults at the holy man of God).[97] Many of these symptoms, from self-mutilation to hurling abuse against authority figures, can of course result from a wide range of disparate causes, some of them pathological and some of them within the range of normal human moods. On occasion, however, TS was assuredly one cause among them, and must have resulted in some of the more seemingly causeless behavioral anomalies that challenged early medieval society.

In modern treatment, the dopamine antagonist haloperidol is the drug of choice.[98] Behavioral treatments have shown some modest success in the short term, but no long-term behavioral cure has been documented.[99] Telling a child not to curse or washing a mouth out with soap are demonstrably ineffective. Tics, however, undergo natural cycles of waxing and waning. Many symptoms lessen on their own in later adolescence or adulthood, and spontaneous remission—lasting only a few days or for many years—is possible.[100] If a person with TS did present at a medieval shrine, any abatement of symptoms from exorcism or from exertions of self-discipline would have been temporary; the person could probably hold out for twenty minutes, at the outside.[101] Modern treatment favors creating an atmosphere in which TS patients are not blamed for their tics, but are allowed safe times and places for the free expression of symptoms. The unique place of the saint's tomb in early medieval Europe may have provided such a protective environment, in which exaggerated expressions of piety as well as blasphemy could exist side by side, and in which the ritual dialogue of exorcism (if a priest was on hand to attempt one) could unfold without subsequent blame attached to the ostensible antagonist. If exorcism could not cure TS, it may have at least provided great relief in allowing someone with severe tics to express them not just openly but vigorously. TS and the broader spectrum of obsessive-compulsive disorders are important for an understanding of demon possession not because the extremes of these conditions are common but because those extremes likely formed an important model for functional possession behavior (in providing an organic precedent for swearing, blaspheming, grunting, growling, and several other manifestations).

Psychosis

Psychosis refers to the experiencing of delusions or hallucinations, the loss of ego boundaries, or impairment in reality which is more severe than simple eccentricity and is unexplained by the normal stresses and demands on an individual.[102] Anyone under tremendous stress can potentially suffer a passing psychotic episode. Alternately, a person with more seriously internalized perceptual or cognitive deficits (for instance, brain trauma or ongoing depression) can labor for years under psychotic ideation. Unlike people with personality disorders, who usually recognize their condition as a disorder and are upset by its consequences, psychotics do not acknowledge the abnormality of their pathological beliefs and behavior.[103] A child's relationship with an imaginary friend, a shaman's journey to the spirit world, a believer's vision of the Virgin Mary, or a survival enthusiast's belief that the government is monitoring him are not considered psychotic if they are integrated within a larger community in which the behaviors make sense, even if the particular experiences are not shared by others. Application of the term "psychosis" implies that the subject's normal functioning is so unacceptable that friends, family members, and medical authorities consider the behavior an illness—that they do not validate the subject's construct of reality as legitimate. The DSM stresses that for psychotic disorders, behaviors can only be considered aberrant in the context of the subject's own culture.[104]

Obviously, this formulation leaves room for a wide range of behavioral anomalies, which will vary among different societies and different times. Some psychoses are dependent on a particular society and lose their contextualized significance outside of it: *latah*, a Malay-Indonesian fright or startle response; *amok*, a dissociative attack marked by violent and even homicidal lashing out, documented in Malaysia and Papua-New Guinea; *pibloktoq*, a sudden seizure in which the person may tear off clothes and roll in the snow, noted among Inuits; and *ebenzi*, a southern African condition of the Shona people, in which the sufferer talks and performs nonsensically (believed to be caused by witchcraft).[105] Other psychoses, such as hallucinations or delusions associated with an identifiable brain lesion, are biological phenomena that can appear in any culture. Since disruptive behavior is only meaningful within the norms of a given society, the community's own assessment of an individual as ill is essential to the identification of a person as psychotic: it makes no sense (as earlier schools of thought attempted) to label the shaman priest as a psychotic, for instance, or to label an entire society as manifesting psychotic impulses. Only the community can define permissible and impermissible reality constructs, although any individual is simultaneously at the nexus of any of a number of diverse and sometimes competing "communities."

The patterns of behavior currently recognized as psychotic in many contexts resemble medieval patterns of demon possession. Brief psychotic disorders are characterized by the sudden onset (generally following trauma or intense stress) of delusions, hallucinations, or severely disorganized or catatonic behavior.[106] The threat of violence to others is not as great as commonly supposed, although suicide rates are elevated. "Delusional disorder" refers to a recurring sense of non-bizarre delusions, such as the belief that one is being covered with insects.[107] Such delusions are recorded for the early Middle Ages: Gregory of Tours writes of a man who believes he is covered with frogs, and who also believes he is openly attacked by demons wielding spears.[108] Given the broad definition of psychosis as either transient or chronic (as a symptom complex rather than a condition) and as dependent upon the interpretation of the surrounding culture, the term can be applied to foreign and past cultures so long as there is enough information to decide what counts as delusional or out of step with common perceptions of reality for that culture. Early medieval writers do not brand those who have visions of heaven or hell as possessed, though we would probably consider someone in a modern, secular context psychotic if he insisted too much on such an experience (or even in a religious context, if the belief is not validated by the broader religious community). In the medieval worldview such experiences fit cultural expectations and fell within the accepted norms of the possible.

With "psychosis" we perhaps reach the limits of our ability to understand the medieval worldview, because while there were clearly visions, perceptions, and experiences that could not have been happening outside of the subject's head, such cases as recorded in the religious writings that were predominate in the early Middle Ages were not considered hallucinatory by observers but revelatory. That is, the reality of the entities putatively assaulting a suffering patient was rarely called into question. According to the (admittedly church-monopolized) writings of the period, these were moments for the testing of moral fortitude or of discerning good spirits from bad, and not of reality testing. Whether this hermeneutic was uniformly shared by everyone in the subject's daily life is hard to say. Spiritually minded people are more inclined to read the world around them as a tapestry of signs and symbols, and to interpret the perceptions resulting from trance-like states of mind (e.g., induced or enhanced through prayer, fasting, group religious experience, or intense emotional introspection) as connections with "deeper" levels of reality. Those who can master their own experiences and regain control were considered saintly (e.g., Cuthbert and Guthlac, if their spiritual struggles against demons were not hagiographic fabrications), while those who could not might eventually be brought to a saint's tomb for help. People shouting or swatting in the air at invisible demons—though these individuals do not necessarily manifest different personalities or speak in the voice of a demon—were brought for exorcism. The demons here are external (in the air or on the body) rather than internal (within the mind or muscles), but fall under the purview of demonic assault because they cause otherwise inexplicable voluntary behaviors on the part of the victim:

> Quidam homo . . . vidit quasi a daemonibus traheretur. Cumque nimia vociferatione ad B. Aldegundem ac sororem ejus S. Waldetrudem clamaret, ut earum meritis & orationibus adjuvaretur; repente de manibus eorum ereptus conticuit, & voces nullas insaniens emisit. Tunc his qui aderant magnopere suggessit, ut ante praesentiam Christi famulae Waldetrudis deportari debuisset.[109]
>
> [A certain man . . . saw it as though he were being dragged around by demons. When he called out in a loud voice for St. Aldegund and her sister St. Waldetrude to help him with their virtues and prayers, suddenly—snatched from (the demons') hands—he became quiet and let out no further insane voices. Then he strongly beseeched those who were there to bring him into the presence of Waldetrude, the servant of Christ.]

There is perhaps not so much difference in this account from Guthlac calling on St. Bartholomew as the saints' biographers would present it: both rely on the perceived support of a stronger spiritual guide to carry them through their difficult moments. In a climate in which the perception of combating spiritual foes is culturally encouraged, it is impossible for us to know when, on occasion, actual compromises in cognitive and perceptual processing were in fact behind the hallucinatory experiences. These qualia would be experientially different though the community was not equipped to differentiate between the two. Hearing voices is an illustrative point: schizophrenics report that the voices they hear are as loud and audible as those of other people in the room. Religiously inspired people sometimes describe their direction as coming from the "voice" of God, though perhaps more as a figure of speech (e.g., to express the clear and compelling nature of the inspiration). These are distinct perceptual phenomena, but they would invisibly blend into the medieval behavioral landscape. Thus breakdowns in reality perception originating from neurological causes could usually be smoothly integrated in a religious worldview. Nonetheless, just as a starter for sourdough bread must periodically be "fed" with flour and warm water to reinvigorate the yeast, the acceptable perimeters of recognized possession behavior could, over time, be periodically reinspired and redefined within a community by the hallucinatory ideation of a person whose consciousness suffers from an organic filtering impairment in reality testing. The onlookers in the Waldetrude episode are not certain about the presence of demons in this case (they specify *quasi*, "as though," and still refer to the man's cries as "insane"), though there is no question that they believe in the reality of demons generally. I use the term "psychosis" then, in deference to the clear reliance of perceptual processing on cognitive structures, and the indisputable fact that these can break down in ways which create individual or social stress. Such breakdowns could elicit a range of communal interpretations, one of which was, on occasion, to be brought to an exorcist for the expulsion of demons.

There are a number of substances derived from plants that can serve as natural neuroleptics (or antipsychotics).[110] The Chinese plant *Ginkgo biloba* has been widely shown to reduce psychotic symptoms, and the root of *Rauwolfia serpentina* has been used in India for centuries as an antipsychotic.[111] A New World analogue is "lizard's tail" (*Saururus cernuus*), a wetland flower common in Florida and the Gulf coast that contains the natural neuroleptic compound manassantin A (but this was apparently not recognized or used by Native Americans). Northern Europe does not seem to have been favored with a comparable naturally appearing phyto-neuroleptic, and in the absence of effective antipsychotics, we should not be surprised if the Anglo-Saxon therapeutic strategy for psychotic complexes focused more on sedation than treatment.

Schizophrenia

Because of its prominent place in the twentieth- and twenty-first-century landscape of serious psychotic disorders, schizophrenia is often cited as a candidate for medieval attributions of demon possession. For this reason, it warrants special attention. Many of its clinical manifestations do indeed resemble in uncanny ways medieval descriptions of demoniacs. The disorder is by no means free of controversy, however. The term "schizophrenia" is a convenient shorthand for a complex of symptoms, many of which appear in early medical descriptions of possession. But whether or not these symptoms of medieval pathology were the manifestations of a coherent neurological disorder—and whether or not this disorder bears a meaningful resemblance to the schizophrenia currently encountered in hospitals and clinics—are subjects of considerable debate.[112]

Manifesting itself in a dizzyingly heterogeneous array of behaviors and mental states, since the term's very inception schizophrenia has defied a precise, universally accepted definition.[113] Since no underlying pathogen has been identified, the condition is diagnosed purely on the basis of observable behaviors.[114] The range of possible symptoms is fairly clear, such as autism or social withdrawal, delusions, hallucinations, emotional flattening, and incomprehensible behavior, but all of these can also occur in other disorders as well. Different models variously prioritize the symptoms as basic or accessory. Eugen Bleuler, who coined the term "schizophrenia" in 1908, implied through the word that a splitting of psychic functions is essential to the disorder (for instance, inappropriate sequences of ideas, or incongruity between ideas and their accompanying emotions).[115] Erik Strömgren tends to view autism (diminished emotional contact with other people) as the definitive characteristic.[116] Alternately, Edward Hare has even suggested that a trait as specific as hearing voices may serve as a defining characteristic: it is common in schizophrenia (occurring in about two-thirds of patients) and relatively rare in other disorders.[117]

Of the three subtypes of schizophrenia generally recognized (paranoid, catatonic, and hebephrenic), today the most common is paranoid schizophrenia—an unremitting delusion of persecution or exaltation. Patients may entertain absurd delusions of grandeur, believing themselves to be individuals of paramount importance or ability. They may perceive themselves to be powerful political or religious figures, or may believe that they have the power to control the weather or communicate with beings from other worlds (in our era, extraterrestrials; in the Middle Ages, demons). Alternately, they may envision themselves to be at the center of widespread, complicated observation and plotting. Often they report feeling as though they have been robbed of their own thoughts and emotions, which have then been replaced by foreign ones. Patients may experience thought insertion (belief that thoughts are being inserted into their heads) or thought withdrawal (belief that thoughts are being removed from their heads). They grow to believe that much of what transpires around them is directed specifically at them, either to confuse them or to influence their thoughts and behaviors.

Paranoid schizophrenics can perceive auditory hallucinations in the form of whistling, humming, or laughing; other times these are vividly perceived as intelligently articulated human speech. The subject often hears voices talking to each other, voices that sustain a running commentary on a subject, criticize behavior, or issue commands. Hallucinated voices may be perceived not only from the vicinity surrounding the patients but even from the patient's own limbs and body parts.[118] The voices are preoccupied with the subject, and are usually critical, antagonistic, curt, and derisive.[119] Such dramatic symptoms are usually even more striking since they often present in a person with an otherwise well-preserved personality and without other significant cognitive or emotional disturbance.[120] In many cases the progression of ideas follows an internal logic opaque to outside observers. Paranoid schizophrenics often speak intelligently, but are building from (perhaps even just a few) private, extraordinary premises. Speech and volitional disturbances are not common in paranoid schizophrenia, and emotions are not flattened as in other forms of the condition: the patient assumes states of anger, fear, and mistrust in response to the perceived external conspiracy or threat.[121] Schizophrenics can become increasingly incapable of adequately caring for themselves as they retreat into an internal world and social mores decrease in priority.

The relationship between many of these symptoms and medieval accounts of demon possession may seem obvious. The schizophrenic feels that his or her emotions and drives are imposed by or compellingly driven in response to perceived external forces. According to the World Health Organization (WHO),

> The disturbance involves the most basic functions that give the normal person a feeling of individuality, uniqueness, and self-direction. The most intimate thoughts, feelings, and acts are often felt to be known to or shared by others, and explanatory delusions may develop, to the effect that natural or supernatural forces are at work to influence the afflicted individual's thoughts and actions in ways that are often bizarre.[122]

There is some question, however, whether or not schizophrenia existed in the early Middle Ages. Edward Hare cautions, "a case may be made both for and against the view that schizophrenia is an ancient disease."[123] On the one hand, a landmark study undertaken by the World Health Organization in the late 1960s and early '70s demonstrated the universal presence of schizophrenic complexes in a number of countries, and across four continents. The findings of the WHO study point to a surprisingly uniform core of schizophrenic symptoms through these various cultures.[124] The implication is that the condition is not merely a social construct—that it is not a phenomenon arising from postindustrial stresses, nor suggested to patients by media or psychoanalysts, for instance—but that it is an organic neurobehavioral disorder. Thus, researchers such as Dilip Jeste et al. are comfortable asserting that "schizophrenia has existed throughout history."[125]

Yet E. F. Torrey, who supplements the data of the WHO schizophrenia project with an impressive collection of studies from almost every corner of the globe, draws a different conclusion from them. While agreeing (and supporting with further data) that schizophrenia is a coherent complex of symptoms, he argues that it is a concomitant of modern industrial civilization, and questions its existence prior to the eighteenth century.[126] If it did exist, he claims, it was extremely rare. It is difficult to calculate the prevalence of schizophrenia in premodern civilizations, however, due to a variety of contaminating factors such as disparate mortality rates, different modes of treatment, and diverse criteria for diagnosis. Richard Warner simply leaves the matter open: "In short, we cannot tell if schizophrenia occurred less commonly in pre-industrial Europe, nor if it occurs less frequently in contemporary pre-industrial settings."[127]

One point on which researchers generally agree is that the symptomological manifestations of schizophrenia have changed notably over the last hundred years, and even within a single generation of clinical observation. Cases of catatonic schizophrenia, for instance, are much rarer than they were early in the twentieth century, while hebephrenic and paranoid varieties have become more frequent.[128] Additionally, researchers comment that the disorder is less serious than it once was, even taking into account the advent of neuroleptic medication. No illness is truly static, after all: viral and bacterial diseases evolve through time, for instance, manifesting themselves variously according to physiological and environmental conditions. Mental and behavioral disorders may be especially sensitive to shifting environmental conditions and cultural contexts. One shift in the nature of schizophrenia of particular importance to a study of demon possession is the changing locus of hallucinatory voices. John Ellard recalls that when he first began clinical observation of schizophrenics in the 1940s, his patients described the voices they heard as emanating from the external environment. In the late 1980s, however, the locus of these voices was primarily internal: the hallucinatory voices had "retreated from the external world into the patients' minds."[129] If Ellard's observation reflects a general trend, earlier generations of schizophrenics may have more readily perceived their auditory hallucinations as external entities (such as demons), rather than describing them as "voices in my head."

Schizophrenia, however, remains a dubious category to apply to the early Middle Ages, since a principal indicator of the condition—hearing voices—is virtually absent in the early medieval possession accounts.[130] In a dialogue over whether schizophrenia existed before the eighteenth century, Edward Hare reported that a search of sources from prior to 1800 yielded no cases of auditory hallucinations in the absence of visual ones: "I can find no account of 'voices' in Burton's *Anatomy*, nor in the main psychiatric treatises of the eighteenth century."[131] A hallucination pattern that seems to be particular to schizophrenia—two or more voices maintaining a conversation audible to the subject—is, to my knowledge, completely absent from the ancient and early medieval accounts.[132] After a systematic review of Greek and Roman sources covering a wide range of genres, an Australian team concluded, "We were unable to identify any descriptions of chronic psychotic disorders in either fiction or accounts of historical figures that would qualify for a diagnosis of schizophrenia according to the DSM-IV (nor for any other major diagnostic criteria used in recent decades) . . . in contrast to schizophrenia, data concerning other mental disorders were readily found."[133] From my own review of early medieval sources, out of 274 specific cases of possession I consulted for which any detailed symptoms are provided, I have found only three possible instances of auditory hallucinations resembling those of contemporary schizophrenia.[134] One is a remark appearing in the Greek *Apothegmata Patrum*: "Abba Poemen said, 'If you have visions or hear voices do not tell your neighbor about it, for it is a delusion in the battle [against demons or against the devil].'"[135] The second is in Gregory of Tours's *Books on the Miracles of St. Martin the Bishop*, where an account of Landulf of Vienne suggests he is suffering from tactile as well as auditory hallucinations:

> Quodsi se subderet terrae, ranarum super eum multitudo horribilis desilire videbatur, sed et voces publice ab eo audiebantur exprobrantium et dicentium: "Martinus, quem expetisti, nihil tibi poterit subvenire, quia nostris es ditionibus mancipatus."[136]
>
> [Whenever he lay on the ground, a horrible swarm of frogs seemed to hop over him, and he heard voices openly reproaching him and saying: "Martin, whom you have openly supplicated, cannot help you because you are under our authority."]

The third instance, already discussed, is that of King Ceolred of Mercia's alleged madness, as related by Boniface in a letter to Ceolred's successor Æthelred. In his rage, Ceolred is said to have "talked to devils" (cum diabolis sermocinans) until his death.[137] This image of the wasted king, raving and babbling to himself as divine punishment for his former transgressions, is strikingly reminiscent of our modern image of paranoid schizophrenics muttering to themselves (if indeed we are not anachronistically imposing a modern visualization of the scene on Boniface's brief allusion). On the whole, though, these three instances are the rare exceptions in a large body of literature documenting a rich spectrum of symptoms and behaviors.[138] I have devoted significant attention to schizophrenia here because it is frequently cited as the cause of demon possession in Anglo-Saxon England and in the Middle Ages more generally.[139] Because of its fluid profile and the relative silence of early sources regarding its most prominent symptom, however, schizophrenia is probably not a fruitful construct to apply to our understanding of pathologies in the early Middle Ages.

Dissociation Disorders and Trauma: Combat Stress and Childhood Sexual Assault

Perhaps the most provocative analogues for demon possession in modern psychiatry are the dissociative disorders. Dissociation, the separating off of some compartments of consciousness from others, is a normal psychological mechanism.[140] Only by fragmenting attention in some controlled way can a person carry on a conversation while peeling potatoes, or sing to the radio while filing documents alphabetically. At all times, even while asleep, numerous levels of consciousness simultaneously filter incoming perceptions, process thoughts and emotions, and coordinate behavior. The compartmentalization of consciousness is attested in late antique sources as a powerful pain management tool:

> Sanctus autem Ammonius et Evagrius, qui eum convenerunt, narraverunt se eum invenisse in talem prolapsum aegritudinem in ipsis locis testiculorum, et penis summum ulcerasse cancrum, qui φαγέδαινα dicitur. Eum, aiebant, invenimus dum a quodam medico curaretur. Et manibus quidem operabatur; et palmae ramos contexebat, et nobiscum etiam loquebatur: reliquo autem corpori manum adhibebat chirurgus. Erat autem Dei gratia, ea praeditus patientia, ut perinde affectus videretur, ac si corpus alterius secaretur.[141]
>
> [Sts. Ammonius and Evagrius, who visited (St. Stephen the Libyan), related that they found him in an advanced state of illness in the location of the testicles, and his penis was greatly ulcerated with the cancer which is called *phagedaina*. "We found him," they said, "being attended by a certain doctor. But nevertheless, he was working with his hands: he was weaving palm leaves and spoke with us. The surgeon attended to the rest of his body. It was through the grace of God, this gift of endurance, that his disposition seemed thus, as though it were someone else's body being cut into."]

Dissociation becomes pathological, however, when the various modes of consciousness are not well integrated or are in direct conflict with one another, as gauged externally by the social conventions of the subject's culture.

Dissociation is implicit in demon possession behavior in which the energumen adopts alternate personae. The term dissociative identity disorder (DID) has replaced multiple personality disorder (MPD) in the DSM, though both are still used in the literature. The prevalence and, indeed, the very existence of DID are disputed, especially following sensationalistic media portrayals and notorious attempts to use DID as a legal defense. Marlene Steinberg believes that the rising prevalence of dissociative disorders in twentieth-century America is the result of post-war changes in family structure, career patterns, and technology; if so, these disorders arise from a combination of social circumstances that may have no adequate historical parallel.[142] Michael Simpson, one of the strongest detractors from the DID hypothesis, comments on the restricted class of patients presenting: they are mostly white women from middle- or upper-class families, and almost all reported cases are in North America. Simpson concludes, "Internationally widespread cultural variants of possession states are not varieties of MPD. On the contrary, MPD is a secular, Western variety of possession state, adapted to the lack of a predominant, single cultural and religious belief structure in North American culture (and some related parts of European culture)."[143] For the time being, however, the American Psychiatric Association endorses the diagnosis by retaining it in the DSM-V.[144] In a review of the literature, David Gleaves et al. conclude that DID meets all the criteria for continued inclusion in the DSM: "the evidence for its construct validity is perhaps greater than that for most mental disorders."[145] Some cases imply malingering (deliberate faking), and others may be iatrogenic (the condition is suggested and reinforced by the caretaker or psychiatrist). In fact, many psychiatrists believe that *all* cases of DID currently reported in the literature are either affected or iatrogenic, but debating the cause of what undoubtedly manifests as a behavioral problem does not make it less of a problem.[146] It is probably not helpful to think in terms of a binary model in which individuals are either "genuinely" dissociating or are faking: there is clearly a spectrum in which different levels of participation in dissociation behavior are accepted and even encouraged in different cultures or in different sectors of society. DID is especially interesting for our purposes because it translates into modern, secular terms perhaps more closely than anything else what is involved in functional possession: the adoption of possession behaviors in the absence of clear organic causes such as epilepsy or brain injury.

Dissociative Identity Disorder is characterized by an alternate or several alternate personalities within an individual, each of whose thoughts and actions are unknown to the other personalities. The individual retains no memory of the episodes during which an alternate personality is in control. Integral to the definition of DID is that the alternate personality or personalities behave consistently: that is, they are well established over time. These criteria distinguish DID from transient psychotic episodes.[147]

The two most common causes of DID are of particular interest here in reconstructing life and experience in Anglo-Saxon England: combat exposure and sexual assault.[148] These are traumatic situations for which stepping out of the self proves a necessary and effective coping mechanism: "DID is a little girl imagining that the abuse is happening to someone else. This is the core of the disorder, to which all other features are secondary. The imagining is so intense, subjectively compelling, and adaptive, that the abused child experiences dissociated aspects of herself as other people."[149] The combination of a strong survival instinct with an intolerable situation leads to the potential creation of alternate personalities. A woman raped once by a stranger, though she may certainly dissociate during the experience ("what is happening to me is not real"), will not necessarily suffer long-term identity fragmentation.[150] A young girl raped periodically by her father, however, must reconcile her feelings of fear and detestation with those of love and attachment. The overpowering emotional confusion leads to cognitive compartmentalization. The girl may later describe that she perceived herself to be floating above the scene, looking down on it—a comment also often heard from survivors of intense combat experience.[151] (The perception of being outside of one's body, floating above and looking down on the scene, has a specific neurologic foundation and can be artificially induced in the laboratory.[152]) Over time the subject may naturally create a persona or a range of personae which provide a safe haven from the brutal reality of her circumstances. She may become adept at retreating to this identity during the ordeal, unaware of what is happening to her "other self" and (often) unable to recall it afterwards. It is the reconciliation of these conflicting identities—especially later in life, when there is no longer a viable need for both identities—that presents difficulties for the subject's emotional, intellectual, and social stability.[153]

Dissociative Identity Disorder has a unique profile: (1) the subject's personality manifests as two or more distinct identities; (2) these identities take control of the patient's behavior alternately; (3) extensive amnesia prevents one identity from being aware of what transpires when another identity is in control (the interval is experienced simply as blackout, or a fugue state); and (4) there is no readily identifiable physiological cause for the fragmentation of consciousness, such as intoxication or seizure.[154] Sometimes the patient may not be aware of the existence of alternate personalities (or "alters"), while in other cases the alters may be critical of one another or be in open conflict.[155] The core of DID—the presence of alters—can be accompanied by a variety of secondary features. Though a number of symptoms overlap with schizophrenia—such as hallucinations, thought insertion, withdrawal, or broadcasting—their etiologies and prognoses are entirely distinct.[156] Colin Ross lists the most prominent secondary features of DID, derived from reviewing a series of 102 cases, finding that referring to the self as "we" or "us" appears in 73.5% of cases—not unlike the Gerasene demoniac episode in the Gospels and a host of medieval analogues afterwards.[157] The DSM also notes that some powerful alters may have the ability to control pain or other physical symptoms, which could appear to onlookers as though one of the personalities is a superior, nonhuman power.[158] This symptomology makes it clear why some researchers believe that possession is simply the variant of DID common in premodern societies, which gains support from the fact that both are not usually prevalent within the same society (or within the same sectors of a society).

It is difficult to determine whether the epidemiological conditions for DID existed in Anglo-Saxon England. Obviously, the clinical manifestations of dissociation will vary widely according to the types of trauma encountered in a given society, and according to what means that society provides the individual for articulating and coping with anxiety. For instance, dissociation is a significant component of what is currently called post-traumatic stress disorder (PTSD).[159] Were Anglo-Saxon soldiers susceptible to post-traumatic stress disorder? Was combat an ordeal which left a lasting psychological scar, which could sometimes result in sleep disorders, nightmares, intrusive thoughts, hypersensitivity, irritability, excessive startle response, blunted affect, detachment, and, ultimately, permanently fragmented compartments of consciousness?

Researchers lament the paucity of data yet assembled for PTSD in traditional societies.[160] Patrick Bracken et al. argue, from theoretical grounds, that extreme caution should be employed in assuming that PTSD, based as it is on the Western concept of the individual as a discreet monadic entity, may not apply to most world cultures. Pittu Laungani argues against applying secular Western categories of trauma to other societies, especially religious ones, and of applying the categories of individualistic cultures to collectivist ones.[161] Nonetheless, negotiating sometimes delicate compromises between Western clinical models and the illness and healing contexts of traditional societies, many researchers are convinced that a common core of trauma-response symptoms is recognizable worldwide. Stamm and Friedman believe that "there is no question that PTSD can be detected among non-Euro-Americans," and provide a list of studies from Southeast Asia, Central and South America, the Middle East, South Pacific islands, Afghanistan, Sri Lanka, and other non-Western cultures in support.[162] Frank Weathers et al. find that, "throughout history the symptoms of war-related PTSD have been readily apparent."[163] Together with somatization, dissociation is a major component of PTSD among non-Western peoples.[164] The oft-anthologized Japanese tale "The Tiger's Whisker" dramatically and un-self-consciously articulates some domestic tensions resulting from PTSD in folkloric terms:

> A young woman by the name of Yun Ok came one day to the house of a mountain hermit to seek his help. . . .
>
> "It is my husband," Yun Ok said. "He is very dear to me. For the past three years he has been away fighting in the wars. Now that he has returned, he hardly speaks to me, or to anyone else. If I speak, he doesn't seem to hear. When he talks at all, it is roughly. If I serve him food not to his liking, he pushes it aside and angrily leaves the room. Sometimes when he should be working in the rice field, I see him sitting idly on top of the hill, looking toward the sea."
>
> "Yes, so it is sometimes when young men come back from the wars," the hermit said. "Go on."
>
> "There is no more to tell, Learned One. I want a potion to give my husband so that he will be loving and gentle, as he used to be."
>
> "Ha, so simple is it?" the hermit said. "A potion!"[165]

Attempts to read PTSD retrospectively into *The Iliad* and *Hamlet* are provocative but hardly diagnostically adequate; a section of *Henry IV Part I*, on the other hand, does present a striking catalog of many of the core features of the condition.[166] Lady Percy is worried about her lord Hotspur; a small sampling will give a sense of the whole:

> Tell me, sweet lord, what is't that takes from thee
> Thy stomach, pleasure, and thy golden sleep?
> Why dost thou bend thine eyes upon the earth,
> And start so often when thou sit'st alone?
> . . . In thy faint slumbers I by thee have watch'd,
> And heard thee murmur tales of iron wars . . .
> Thy spirit within thee hath been so at war . . . [167]

Hotspur's social and emotional worlds have shrunk; his ability to eat, sleep, and enjoy relations with his wife has been disturbed; and he relives battlefield stress in a way that estranges him from others. The exaggerated startle response is especially telling, and Lady Percy catches him frequently breaking out in sweat at night in bed.[168]

Recent studies tend to support the universality of PTSD as a psychological symptom complex with at least some hardwired components.[169] Intrusive and hyperarousal symptoms seem to have more universality than others (such as avoidant/numbing symptoms) and so may have a common psychobiological basis.[170] The amygdala and the hippocampus—areas of the limbic system key in evaluating external stimuli and assigning emotional and behavioral response—have drawn particular attention. For instance, the hippocampus is markedly smaller in PTSD sufferers: studying Vietnam veterans, Bremner et al. found an 8% reduction in right hippocampal volume, while Gurvitz, Shenton, and Pitman found a 26% shrinkage in the left hippocampus and a 22% shrinkage in the right hippocampus in those suffering severe PTSD from intense combat exposure.[171] Stein et al. record a 7% hippocampal volume reduction in women with PTSD resulting from repeated childhood sexual abuse.[172] It has been hypothesized that increased release of glucocorticoids, excitatory amino acids, and serotonin may be associated with damage to the hippocampus.[173] The hippocampus relates incoming stimuli with stored memories and assesses the stimuli for their associations with reward or punishment.

Joseph LeDoux has found that emotionally negative conditioning prevents the subsequent realignment of appropriate fight-or-flight responses. The amygdala, which plays a critical role in attaching emotional significance to incoming stimuli, may be permanently modified by even a single traumatic experience. Even one or two training trials can leave an indelible imprint on the subject, an imprint which can be submerged but never permanently erased.[174] It is also possible that a single head wound can result in PTSD symptoms, independently of any anxiety associated with a traumatic environment—that is, that even when a subject is not overly stressed in battle (for instance), a blow to the head can itself upset the hormonal balance of brain chemistry.[175] After the physiological effects of trauma are better understood, it may be possible to point to more definitively biological (and therefore universal) results of trauma.[176] So far, though, it seems clear that extreme trauma is capable of permanently altering some of the most fundamental brain structures and their functioning, and of inhibiting the normal integration of stimuli and categorization of experience.

Marten DeVries indicates that, "cultural social roles, shared values, and historical continuity will act as key stress managers."[177] Indeed, DeVries argues that the very function of culture is to provide stability and predictability for the individual and group, by offering a stable construction of reality through custom, history, myth, and ritual. These cultural narratives affirm such positive aspects as the survival of the community and the existence of privileged links with the spirit realm.[178] According to DeVries, culture is a protective shield against the inherent stresses, pains, and catastrophes that can potentially befall individuals and communities in any era or region. Implicit in DeVries's account is the premise that vulnerability is an inherent element of the human condition, and presumably no culture can shield all its members perfectly from the potential for deep-rooted emotional damage.

What sorts of experiences count as traumatic will sometimes differ widely among cultural contexts: one has only to contrast pederasty in classical Athens (a sign of social status) with pederasty in the modern world (a criminal pathology). Violent, nonconsensual wounding is assuredly universal as a pain or stressor, however. Even when cultures incorporate pain into certain rituals (asceticism, initiation rites, self-mortification, etc.), the positive channeling of violence still attests to its universality and power—that is, the fact that pain is used to distinguish or transform the individual confirms that the individual is not immune to or unaware of the physical sensation.[179] Warrior societies worldwide often develop intricate "age-sets" (gradated phases within the life cycle) and mutilation rites (such as piercing, tattooing, scarring, or circumcising), which serve, above all, to eliminate ego-identity in the individual and enforce group identity.[180] DeVries notes, "culture cannot . . . blunt the immediate physical power of violence and the emotional shock of betrayal."[181] As Royal Hassrick writes of the Sioux, "it is likely that they credited bravery and flaunted danger to cover an innate normal fear."[182] Thus we cannot dismiss out of hand the notion of an individual suffering from combat-related trauma in a premodern warrior society, since these societies expended formidable energies and resources addressing that very danger. In fact, these societies are largely predicated on the transformative power of an individual's fear of traumatic pain and of death.

Soldiers who perform bravely and competently are not, for all that, utterly fearless (as legend portrays the Germanic *berserkr* and Celtic *riastradh*). Complete fearlessness is pathological and is of little tactical service to an individual or to his comrades: as Alcuin writes to Charlemagne, "praeceps pugnantium praesumptio saepe in periculum cadit" (rash boldness in battle often brings danger).[183] The uneasy marriage of self-preservation instinct and military obligation explains the intense focus on courage and loyalty in the art and literature of warrior societies: the very pervasiveness of this focus suggests a continual need to affirm bravery and sacrifice in the individual, despite very natural feelings of fear. The heroic elements of *The Battle of Maldon* which Roberta Frank and Gerald Morgan point out as universal among the heroic literatures—courage and loyalty, a noble death for a transcendent cause, a staunch refusal to leave the battlefield after the chief is dead or to leave the fallen chief unavenged—encourage these culturally imposed attitudes in individuals who are otherwise the farmers and fathers of a community's day-to-day life.[184] Modern commentators dwell on Byrhtnoth's controversial *ofermod* and debate the wisdom of his decision to allow the Vikings passage across the ford, but the *Maldon* poet is manifestly more interested in the dynamics of loyalty to the leader under duress than in Byrhtnoth's tactical decisions.[185] Loyalty is also the principal tension of the climactic scene in *Beowulf*, when many of Beowulf's retainers abandon him in his hour of need.[186] As Janet Bately concludes in a close reading of terms for "bravery" in Old English epic poetry, words for bravery are linked more with expectations or with failed ideals than with descriptions of bravery in action. "Brave" (e.g., *unearh*, *unforht*, *cene*, *snell*, *modig*) is "not what people are, but what they need to be."[187] The maxims repeated in wisdom literature as well as heroic literature are designed to impose order on a situation with implicit potential for chaos.[188] Paul Cavill compares three proverbs from *Maldon* and *Beowulf*:[189]

> Ne mæg na wandian   se þe wrecan þenceð
> frean on folce,   ne for feore murnan.[190]
>
> [He who intends to avenge his people's lord can never pause, nor care for his own life.]

> A mæg gnornian
> se ðe nu fram þis wigplegan   wendan þenceð.[191]
>
> [He who intends to turn now from this battle will always lament it.]

> Swa sceal man don,
> þonne he æt guðe   gegan þenceð
> longsumne lof,   na ymb his lif cearað.[192]
>
> [Thus should a person act when he hopes to gain enduring praise in battle; he does not worry about his life.]

As a group these solemn adages, according to Cavill, "locate the threat to the community in the mental realm," and it is the "mental concentration of the warriors" that they seek to direct toward undistracted patriotic fighting spirit.[193] Christian or pagan, societies galvanized for war must marshal their resources to elicit a strong group identity and to foster a sense of fortitude, sacrifice, and a greater cause in their fighting men.

A late seventeenth- or early eighteenth-century Japanese treatise on the code of the Samurai opens, "One who is supposed to be a warrior considers it his foremost concern to keep death in mind at all times, every day and every night, from the morning of New Year's Day through the night of New Year's Eve."[194] Halfway across the world, the intricately encoded system of Sioux battle rites—which included a choreographed ritual of multiple "coups" (close-quarter touches or wounds) on a single victim by multiple warriors, and which resulted in an economy of social prestige expressed in war trophies (scalps and especially horses)—"suggests that these features may actually have been institutionalized as a mechanism to prevent flinching" when faced with intense fear or danger.[195] Hassrick argues that such elaborate constructs reveal the potential anxiety of being in danger, and the "helplessness of the individual fully to cope."[196] Social mechanisms that channel the impulses of the individual into sacrifice for the group cannot hope to achieve complete success, else there would be no need for such deeply invested proverbs and rituals.

Katherine O'Brien O'Keeffe draws attention to the disparity between literary ideal and historical reality in Anglo-Saxon heroic society, and, citing Æthelred's law code (ca. 1008), suggests that battlefield desertion may have been a common occurrence.[197] Battlefield desertion is certainly a pervasive anxiety throughout Old English poetry. In a speech before the Battle of Maldon the trusty thane Offa correctly predicts that boasts will not be honored and that the courage of many will fail on the battlefield.[198] In *The Anglo-Saxon Warrior Ethic* John Hill draws further attention to the disparity between literary portrayal and social reality in Old English literature. He denies any sort of "coded" fighting instinct in the Anglo-Saxon warrior, such as not leaving a battlefield after the lord has fallen.[199] The heroic literature of Anglo-Saxon England, he argues, was designed to encourage such heroic instinct, not to depict it. Physical pain and the fear of imminent death are potentially traumatic, even to warriors of the early Middle Ages.

We know that an Anglo-Saxon warrior occasionally lost nerve and ran from the battlefield, but what is less well documented (by its very nature) is the anxiety potentially experienced later in life by a warrior who stood his ground. It appears that recovery from trauma relies far more on communal solidarity and social support networks than on internal neurophysiological processes.[200] Jonathan Shay surmises that the psychic numbing so evident in Vietnam veterans results largely from the lack of communal expressions of grief, and that rituals such as overt communal mourning are integral in preventing a permanent sense of dissociation and "taint."[201] Anglo-Saxon veterans could have presumably expected strong emotional encouragement from their family and compatriots—at least, those who returned to friends and family could have. Many may not have had a home to which to return. War disrupts families and scatters villages, and the *Anglo-Saxon Chronicle* documents chillingly the destruction of entire communities:

> (1065) þa Ryðrenan dydan mycelne hearm abutan Hamtune . . . ægþær þæt hi ofslogon menn ⁊ bærndon hus ⁊ corn ⁊ namon eall þæt orf þe hig mihton to cuman, þæt wæs feola þusend, ⁊ fela hund manna hi naman ⁊ læddan norð mid heom, swa þæt seo scir ⁊ þa oðra scira þæ ðærneah sindon wurdan fela wintra ðe wyrsan.[202]
>
> [the (Vikings) perpetrated great harm around Northampton . . . in that they killed people and burned houses and grain, and seized all the cattle they could get to—that was many thousands—and they seized many hundreds of people and took them north with them.]

Individuals might be taken as prisoners of war or sold into slavery, in many cases never to see a familiar place again. Furthermore, a warrior surviving his lord or experiencing shame at some other loss or breach of duty may have had to live in exile.

Exile is among the more pervasive themes of Old English poetry, from Grendel's brooding exclusion from the mead-hall to such elegiac poems as *The Seafarer*, *The Wanderer*, *Deor*, and *The Wife's Lament*.[203] Though ultimately consolatory in tone, the poetic voice in this cycle laments displacement, banishment from normal social activity, and the futility of trusting in worldly comforts. The narrator of *The Wanderer* has suffered the loss of his lord, and thereby his home and companions. The narrator of *The Wife's Lament* succinctly states, "A ic wite wonn minra wræcsiþa" (I perpetually suffer hardship from my cruel wanderings).[204] These poems express the pain of solitude and sometimes of betrayal; the narrators are trapped in the prison of memory.[205] While most surviving Old English poetry is devotional and expresses the comforts of faith, the elegies and elegiac passages reflect an important thread that reveals anxiety over solitude, frustrated opportunities to fraternize or to socialize through communal ritual, and an inability to progress emotionally—all of which bear some resemblance to the trauma now well-known to accompany war- or catastrophe-related loss. Battle in the early Middle Ages was brutal and done in close quarters, and often the stakes were high (protection of family and village). It is sometimes explicitly mentioned that early medieval demoniacs were soldiers (e.g., a *scutarius* in Jerome's *Life of Hilarion* or the *miles* Avitianus in Eugippius's *Life of Severin*), though in an era of levied militias rather than standing armies, "soldier" was not necessarily a defined profession that would be used to identify a man.[206] With that in mind, it is notable that one of our few cases of Anglo-Saxon possession does indicate the demoniac is a soldier: Ecga, the *comes* accompanying King Æthelbald in exile, must have fought in a number of engagements and endured other hardships by the time he is brought to Guthlac for healing. By this time, he does not know himself any longer.[207]

Aside from combat experience, the other major stressor commonly associated with dissociation in the modern world is childhood sexual assault (CSA). In fact, CSA is the single most common predictive criterion for DID.[208] In this respect, CSA can offer an intriguing complement to combat survival, as each affects a different demographic: male versus female. The lack of data, however, makes it difficult to assess the prevalence of CSA in Anglo-Saxon England. Furthermore, dissociation resulting from childhood trauma (such as incest) is far more complicated symptomatically than adult trauma (such as combat), making it even more difficult to isolate specific signs later in life indicative of early abuse. Whereas combat experience is a source of honor in warrior societies, childhood sexual experience in premodern European culture—in pagan and Christian areas alike—was stigmatized, and a source of shame with little hope for extensive communal support networks or even public acknowledgment of the crime.[209] The question of whether or not children were sexually abused in Anglo-Saxon England is perhaps indeterminable, so unlikely is it that cases would have been recorded in the historical sources. Even in our own modern culture, the problems of acknowledging widespread childhood sexual abuse are so pervasive that we were in denial until very recently.

Historians are uncertain about the history of child abuse. On the one hand, Lloyd DeMause offers a bleak history in which children have been the abject, servile victims of parental neglect and violence since the earliest periods of human history. Child abuse does not appear much in the documentary record, then, only because it was the norm and would have been taken for granted.[210] Though DeMause collects a wide range of sources supporting this view, they are nonetheless selectively chosen: he virtually ignores the vast documentary testimony of parental kindness and empathy. Diane Schetky agrees that child abuse is "nothing new"; we have simply become more aware of a problem that has always existed.[211] Others draw attention to the changing circumstances of family and culture in the industrialized West and posit that child abuse may indeed be a relatively new problem, at least in the forms and the extent to which we know it. The unstable nuclear family, the declining role of religion, the sexual revolution, and changes in work and child supervision habits, for instance, may affect the nature and prevalence of CSA in the developed world.[212] On this reading, children in previous eras may have been more protected from adult sexuality than ours are. These evolutionary models have been further nuanced with a variety of social construction theories—models which consider "abuse" a construct of twentieth-century values and concerns, and therefore a creation of the twentieth century.[213] Rex Stainton Rogers muses, for instance, that our current notions of "the best interests of the child" and of "child abuse" may seem as morbidly curious to future generations as the nineteenth-century medical evaluation of masturbation as self-abuse is to us.[214] It is at least clear, then, that no linear progression can be traced that will be applicable to all cultures throughout human history, and that child abuse must be evaluated afresh for any given historical group.

DeMause's widely influential book *The History of Childhood* pictured all childhood prior to the seventeenth century as "a nightmare," rife with children being more frequently "killed, abandoned, beaten, terrorized, and sexually abused" the further one goes back in history.[215] This relatively common generalization has been effectively discredited, at least for the Middle Ages.[216] Speaking of child abuse without specific reference to sexual abuse, recent historians believe that children in early medieval Europe suffered neither widespread violence nor neglect from their parents. Eleanora Gordon only finds five instances of child abuse in the 216 cases of children's illnesses and injuries reported at five twelfth-century English shrines.[217] She concludes, "although children were certainly neglected, abandoned, and abused, as they are today, the records in this study show that those parents who invoked the saints' aid for their children were deeply devoted to their offspring."[218] David Nicholas offers evidence for care and affection bestowed upon children from infancy through adolescence, finding that, "Just as it is true today, many children were abused and many others were loved, even pampered."[219] Speaking specifically of Anglo-Saxon England, Mathew Kuefler concludes, "The sources . . . record the harshness of life generally, and so indicate that by modern standards life was cruel for all, even if children were not especially maltreated."[220] Thus, though we can no longer credit generalized stereotypes of the Middle Ages as an arena for rampant domestic brutality, the consensus that childrearing practices in the Middle Ages resembled modern ones in many particulars also leaves open the possibility of medieval child sexual assault, as that is well-attested in our own day. The question is not whether medieval parents were more violent than modern ones but whether they were *as* violent. This fact would be sufficient to accept that the primary environmental factor in the etiology of DID, as it is known today, also existed in Anglo-Saxon England.

As with child abuse, opinions concerning rape in the Middle Ages are conflicting and often extravagant. G. Rattray Taylor evaluates the situation in early England recklessly: "rape and incest characterize the sexual life of the English in the first millennium of our era."[221] Yet the archaeological record is of little help regarding rape in Anglo-Saxon England. Hawkes and Wells believed they had found evidence of brutal rape in the skeletal remains of a sixteen-year-old girl in the Worthy Park graveyard of Kingsworthy, Hampshire: a slight thickening of the right femur at the pelvis joint consistent with hemorrhaging of torn thigh muscles. They vividly reconstruct a putative cause of this slight femoral bony growth: "Tearing of their tendons, which is very uncommon in young persons of this age, is almost invariably due to violent separation of the thighs whilst trying to resist this and bring them tightly together. In a sixteen-year-old girl the effort to draw her thighs together, and perhaps cross her legs, whilst a powerful man was forcing them apart, could easily produce the injury we find here."[222] They likewise interpret a lesion on the left femur as "due to a direct injury during the hurly-burly of her violation," and the unusual posture in the grave as evidence of live burial after the community had discovered her pregnancy some five to six months following the rape.[223] The details the authors proceed to spell out of both the alleged rape itself and her subsequent death rites read more like a deranged fantasy on their part than a rigorous archaeological analysis: building on the premise that "lust, rapine, blood and vengeance stalked across Early Saxon England," they conclude that, "naked, bound, lacerated and perhaps still alive, with the howl of human jackals in her ears, her passport to oblivion is likely to have been the slime and mire of this chalky trench."[224] In any event, their forensic reconstruction has been effectively discredited: the femoral lesions in question can be caused by any of a number of accidental causes.[225] Sam Lucy comments further that such interpretations of skeletal posture—after so much time, in which materials deteriorate at different rates and items shift within the grave—are unwarranted.[226]

Documentary records offer a wide range of provocative statements about women and violence, though it is often difficult to evaluate such statements contextually.[227] Legal and penitential texts can provide a point of orientation. Whereas rape only appears in Roman law relatively late and is primarily a question of property devaluation, the Anglo-Saxon legal tradition drew more attention to rape as an injury against an individual.[228] Early Germanic law codes were intimately concerned with violence against women; they catalog in great detail nonconsensual contact with various parts of a woman's body.[229] By the time of Alfred, at least, the woman's consent or lack thereof is a relevant factor in determining the seriousness of the crime (as in Alfred 18, and later on II Cnut 73.2).[230] Alfred's code details various tiers of social class and severity of assaults, and explicitly mentions the rape of underage girls: "Gif mon ungewintrædne wifmon to niedhæmde geðreatige, sie ðæt swa ðæs gewintredan monnes bot"[231] (If someone threatens [or attacks] an underage woman with rape, may that carry the same compensation as for a mature woman). Theodore's Penitential addresses the age at which a parent can no longer choose a daughter's spouse against her will, referring explicitly to the young woman's "power" or "control" of her body: "puella autem XIV annorum sui corporis potestatem habet" (a girl of fourteen years has control over her own body).[232] A Latin directive from the tradition of Halitgar's Penitential provides a reminder of the extreme circumstances in which a young woman could find herself in the early Middle Ages:

> Si puella aliqua desponsata sit, et interea in captivitatem ducta fuerit, vel causa aliqua ab eo erepta, cui desponsata erat, et postea acciderit, ut alter in alterius viciniam veniat, cum venia conjungi possunt, quia ab eo invita aberat.[233]
>
> [If a girl is betrothed, and in the meantime she is carried off in captivity or is taken from him to whom she had been promised by whatever means, and if it should then befall that one happens into the vicinity of the other, they may still be married, if they want to, since she had gone away from him unwillingly.]

The *Anglo-Saxon Chronicle* and the *Life of Alfred* allude hauntingly to convents being raided by Vikings and all the nuns being taken.[234] The fate of female slaves in the early Middle Ages can often be a grim one, as an account in Cogitosus's *Life of Brigit* reminds us: a wealthy man plots to reduce a woman to slavery (a neighboring woman of his own people, whom he desires), specifically so that he "postea uteretur, ut vellet, amplexibus" (then might have use of her, as he wished, in sexual embraces).[235] II Cnut attempts to discourage men from having sex with their own slaves (*wyln*, "female slave")—at least, it attempts to discourage married men (*wiffæst wer*) from doing so.[236] Finally, we should recall that boys might be potential subjects of sexual attention as well as girls, if the Anglo-Norman Rule of Lanfranc for the monks of Christ Church, Canterbury is any indication. Great care is taken to prevent monks from having undue contact with young men (*iuvenes*).[237]

While rape is a crime, incest is taboo: a defiling of the proper order of family and a crime against God.[238] It is also an unequivocal danger in many societies modern and premodern; Freud argues that the prevention of the possibility of incest is the unspoken rationale behind the intricate rules of who may be alone with whom in many cultures ("laws of avoidance").[239] In this light, father-daughter incest is suspiciously absent in Theodore's Penitential, which otherwise sets up a categorical list of incestuous offenses:

> 2.16. Si cum matre quis fornicaverit, XV annos peniteat et nunquam mutat nisi dominicis diebus. Et hoc tam profanum incestum ab eo similiter alio modo dicitur, ut cum peregrinatione perenni VII annos peniteat.
> 2.17. Qui cum sorore fornicaverit XV annos peniteat eo modo, quo superius de matre dicitur.[240]
>
> [2.16. If someone fornicates with his mother, he must do penance for 15 years and may not change except on Sundays. And this is such an unholy form of incest, the same matter is spoken of in another way: that he must do penance for seven years, with continual pilgrimage.
> 2.17. He who fornicates with his sister must do penance for 15 years, just as was said above about the mother.]

The text goes on to consider brother committing incest with brother (2.19) and a mother "imitating incest" with her "small son" (2.20), but nowhere is father-daughter incest mentioned—though presumably, this is far more obviously a danger than these others.[241] These lists of provisions are repeated more or less as a unit in a variety of Anglo-Saxon penitentials such as the *Canons of Gregory* and the Penitential of Bede.[242] It is only in the Penitential of Egbert that a provision is added for father-daughter relations: "si cum filia vel sorore [fornicaverit], XII annos peniteat" (if one has fornicated with his daughter or sister, he is to do penance for twelve years).[243] We should keep in mind that many of these provisions are in texts manifestly of exotica rather than honest confrontations of dangerous social ills—and this is precisely why it is unnerving that father-daughter incest is absent throughout most of this tradition. Why was father-daughter incest usually passed over in such otherwise completist texts?

I have not come across any evidence in the literary record of incestuous sexual abuse within a household in Anglo-Saxon England in the literary record, but for such a notoriously elusive practice, the silence of the written record is hardly the final word. The implicit communal conspiracy of silence that can shroud such practices is by now well-documented, even in traditional societies.[244] The (late) Old English translation of *Apollonius of Tyre* contains a description of father-daughter rape, one of the few in the Anglo-Saxon literary record.[245] This is not a description of a contemporary or recent event in England itself, but the dramatic opening scene of a Mediterranean romance that predates the period of Anglo-Saxon letters by several centuries. King Antiochus of the city of Antioch sends all the servants away from his daughter's chamber one morning and takes her by force:

> Đa gelamp hit sarlicum gelimpe: þa ða se fæder þohte hwam he hi mihte healicost forgifan, þa gefeol his agen mod on hyre lufe mid unrihtre gewilnunge, to ðam swiðe þæt he forgeat þa fæderlican arfæstnesse and gewilnode his agenre dohtor him to gemæccan, and þa gewilnunge naht lange ne ylde, ac sume dæge on ærnemergen þa he of slæpe awoc, he abræ into ðam bure þar heo inne læg and het his hyredmen ealle him aweg gan, swilce he wið his dohtor sume digle spæce sprecan wolde. Hwæt he ða on ðare manfullan scilde abisgode and þa ongeanwinnendan fæmnan mid micelre strengðe earfoðlice ofercom, and þæt gefremede man gewilnode to bediglianne.[246]
>
> [Then a grievous thing happened: when the father reflected on the highest-ranking person whom he could wed, his own heart turned to desire for her (his daughter) with wicked passions—so much that he forgot his paternal duty and wished for his daughter to be his mate. He did not delay in that desire very long, but one day at daybreak when he woke up, he broke into the chamber where she lay and ordered all the servants to go away, since he wanted to have some words with her

> in private. Alas! He then busied himself with that wicked crime and, with great strength, overpowered the resisting woman. He wished to conceal the crime he had committed.][247]

Peter Goolden points out that the description of the rape is "unusually heavily paraphrased" from the Latin original—"no doubt," he concludes, "the subject-matter was too unpleasant for exact translation."[248] By contrast, the subsequent passage adheres closely to the Latin original. When the girl's foster-mother comes in, the girl stolidly tells her about the misdeed:

> Ða gewearð hit þæt þæs mædenes fostormodor into ðam bure eode and geseah hi ðar sittan on micelre gedrefednesse and hire cwæð to: "Hwig eart þu, hlæfdige, swa gedrefedes modes?" Þæt mæden hyre andswerode: "Leofe fostormodor, nu todæg forwurdon twegen æðele naman on þisum bure." Seo fostormodor cwæð: "Hlæfdige, be hwæm cwist þu þæt?" Heo hyre andwirde and cwæð: "Ær ðam dæge minra bridgifta ic eom mid manfulre scilde besmitan." Ða cwæð seo fostormodor: "Hwa wæs æfre swa dirstiges modes þæt dorste cynges dohtor gewæmman ær ðam dæge hyre brydgifta and him ne ondrede þæs cyninges irre?" Ðæt mæden cwæð: "Arleasnes þa scilde on me gefremode." Seo fostormodor cwæð: "Hwi ne segst þu hit þinum fæder?" Ðæt mæden cwæð: "Hwar is se fæder? Soðlice on me earmre is mines fæder nama reowlice forworden and me nu forðam deað þearle gelicað."[249]
>
> [Then it happened that the maiden's foster-mother came into the chamber and saw her sitting there in great distress and said to her, "Lady, why are you so troubled in spirit?" The maiden answered her, "Dear foster-mother, today two valuable names have just been ruined in this room." The foster-mother said, "Lady, about whom are you speaking?" She answered her and said, "I have been defiled with a wicked crime, even before my wedding day." Then the foster-mother said, "Who was ever so presumptuous that he dared defile the king's daughter before her wedding day, without fearing the king's wrath?" The maiden said, "Wickedness has committed this crime against me." The foster mother said, "Why don't you tell your father?" The maiden said, "Where is 'the father'? Truly, my father's name is pitifully ruined for me, and now because of that, death is all that's left me."]

The conversation becomes a game of riddles, almost, with the foster-mother asking practical, simple questions and the girl parrying with enigmatic evasion and metaphor. The girl is evidently unable to confront the situation explicitly. Old English (like Old Norse) is famous for understating affective content, and suggesting powerful emotions through minimalist language. As the story evolves in the later Middle Ages, the poignant sense of hurt and betrayal becomes more explicit, along with the language of physical wounding. A fourteenth-century version of the Apollonius story reads:

> stimulante furore libidinis diu repugnanti filiae suae nodum virginitatis eripuit. Perfectoque scelere evasit cubiculum. Puella vero stans dum miratur scelestis patris impietatem, fluentem sanguinem coepit celare: sed guttae sanguinis in pavimento ceciderunt.[250]
>
> [Aroused by the fury of his lust, he tore away the knot of his daughter's virginity,[251] though she resisted for a long time. Having completed this wickedness, he fled the chamber. As the girl stood there, astonished by the blasphemy of her vicious father, she hid the stream of blood: but drops of blood fell to the floor.]

The incestuous father motif is common in folklore and in the mythologies of many peoples, and its value may be more symbolic than descriptive.[252] Certain recurring elements in medieval romances suggest literary patterning: for instance, the incest victim is invariably an only child and an heiress, and the father is subsequently urged to marry her by his counselors.[253] In all of this pattern's versions, furthermore, only a single rape incident is mentioned in each case, and not the ongoing incestuous abuse that is often the pattern in modern families. Still, it is disturbing when one occasionally finds a vivid detail added to the incest scene, such as the drops of blood above or the violent visualization provided by Chaucer's Man of Law:

> How that the cursed kyng Antiochus
> Birafte his doghter of hir maydenhede,
> That is so horrible a tale for to rede,
> Whan he hir threw upon the pavement.[254]

The king does not throw his daughter onto the floor in any version of the tale, Latin or vernacular, prior to Chaucer; one hopes the Man of Law has no experience in the matter and has invented the detail simply to rhyme with the subsequent *avysement*.[255] He categorically states, in any event, that he will not include such "unkynde abhomynacions" in his own tale of Constance.[256] Behind the literary topos lingers the possibility of disturbing realities, from which authors shy away even as they promulgate the narrative tradition. As provocative as the incident in *Apollonius* is, however, it remains an isolated instance of incest in the Old English corpus, perhaps too rooted in literary precedent to give us much insight into contemporary social issues.

Finally, Ælfric and Wulfstan may provide us with refracted hints of incest as a social anxiety in late Anglo-Saxon England. The Old Testament itself contains numerous cases of incest, some of which inevitably make their way into Old English literature (such as the Exeter Book riddle whose solution is Lot).[257] Ælfric is uneasy with these passages, and in his "Preface to Genesis" he expresses concern that certain customs apparently sanctioned in the Old Testament may be potentially dangerous if translated into the vernacular for contemporary audiences: "ic ondræde, gif sum dysig man þas boc ræt oððe rædan gehyrþ, þæt he wille wenan, þæt he mote lybban nu on þære niwan æ, swa swa þa ealdan fæderas leofodon þa on þære tide" (I dread that if some ignorant person reads the book or hears it read, he might imagine that it is alright for him to live now, under the new law, the same way that the old fathers lived then, in that time).[258] Out of the many alien and sometimes disturbing themes that abound in the Old Testament, here Ælfric singles out incest and polygamy as the most sensitive and volatile: "On anginne þisere worulde nam se broþer hys swuster to wife and hwilon eac se fæder tymde be his agenre dehter" (In the beginning of this world, brothers took their sisters as wives and fathers sometimes had children by their own daughters).[259] Wulfstan goes even further, studiously omitting from his own version of Ælfric's *De falsis diis* references to father-daughter incest among the pagan gods. By contrast, Wulfstan seems to harbor no qualms about including brother-sister incest.[260] As in the vernacular translation of *Apollonius*, father-daughter incest is an uncomfortable theme for both Ælfric and Wulfstan. Perhaps, then, it is not a purely fossilized literary motif for these translators, but a perceived source of potential danger.

For heartrending scenes of pillage and criminal violence more generally, one need look no further than Wulfstan's celebrated *Sermo Lupi ad Anglos*. This paints a gruesome picture of a tumultuous society in which violence to women is an ever-present possibility. Wulfstan alleges that bands of corrupt English men pool together to buy a woman, use her for sex, and then sell her into slavery abroad:

> scandlic is to specenne þæt geworden is to wide ⁊ egeslic is to witanne þæt oft doð to manege þe dreogað þa yrmþe, þæt sceotað togædere ⁊ ane cwenan gemænum ceape bicgað gemæne, ⁊ wið þa ane fylþe adreogað, an after anum ⁊ ælc æfter oðrum, hundum gelicost þe for fylþe ne scrifað, ⁊ syððan wið weorðe syllað of lande feondum to gewealde Godes gesceafte.[261]
>
> [It is shameful to relate what has happened too often, and it is terrible to realize what too many often do when they perpetrate a certain wrong: they join together and buy one woman as a common purchase, and commit unclean sin with the same woman one after another—each after the other!—just like dogs who pay no regard to uncleanness. Then they sell the creature of God for a price abroad, into the hands of enemies.]

This was perhaps too charged and potent a scene for many readers: the passage only appears in two of the five manuscript copies of the *Sermo*. It is not entirely clear whether Wulfstan is here alleging what we would think of as gang rape or whether the woman is simply passed along from one of the joint owners to the next in succession, but in either case—if Wulfstan's accounts are accurate and he is not indulging in the hyperbolic rhetoric common in homilies (and especially common in Wulfstan's homilies)—we must imagine an appalling ordeal for the woman. A little further, he describes an equally horrific situation; here it is clear that the gang activity (this time by Viking marauders) occurs in a single place and time: "Oft tyne oððe twelfe, ælc æfter oþrum, scendað to bysmore þæs þegenes cwenan ⁊ hwilum his dohtor oððe nydmagan þær he on locað"[262] (Often ten or twelve, one after another, shamefully insult the thane's wife—and sometimes his daughter or other female relative—while he looks on). The mention of a daughter—though not specifying age at all in this instance—leaves plenty of room to acknowledge that girls were potentially exposed to ghastly experiences in this turbulent age.[263]

We are thus left with only tantalizing glimpses and clues into the possible sexual violence against Anglo-Saxon women and girls, without the means of directly verifying or corroborating our suspicions. Considering international prevalence rates in the modern world, David Finkelhor argues that CSA has been identified in "a large fraction of the population" of over twenty countries.[264] A recent study conducted in Turkey helps illuminate how such father-daughter incest can function. Most of the fathers of sexually abused girls in this study were their biological fathers, implying that the practice does not necessarily result from the breakdown of the nuclear family.[265] Of the sexually abused girls only one-third had been penetrated vaginally, and even in the cases of penetration, three-quarters did not have ruptured hymens—indicating a carefully gauged level of contact designed to preserve virginity.[266] Yüksel comments, "The importance of virginity is generally very high, especially in the traditional region. In many places the absence of virginity may mean that a young girl loses her chance for marriage. If the situation is known, she loses her prestige within the family as the family loses it in their close neighborhood. . . . Sexual abusers seem to pay attention to this issue."[267] The experience is no less damaging for all that; the women in the study were specifically selected because of their presentation of a wide range of psychiatric problems. For instance, one of the conditions most strongly correlated with childhood sexual abuse was self-mutilation, a commonly reported symptom of medieval demon possession (though of course there is a wide range of potential causes for such behavior).[268]

Sexual attention from a parent figure covers a wide spectrum and degree of severity, not all of which will be equally traumatic to a child. There is reason to think, however, that if such practices existed, they would have the potential to be profoundly traumatic to an Anglo-Saxon girl—arguably, perhaps, more so than today, since Anglo-Saxon England stressed virginity far more than twentieth- and twenty-first-century societies in the developed world. An earlier age may have compounded the victim's psychological difficulties with the onus of "pollution" in the religious sense, a dimension which is largely atrophied or sublimated in the modern secular world. There was no public discourse of rape awareness, although there may well have been support networks among women. Support (or lack thereof) from family members especially, according to Finkelhor, is "the most consistent predictor of impact of sexual abuse on a child."[269] In the absence of these healing mechanisms, a girl may have been at high risk for a permanently fractured identity.

Occasionally, medieval narratives provide details that suggest the very real possibility of abuse within the family or household. The *Life of Caesarius of Arles* includes the account of a servant or slave woman (*ancilla*), from an estate called Luco, that on a certain reading, links violence or abuse with demon possession. The lady Eucyria brings her servant to Caesarius, claiming that she is regularly harassed by a demon (the demon Diana, according to locals: "daemonium quod rustici Dianam appellant").[270] Eucyria explains that the girl is so possessed that "paene omnibus noctibus assidue caedatur" (almost every night she is constantly beaten) and she is continuously heard crying.[271] Caesarius asks to examine the servant's wounds, and the narrator (a cleric accompanying Caesarius) records:

> Si mihi fideles credunt, coram deo dico, oculis meis vidi plagas, quas ante aliquos dies in dorsum et in scapulas acceperat, ad sanitatem venire; pridianas autem et in ipsa nocte impressas recentes inter illas intextas.[272]
>
> [If the faithful believe me, I assert in the presence of God that I saw with my own eyes some blows that were healing, which she had received on her back and shoulders a few days before. Recent wounds, however, inflicted the previous day and on the night before, were woven among them.]

She is, of course, fully healed by the good bishop. Part of the wonder behind this miracle story is that the violence delivered by demons is nonetheless real, physical violence that leaves tangible wounds on the body. If we subtract demons from the equation, however, we are left to question how such marks really did get there. A frightful picture suggests itself of the life of this slave girl. Even though sexual violence is not mentioned in this account, the scene reminds us how helpless certain sectors of early medieval society were, how the clergy could serve the important role of providing a sympathetic ear and a heartfelt prayer, and how those very pastors—and the community at large—could be complicitous in perpetuating a public narrative that helped conceal and enable the abuses that had been brought forth. The text states that the bishop blessed the slave girl and left her with some holy oil with which she should be anointed at night. It further states that, as a result, she was never troubled by the demon again (but perhaps the bishop was not in a position to know what actually happened to the girl once he and his entourage moved on). What is intriguing, however, is the particular strategy employed here: Caesarius leaves Eucyria with oil for anointing the slave girl nightly. The healing touch of her mistress may well have been of comfort to the girl. Beyond this, though, the strategy shrewdly ensures at least two things: first, that the girl remains more closely under Eucyria's supervision, in specifying that this process be conducted nightly; and second, that it places Eucyria in intimate contact with the girl's body, thus allowing her to gauge exactly when and where such marks appear. Lady Eucyria is thus granted the authority to take closer, more personal control of the situation. This arrangement would perhaps dissuade whoever is surreptitiously responsible for the wounds from harassing the girl further.

Aside from combat violence and sexual abuse, Anglo-Saxons suffered traumas of others sorts. We are only beginning to realize the impact of war and war-related loss on children, and war was a pervasive fact of life, in one location or another, throughout virtually all generations of the Anglo-Saxon period. Researchers have learned that repeated exposure to trauma does not necessarily "harden" a child: coping reserves are depleted rather than strengthened by repeated trauma, traumas of different sources, and/or multiple traumas coinciding with one another temporally.[273] The ordeal of witnessing violence, losing loved ones, or becoming displaced can easily lead to psychotic symptoms.[274] We can be sure that Anglo-Saxons suffered trauma of some sort or other—they were neither above nor beneath the human condition—and presumably they coped with it to some extent using dissociative mechanisms; but without records of the patients' phenomenological perception of the condition, or of the response from friends and family, it is difficult to draw any clear connection between trauma victims and any demoniacs who may have presented at Anglo-Saxon shrines or to holy men and women.[275]

The point of the remarks in this chapter has not been to read particular anecdotes in medieval hagiography as literal records of actual events, nor to map them directly onto currently recognized pathologies in any one-to-one sense. The anecdotes can rather serve, on the whole, to indicate the sorts of conditions that were possible and can help us understand what sorts of responses these conditions potentially elicited from the community and from healers. We have had to search far afield in time and place (in continental sources, as well as in classical and late medieval ones) to supplement the scant materials left from Anglo-Saxon England, with the tacit understanding that the further afield we search, the less certain our conclusions will apply. We are left, though, with a final picture of a society with a wide array of potential assaults on the individual, both from within (such as organic neurological conditions) and without (such as trauma-induced psychiatric damage)—though the most sensational of possible symptoms would have presented only very rarely. Nonetheless, these conditions would conceivably have presented behaviors challenging both to the economic integrity of the small community (which relies on the labor of everyone), and beyond that, perhaps challenging to a worldview premised on the effective intermediacy of church representatives and on a sense of personal identity that presumes the indivisible integrity of the human will.

NOTES

1. Quoted in John Bamberger, *Evagrius Ponticus*, p. 67.

2. *Miracula Sancte Ætheldrethe* 3 (Goscelin, *Hagiography*, p. 110). This work is edited and extracted by Rosalind Love from the composite narratives relating to St. Æthelthryth in CCCC 393 and Dublin, Trinity College, MS 172 (B.2.7); Love argues for its independent existence and dubs this the *Miracula Sancte Ætheldrethe* (pp. lx–lxi). The work cannot be dated, however, with any more precision than between the late tenth and early twelfth century (pp. lxv, lxxi). The work may or may not be by Goscelin; the most recent editor leans away from this ascription (p. lxv).

3. *Vita Cuthberti* 4.17 (Colgrave, *Two Lives*, pp. 136–38).

4. Bede, *Vita Cuthberti* 45 (Colgrave, *Two Lives*, p. 299). On paralysis, see Bonser, *Medical Background*, pp. 413–16.

5. Bede, *HE* 3.11, p. 248.

6. *Vita Genovefae* 47 (Krusch, *Passiones* [MGH, SRM 3], p. 234).

7. Gregory of Tours, *Liber vitae partum* 8.8 (Krusch, *Miracula et opera*, p. 249).

8. Norman Moore, *Book*, p. 47.

9. Clarke, *Mental Disorder*, p. 70.

10. Borderline personality disorder (BPD) bears a close resemblance to certain aspects of possession (erratic behavior, unstable identity, and potential for violence). BPD is characterized by an unstable sense of self, short (but intense) relationships, and impulsiveness. Often manipulative and demanding of attention, BPD patients have difficulty forming lasting friendships and relationships. They are unusually preoccupied with gaining approval from others, because of low self-esteem and an inability to act independently (e.g., to commit to long-term goals). Subjects often suffer from depression punctuated by outbursts of anger, panic, or despair that can result in violent and self-destructive behavior. Self-mutilation and suicide attempts are common (DSM-IV, p. 651; Clarkin, Marziali, and Munroe-Blum, *Borderline Personality Disorder*). However, unlike demon possession, there is no true fragmentation of the self in BPD: the subject does not claim to be someone else. Most importantly, BPD may be a uniquely modern condition: patients express a profound sense of boredom, inner emptiness, and identity confusion (such as gender identity and value), all of which are especially prominent in postindustrial societies. There is reason to believe that BPD may be correlated with increasing rates of substance abuse and changes in family life and leisure habits—in short, that modernization is a requisite for BPD as it is commonly understood (Millon, "Borderline Personality," pp. 197–210; Paris, "Personality Disorders," pp. 32–33).

11. Conn, Borer, and Snyder, *Current Diagnosis*; Tierney, McPhee, and Papadakis, *Current Medical Diagnosis*.

12. The definitive history of epilepsy is Temkin, *Falling Sickness*; see also Eadie, "Understanding," pp. 1–12; Eadie, *A Disease Once Sacred*; von Storch, "Essay," pp. 614–50.

13. The inference has to be made from analogy, since the actual motives behind prehistoric trepanation are irretrievable. In places as diverse as Melanesia and Yugoslavia, trepanation was practiced for epilepsy, headache, insanity, and mental or nervous disorders in general until the late nineteenth century (Lisowski, "Prehistoric and Early Historic Trepanation," p. 658). Medieval authorities only seem to recommend the procedure for head wounds, however, and the motives for Anglo-Saxon trepanation are unknown (Parker, "Skulls," pp. 73–84).

14. J. V. Kinnier Wilson and Reynolds, "Translation," p. 189.

15. An unambiguous attack on popular superstition, *On the Sacred Disease* remains one of the most important milestones of Greek medicine (Temkin, *Falling Sickness*, p. 4). The term "Hippocratic" here refers to the school of medicine in which numerous writings were inevitably attributed to the eponymous doctor, though in this case even Galen rejected the text's authenticity. The treatise notes that epilepsy is genetic and states that epilepsy is a problem with humoral brain chemistry rather than spirit possession. The treatise was unknown to the Latin Middle Ages (5). The text is edited and translated in Hippocrates, "Sacred Disease," pp. 127–83.

16. Lennox, *Epilepsy*, pp. 707–8. The attribution to Alfred undoubtedly refers to his mysterious illness described in chap. 74 of the *Life of Alfred* (see above, in the introduction). Other figures who have had epilepsy ascribed to them include Pythagoras, Amenhotep, Socrates, Buddha, Caesar, St. Paul, Plotinus, and Mohammed (Lennox, *Epilepsy*, pp. 707–8).

17. Gregory of Tours, *Liber de virtutibus S. Martini* 2.18 (Krusch, *Miracula et opera minora*, p. 165).

18. Kindschi, "Latin-Old English Glossaries," p. 58.

19. Bede, *HE* 3.11, p. 248.

20. *Vita Cuthberti* 2.8 (Colgrave, *Two Lives*, p. 90).

21. It is hard to know what *færlicre adle* (sudden sickness) might mean—it has usually been taken to mean seizures (as in Grattan and Singer, *Anglo-Saxon Magic*, p. 147, and in the *DOE*); but is overall too vague for reconstruction (*Lacnunga* 66 [Pettit, *Anglo-Saxon Remedies*, 1:56, and see 2:93]). Grattan and Singer also translate *onfeall* as "sudden seizure" (*Anglo-Saxon Magic*, p. 34, when speaking of recipes in *Leechbook* 1.39 [Cockayne, *Leechdoms*, vol. 2, pp. 98–104]; others, such as Bosworth-Toller, translate this as "swelling").

22. Bonser, *Medical Background*, p. 415; Stephen of Ripon, *Vita Wilfridi* 37 (Colgrave, *Wilfrid*, p. 74).

23. Temkin, *Falling Sickness*, p. 100. For more on dancing manias, see the conclusion, below.

24. Marsden and Reynolds, "Seizures," p. 153.

25. Dreifuss, "Classification," pp. 79, 83.

26. Marsden and Reynolds, "Seizures," p. 152.

27. Caelius Aurelianus, *Acute Diseases*, p. 479.

28. See, for instance, fol. 3v of the *Canterbury Psalter* (Paris, Bibliothèque nationale de France, MS lat. 8846), reproduced in Strickland, *Saracens*, p. 80; fol. 24r of the fourteenth-century *Holkham Bible Picture Book* (London, British Library, MS Add. 47682), reproduced in Doob, *Nebuchadnezzar's Children* (pl. 2); fol. 91r of the ninth-century Drogo Sacramentary of Metz (Paris, Bibliothèque nationale de France, MS lat. 9428); and page 43 of Washington, Freer Gallery of Art, MS 32.18 (an Armenian Gospel book), reproduced in the *New Catholic Encyclopedia*, 4:839 (s.v. "Diabolical Possession"). See also 5:748 (s.v. "Exorcism").

29. Kaviratna, *Charaka-Samhita*, p. 212; and see Haldipur, "Madness," pp. 335–44.

30. Marsden and Reynolds, "Seizures," p. 151.

31. Dreifuss, "Classification," p. 79.

32. Murdoch, "*Peri Hieres Nousou*," p. 149. He continues, "The charm might indeed have helped. The details of first aid provided by the modern Epilepsy Association include keeping calm, clearing a space round the patient, not giving food or drink, and speaking reassuringly to the patient after the attack" (149).

33. For lupines, see Dendle, "Lupines." For peony, see Tsuda et al., "Protective Effects," pp. 518–25; and Sugaya et al., "Inhibitory Effects," pp. 65–77.

34. Alarcón, Foulks, and Vakkur, *Personality Disorders*, p. 105; and also Alarcón, "Cross-Cultural Issues," pp. 561–78.

35. See Alarcón, Foulks, and Vakkur, *Personality Disorders*, p. 114; Krippner, "Cross-Cultural Treatment Perspectives"; Morris, *Anthropology*; Shweder and Bourne, "Does the Concept," pp. 97–137.

36. Kirmayer, "Pacing," p. 106.

37. Paris, "Personality Disorders," p. 29.

38. Alarcón, Foulks, and Vakkur, *Personality Disorders*, p. 110; see also pp. 71–72.

39. Alarcón, Foulks, and Vakkur, *Personality Disorders*, pp. 108–9, 221; and see also p. 171: "The diagnosis and classification of personality disorders across cultures, although difficult, are not impossible."

40. For personality disorders, see Akhtar, *Broken Structures*; First and Tasman, *DSM-IV-TR*; Kantor, *Diagnosis*; Manfield, *Split Self/Split Object*; Turkat, *Personality Disorders*.

41. First and Tasman, *DSM-IV-TR*, pp. 739–40.

42. DSM-IV, p. 341.

43. Thus Kate L. Harkness and Scott M. Monroe: "severe sexual abuse, sexual abuse, antipathy, and neglect, as well as both high and lax levels of supervision and discipline, were significantly associated with endogenous versus nonendogenous depression.... Sexual abuse was also associated with more severe depression and higher levels of suicidal ideation" ("Childhood Adversity," p. 390). "Endogenous" refers to depression not sparked by obvious external causes or life events.

44. Cross-National Collaborative Group, "Changing Rate," pp. 3098–105; First and Tasman, *DSM-IV-TR*, p. 750; Klerman and Weissman, "Increasing Rates," pp. 2229–35.

45. For a sample critique—of which there are many—of the concept of depression as applied to other cultures, see Jadhav, "Cultural Origins," pp. 269–86.

46. Goodwin and Jamison, *Manic-Depressive Illness*, p. 242.

47. First and Tasman, *DSM-IV-TR*, pp. 804–5.

48. John Cassian, *Conlationes* 4.2 (Petschenig, *Iohannis Cassiani Conlationes*, p. 98). On John Cassian, see Lake, "Knowledge," pp. 27–41.

49. For example, demons visit the hermit Guthlac, cajoling him to fast for a full week rather than for shorter periods (Felix, *Vita Guthlaci* 30; Colgrave, *Felix's Life*, pp. 98–100). Guthlac sees through this demonic ruse and considers the suggestion "vain" (*ydele*, in the OE translation; Gonser, *Das angelsächsische*, p. 126). After driving the demons away with a psalm, he eats his daily ration right away to spite them.

50. Stanley Jackson, *Melancholia and Depression*, p. 51. See also Langslow, *Latin Alexander*.

51. *Enchiridion*: Baker and Lapidge, *Byrhtferth's Enchiridion*, p. 12; *Ramsey Medical Treatise*: Hart, *Learning*, 2:443–61. Debbie Banham cautions against the "tendency to overestimate the sophistication of Anglo-Saxon medicine of the tenth century" ("A Millennium," p. 231), pointing out that there is very little explicit theory prior to the eleventh century (234). Cameron notes, "the Anglo-Saxons in their medicine paid lip service to the humoral theory but do not seem to have grasped its full implications" (*Anglo-Saxon Medicine*, p. 161). For an exception, see the treatment of humors in a recipe for cough (*Lacnunga* 173; Pettit, *Anglo-Saxon Remedies*, 1:121); see also Jolly, *Popular Religion*, p. 108.

52. Stryker, "Latin-Old English Glossary," pp. 303, 311.

53. Aldhelm, *De virginitate*, ch. 32 (Gwara, *Aldhelmi Malmesbiriensis*, vol. 2, p. 427).

54. Stryker, "Latin-Old English Glossary," p. 70. For a nuanced reading of the multivalent nature of this phenomenon in its early developmental use, see Crislip, "Sin of Sloth."

55. John Cassian, *Institutes* 10.1–2 (Petschenig, *Cassiani Opera*, pp. 173–74).

56. Evagrius, *Praktikos* 12 (John Bamberger, *Evagrius Ponticus*, pp. 18–19; cf. p. 23).

57. Bloomfield, *Seven Deadly Sins*, p. 72.

58. Scragg, *Vercelli Homilies*, p. 74.

59. Ælfric of Eynsham, *Dominica in media Quadragesima* (*Catholic Homilies* 2.12; Godden, *Second Series*, pp. 124–25). The distinction between a productive and a destructive sense of "sadness" is biblical (2 Corinthians 7:10).

60. Crislip lays out some problems with identifying early models of *acedia* with current clinical notions of depression ("Sin of Sloth," p. 158n90).

61. The second diagnostic criterion for a major depressive episode reads: "markedly diminished interest or pleasure at all, or almost all, activities most of the day, nearly every day" (First and Tasman, *DSM-IV-TR*, p. 739).

62. Wenzel, *Sin*, p. 165.

63. Seabourne and Seabourne do not mention that demonic instigation is listed as an explicitly stated cause in the Eyre suicide records for England from the twelfth to fourteenth centuries. Mental illness leading to suicide is represented there as *demens*, *in frenesi*, or *furore detentus* ("Suicide," p. 43). Regarding methods of suicide (in the two hundred or so cases they collected), the authors found that "hanging is the most common method of self-killing in both men and women, drowning is the next most common in men and women and the use of sharp objects is an almost exclusively male method of self-killing" (44). In modern major depressive disorder, up to 15% of subjects die by suicide (DSM-IV, p. 340).

64. Seabourne and Seabourne, "Suicide," p. 45. Men continued to outpace women in self-killing rates throughout Tudor, Stuart, and Victorian times (45).

65. Williams, *Two Lives*, p. 68.

66. Williams, *Two Lives*, p. 68.

67. Even here, however, the cases most resembling demon possession are extreme cases: "Most people with the syndrome are not exceptional. Those who have mild Tourette syndrome (the majority) live quite unnoticed in their communities, pursuing their daily business in all walks of life" (Robertson and Baron-Cohen, *Tourette Syndrome*, p. 40).

68. Leckman and Cohen, *Tourette's Syndrome*, p. 11.

69. Berecz, *Understanding Tourette's Syndrome*, p. 1.

70. Howard Kushner traces the competing schools of organic versus psychoanalytic schools of thought in *A Cursing Brain*.

71. Staley, Wand, and Shady, "Tourette Syndrome," p. 14. Shapiro et al. identify the "refocusing from a psychological to an organic central nervous system etiology" as one of the principal achievements in TS studies of the last quarter century (*Gilles de la Tourette Syndrome*, p. 26).

72. The pathogenesis of TS is still poorly understood, though the breakdown of behavioral inhibitions implicates the limbic system in addition to the obvious motor function systems.

73. Comings, *Tourette Syndrome*, p. 25; Zohar et al., "Epidemiological Studies," p. 190. Felix Y. Attah Johnson is perhaps overzealous in claiming it has been described "in all racial groups" ("Gilles de la Tourette Syndrome," p. 129). Earlier studies suggesting a higher prevalence of TS among people of Eastern European or Jewish background have not been consistently replicated (Shapiro et al., *Gilles de la Tourette Syndrome*, pp. 74–78).

74. Robertson and Baron-Cohen, *Tourette Syndrome*, p. 20. Staley, Wand, and Shady compare studies across a range of countries, concluding that today TS has a globally consistent distribution with a similar range of symptoms: "A strikingly similar pattern emerges from descriptions of TS documented in reports from both North America and Europe and

other regions and cultures of the world" ("Tourette Syndrome," p. 13). Coprolalia varied greatly, however, from 4% in Japan to 60% in Hong Kong (11).

75. Freeman et al., "International Perspective," pp. 436–47. Age of onset and a link between anger control and comorbidity were both consistent across the study sample, while the prevalence ratios between males and females showed the greatest variation. Shapiro et al. discuss contaminating factors (e.g., the greater likelihood of bringing in males for treatment; and the greater urgency associated with symptoms such as rage, which have higher prevalence among male TS patients), yet after accounting for those factors, still conclude that "the higher male to female ratio in Tourette's disorder appears to be real" (*Gilles de la Tourette Syndrome*, p. 73).

76. Robertson and Baron-Cohen, *Tourette Syndrome*, p. 20; Zohar et al., "Epidemiological Studies," p. 192.

77. Shapiro et al., *Gilles de la Tourette Syndrome*, p. 2.

78. Comings, *Tourette Syndrome*, p. 17.

79. In fact, coprolalia presents in less than a third of the clinically reported cases of TS (Comings, *Tourette Syndrome*, p. 163), and because of the nature of the symptom, this may be significantly higher than the number of cases of TS subjects overall—that is, it may be this symptom which finally causes many families to finally seek professional help, and so it may be reported disproportionately to its actual prevalence. Robertson and Baron-Cohen estimate 10% coprolalia in TS sufferers overall (*Tourette Syndrome*, p. 21).

80. Described by diagnosing physician Earls in "Psychosocial Factors."

81. Shapiro et al., *Gilles de la Tourette Syndrome*, p. 151.

82. Shapiro et al., *Gilles de la Tourette Syndrome*, p. 153.

83. "It's noteworthy that TS-OCD always pushed the person in precisely the direction proscribed—with such incredible exactness that individuals feel compelled to yell 'Hijack!' in an airplane, and 'Fuck!' in church, but not vice versa"; Berecz, *Understanding Tourette Syndrome*, p. 55. Another TS sufferer had FBI agents show up at his door, after saying there was a bomb on the plane when ordering tickets over the phone from his travel agent. The same patient is also in constant danger of yelling out to a woman "I want to rape you" in the midst of casual conversation (Kushner, *Cursing Brain*, p. 2).

84. Berecz, *Understanding Tourette Syndrome*, pp. 102–4.

85. Berecz, *Understanding Tourette Syndrome*, p. 90.

86. In fact, markets and fairs in Anglo-Saxon England may well have taken place on Sundays and on feast days, while people were gathering for church service. This, in any event, is Peter H. Sawyer's best guess in a review of the (admittedly slight) evidence ("Fairs," pp. 153–68); see also Blair, *Church*, pp. 335–36.

87. Shapiro et al., *Gilles de la Tourette Syndrome*, p. 153.

88. Walafrid Strabo, *Vita Galli* 2.23 (Krusch, *Passiones* [MGH, SRM 4], p. 328).

89. Boniface, Letter 73 (Tangl, *Die Briefe*, p. 153).

90. Earls, "Psychosocial Factors," p. 58.

91. Robertson, "Self-Injurious Behavior," pp. 105–14.

92. Cyprian, *De lapsis* 24 (Bénevot, *De lapsis*, p. 37); Sulpicius Severus, *Dialogi* 1.22 (Halm, *Sulpicii Severi*, p. 175); *Miracula Austrebertæ* 15 (*Acta Sanctorum*, February 10, p. 425).

93. *Vita Cuthberti* 2.8 (Colgrave, *Two Lives*, p. 132); Felix, *Vita Guthlaci* 41 (Colgrave, *Felix's Life*, p. 128).

94. See, for instance, the possessed women crying so loudly in the Basilica of St. Hilary that the edifice shakes, in Baudonivia's *Vita Radegundis* 27 (e.g., *Vita Radegundis*, book 2) (Krusch, *Fredegarii*, p. 394).

95. Paulinus of Milan, *Vita Ambrosii*, p. 33 (PL 14: col. 38D).

96. *Vita Caesarii ab eius familiaribus scripta* 1.43 (Morin, *Sancti Caesarii Episcopi Arelatensis*, p. 313).

97. Palladius, *Historia Lausiaca* 26 (PL 73: col. 1123D); Gregory of Tours, *De passione et virtutibus Iuliani* 30 (Krusch, *Miracula et opera*, p. 126).

98. Tourette's symptoms resemble those for schizophrenia, and in fact dopamine blockers reduce symptoms for both conditions (Leckman and Cohen, *Tourette's Syndrome*, p. 5; Erenberg, "Treatment," pp. 241–43; Shapiro and Shapiro, "Neuroleptic Drugs," p. 353). Stimulants exacerbate symptoms, while depressants (including alcohol) can subdue them. Depressive symptoms may result from serotonin deficiencies (most antidepression treatments increase serotonin levels). Suicide, aggression, and impulsivity are correlated with low serotonin. Lithium (like shock therapy) leads to increased serotonin production and inhibits aggressive behavior. Dopamine and serotonin are linked, in that genetic defects that decrease brain serotonin metabolism also decrease dopamine metabolism, and vice versa (Comings, *Tourette Syndrome*, p. 510).

99. King et al., "Psychosocial and Behavioral Treatments," p. 346.

100. Bruun and Budman, "Natural History," pp. 34–35. After a review of the literature the authors conclude that "the core symptoms of TS (vocal and motor tics) tend to disappear or diminish in adulthood" (35), and state that around a third of cases remit completely in late adolescence, another third will show significant improvement during that time, and the final third will continue tic behavior through adulthood (36).

101. Mary Lou Reaver, personal communication to author, July 14, 2003 (Executive Director of the Pennsylvania Tourette Syndrome Association). Reaver is of the opinion that exorcism could not be enduringly effective against TS symptoms, regardless of religious convictions or susceptibility to suggestion.

102. DSM-IV, pp. 273–315; DSM-V, p. 87.

103. Marcus, *Psychosis*, pp. 57–58.

104. DSM-IV, p. 296; DSM-V, p. 87.

105. See Lebra, *Culture-Bound Syndromes*; Simons and Hughes, *Culture-Bound Syndromes*. For a scathing attack on constructs of culture-specific disorders, see Bartholomew, *Exotic Deviance*.

106. DSM-IV, pp. 302–14; DSM-V, pp. 94–96.

107. "Non-bizarre" delusions are those which are possible but simply untrue (e.g., that the government is tracking the subject's every step). A "bizarre" delusion, by contrast, is "clearly implausible" or even "not understandable": for instance, a subject's conviction that all his organs have been surgically removed and then replaced with someone else's, without leaving traces or scars (DSM-IV, pp. 275, 296; DSM-V, p. 87).

108. Gregory of Tours, *Libri de virtutibus sancti Martini episcope* 2.18 (Krusch, *Miracula et opera*, p. 165).

109. *Vita Waldetrude* 3 (*Acta Sanctorum*, April 9, p. 841).

110. The discovery of antipsychotics in the 1950s revolutionized the mental health care industry, and, in many respects, altered both professional and popular attitudes toward mental health in general. The discovery has refocused attention to neurochemical, rather than social, causes, both for psychoses (especially schizophrenia) and for many disorders. The antipsychotics (or neuroleptics) currently used to treat schizophrenia were discovered by accident in 1952 by Henri Laborit, a French surgeon working on antihistamines. Observing that certain chemicals induced tranquility without loss of consciousness, he synthesized the first antipsychotic—chlorpromazine. The resulting drugs have proven clinically

effective in a large number of cases, especially for positive symptoms (e.g., hallucinations, delusions, and bizarre behavior, as opposed to negative symptoms such as affective flattening, apathy, and attention impairment; Tamminga, "Principles," p. 272). It is not entirely certain how antipsychotics work neurochemically, though one recently popular theory has focused around the fact that all neuroleptics developed so far block dopamine receptors. The implication is that schizophrenic behavior (and psychotic behavior in general) can result from overstimulation of the dopaminergic system (Carlsson, "Dopamine Theory," pp. 379–400; McKenna, *Schizophrenia*, pp. 135–63; Siegel et al., *Basic Neurochemistry*, p. 865; Waddington, "Clinical Psychopharmacology," pp. 341–57). The dopamine hypothesis is losing some ground, however, since many of the studies supporting it are circumstantial, conflicting, and confounded by the additional factor of neuroleptic treatment (Kerwin, "Neuropharmacology," p. 42).

111. It was the isolation of reserpine, the active compound in *Rauwolfia*, which initially sparked serious interest in the therapeutic possibilities of botanical folk medicine in the scientific community in the 1950s.

112. In fact, not all researchers agree that schizophrenia is a term that meaningfully describes a coherent class of behavioral abnormalities (Kendell, "Schizophrenia," p. 60). Some argue that the term clumsily serves to clump together inappropriate social and cognitive behavior, without adhering to the normal scientific requirements for identifying a pathogen or syndrome. Emphasizing that his own clinical experience leaves him with a sense of a wide range of abnormal mental states and behaviors that are almost always custom-tailored to the particular anxieties and social environment of each patient, Theodore Sarbin writes, "the fact that two (or 200) persons who exhibit no absurdities in common may be tagged with the same label demonstrates the vacuity of the concept" (Sarbin, "Social Construction," p. 191; see also Fabrega, "On the Significance," pp. 45–65). Sarbin charges that the term is a "moral verdict" rather than a medical diagnosis ("Social Construction," p. 194). Morton Wiener questions whether all of the regularly cited symptoms of schizophrenic disorientation really classify as medical symptoms: "Does discomfort or disruption of any kind (e.g., being lost in an unknown city) constitute pain and suffering in a medical sense, and is it therefore a disease?" (Wiener, "Schizophrenia," p. 204). Despite these reservations, the American Psychiatric Association and the National Institutes of Health treat schizophrenia as a mental health problem of paramount importance. While most agree that there is no single underlying pathogen or cerebral malformation, researchers generally acknowledge an immediately recognizable pattern among both their own schizophrenic patients and those in the literature and are comfortable referring to a coherent complex of "schizophrenias" or "schizophrenia spectrum disorders." Robert Kendell notes that while most psychiatrists concede that the term "schizophrenia" may no longer be in use in fifty years' time, for the present it remains an indispensable diagnostic model for responding to pathological behavior and deciding on a course of treatment. For tortured patients and exasperated physicians, the model provides a constructive approach to a particularly obstinate malady, and neuroleptics (medication developed within the constructs of the "schizophrenia" model) have provided tangible solutions in a large number of cases.

113. DSM-V, pp. 100–105.

114. In fact, an abundance of physical processes have been associated with schizophrenia, such as ventricular enlargement, altered dopamine activity, prominent cortical sulci, smooth pursuit eye movement abnormalities, and altered glucose metabolism. None of these have gained general acceptance as particular features of schizophrenia, however, or yielded any positive course of treatment. Richard Lewine considers it strange to treat the condition as

a brain disease, when no single brain abnormality characterizes more than 20–33% of any given sample ("Epilogue," p. 499).

115. Eugen Bleuler, "Die Prognose," pp. 436–64. His classic presentation of the subject followed: "Dementia Praecox" (English translation in Zinkin, *Dementia Praecox*).

116. Strömgren, "Autism," p. 42.

117. Hare, "Commentary One," p. 316.

118. The speaker of the voice is usually unknown to the subject, but the sex of the voice is nearly always identifiable (Cutting, "Descriptive Psycopathology," p. 17).

119. Straube and Oades, *Schizophrenia*, p. 8.

120. Mary Coleman and Gillberg, *Schizophrenias*, p. 22.

121. Warner and de Girolamo, *Schizophrenia*, p. 114.

122. Warner and de Girolamo, *Schizophrenia*, p. 111.

123. Hare, "Commentary One," p. 316.

124. Sartorius et al., "Early Manifestations," p. 927; and Jablensky et al., *Schizophrenia*. See also Stefanis, "On the Concept," p. 42.

125. Jeste et al., "Did Schizophrenia Exist," pp. 493–503.

126. Torrey, *Schizophrenia*, pp. 39–40. See also Ellard "Did Schizophrenia Exist"; and Hare, "Commentary One."

127. Warner, "Commentary Two," p. 318.

128. Manfred Bleuler, "Concept," pp. 1–15; Strömgren, "Autism," pp. 38–39. The World Health Organization's pilot study of international schizophrenia also found that catatonic manifestations were more prevalent in the developing world than in the developed world (Sartorius et al., "Early Manifestations," p. 920).

129. Ellard, "Did Schizophrenia Exist," pp. 308–9. Dr. Ellard reiterated this observation to me in a personal communication, July 4, 2005.

130. See Kroll and Bachrach, "Medieval Visions," for speculation that schizophrenia may have altered its profile from medieval to modern times, manifesting increasingly as auditory hallucinations rather than visual ones (esp. pp. 713–16).

131. Hare, "Commentary One," p. 316.

132. Dendle, "Schizophrenia," p. 522.

133. Evans, McGrath, and Milns, "Searching," p. 327.

134. Hearing voices in schizophrenia is dysfunctional because the voices are considered alien and unwelcome by both the individual experiencing them and the community watching on. Thus, the socially sanctioned auditory hallucinations perhaps experienced by Greek oracles, mystics such as Joan of Arc, or Saami shamans ("He spoke in the woods to himself as if he had been accompanied by eighty persons" [Svenska Landsmal, quoted in Hultkrantz, "Aspects of Saami (Lapp) Shamanism," p. 141]) are, by definition, not "symptoms" of a disease at all. The positive hallucinations of Christian mysticism (hearing the voice of God or of Mary) did not become common until the later Middle Ages, so far as the historical record permits us to determine.

135. Benedicta Ward, *Sayings*, p. 187 (item 139).

136. Gregory of Tours, *Libri de virtutibus sancti Martini episcopi* 2.18 (Krusch, *Miracula et opera*, p. 165).

137. Boniface, Letter 73 (Tangl, *Die Briefe*, p. 153).

138. Dendle, "Schizophrenia," p. 522.

139. Anglo-Saxon England: Meaney, "Anglo-Saxon View," p. 17. Middle Ages: Kemp, "'Ravished of a Fiend,'" p. 75; Kroll and Bachrach, "Medieval Visions," p. 709; and Newman, "Possessed by the Spirit," p. 768.

140. The term "dissociation" was used as early as 1845, by Moreau de Tours, though it was Pierre Janet who developed and popularized the concept of compartmentalized layers of consciousness (Rothschild, *Body*, p. 66).

141. Palladius, *Historia Lausiaca* 30 (PL 73: col. 1131D).

142. Steinberg, *Handbook*, p. 172.

143. Michael Simpson, "Gullible's Travels," p. 115. In some studies women make up more than 90% of DID cases (First and Tasman, *DSM-IV-TR*, p. 1031).

144. DSM-V, pp. 292–98.

145. Gleaves, May, and Cardeña, "Examination," p. 602; results accepted in Maldonado and Spiegel, "Dissociative States," p. 500.

146. The cross-cultural evidence, especially as DID relates to cultural paradigms of spirit possession, is reviewed in Golub, "Cultural Variations," pp. 285–326. For an interesting debate on the existence of DID, see McHugh and Putnam, "Resolved," pp. 957–63. McHugh argues that MPD is a "socially created artifact—in distressed people who are looking for help" (959), while Putnam counters that even this represents a pathology: "the simplistic argument that MPD is individually and socially caused 'hysteria' evades the much more important question of what is the best approach to helping these patients" (961).

147. Thigpen and Cleckley, "On the Incidence," p. 64.

148. Maldonado and Spiegel, "Dissociative States," p. 498.

149. Ross, *Dissociative Identity Disorder*, p. 59.

150. Dancu et al., "Dissociative Experiences," p. 263.

151. Incest survivors, traffic accident victims, and combat veterans report "mentally leaving their bodies at the moment of the trauma and observing what happens from a distance" (Van der Kolk, Van der Hart, and Marmar, "Dissociation," p. 307). Dissociation at the time of the trauma is among the single most reliable predictors for dissociative behavior in later life (314).

152. Electrical stimulation of the right angular gyrus consistently produces a sensation in which a subject reported, for instance, floating "two metres above the bed, close to the ceiling," looking down on herself; Blanke et al., "Stimulating Illusory Out-of-Body Perceptions," p. 269. Such experiences are reported as "in colour, and . . . visually clear and very realistic" (Blanke et al., "Out-of-Body Experience," p. 247); see also Blanke and Thut, "Inducing," pp. 425–39. For an organic description of out-of-body experiences, see Bünning and Blanke, "Out-of-Body Experience," pp. 331–50.

153. Though some psychiatrists implicitly identify dissociation with repression—as though the alters are repressed emotions surfacing—many intentionally avoid a commitment to Freudian psychology by distinguishing the two (perhaps the most famous is Hilgard, *Divided Consciousness*). Steinberg distinguishes the two by the source of pain: repression distances pain arising from within the individual, while dissociation distances pain from without (*Handbook*, p. 26). Parts of the psyche that are simply repressed, however they may surface, do not usually take on identities of their own. For a critique of the connection normally assumed between trauma (including childhood sexual abuse) and dissociation, see Tillman, Nash, and Lerner, "Does Trauma Cause," pp. 395–414.

154. DSM-IV, p. 487; DSM-V, p. 292.

155. DSM-IV, p. 484; DSM-V, p. 293.

156. Ellason and Ross, "Positive and Negative Symptoms," pp. 236–41; Steinberg, *Handbook*, pp. 283–84.

157. Ross, *Dissociative Identity Disorder*, p. 137. The indwelling persona has a different name in 70.6% of cases.

158. DSM-IV, p. 485; DSM-V, p. 293.

159. Brett, "Classifications," pp. 191–204.

160. DeVries, "Trauma," p. 399.

161. Laungani, "Culture," pp. 119–43. Harvey Whitehouse advocates a balanced position, in which the brain processes are developed and expressed through socially regulated patterns of thought and behavior ("Cultural Cognition," pp. 17–30).

162. Stamm and Friedman, "Cultural Diversity," p. 73. Alexandra Argenti-Pillen reviews further studies, confirming that traumatic stress responses transcend political and religious boundaries ("Discourse," p. 88).

163. Weathers, Litz, and Keane, "Military Trauma," p. 105.

164. Stamm and Friedman, "Cultural Diversity," p. 73.

165. Courlander, *Tiger's Whisker*, pp. 9–10. The hermit tells her he needs her to procure a tiger's whisker for the "potion" he intends to make, and in the exercise of approaching the ferocious tiger tenderly and obsequiously, she learns also to approach her volatile husband.

166. Achilles: Shay, "Learning" (Shay's arguments are further developed in his monograph, *Achilles in Vietnam*); Hamlet: Sonnenberg, "Transcultural Observation," pp. 58–59; Hotspur: Weathers, Litz, and Keane, "Military Trauma," p. 104.

167. Shakespeare, *First Part*, p. 857.

168. Weathers, Litz, and Keane, "Military Trauma," p. 104.

169. Sack, Seeley, and Clarke, "Does PTSD Transcend," pp. 49–54.

170. Stamm and Friedman, "Cultural Diversity," p. 78.

171. Bremner et al., "MRI-Based Measurement," p. 978; Gurvitz, Shenton, and Pitman, "Reduced Hippocampal Volume," pp. 232–33. For discussion see Bremner et al., "Does Stress," pp. 797–805.

172. Stein et al. "Neuroanatomical and Neuroendocrine," cited in Van der Kolk, "Body," p. 232. On the debate regarding hippocampal shrinkage in PTSD, and the range of possible explanations for it, see Roger Pitman, "Hippocampal Diminution," pp. 73–74.

173. Bremner et al., "MRI-Based Measurement," p. 979; Southwick et al., "Neurobiological and Neurocognitive Alterations," pp. 27–58.

174. LeDoux, "Emotion," p. 279; Rauch et al., "Exaggerated Amygdala Response," pp. 769–76.

175. Harvey, Kopelman, and Brewin, "PTSD," pp. 230–46.

176. De Bellis, Hooper, and Sapia, "Early Trauma Exposure," pp. 153–77; Giller, *Biological Assessment*; Khouzam, Ghafoori, and Hierholzer, "Progress," pp. 1–28; Orr and Kaloupek, "Psychophysiological Assessment," pp. 69–97; Van der Kolk and Greenberg, "Psychobiology," pp. 63–87.

177. DeVries, "Trauma," p. 401.

178. DeVries, "Trauma," pp. 400–401.

179. Pain (emotional as well as physical) is an integral part of such initiation rites: "The experience of pain is common in rituals of maturity, often accompanied by the teasing or terrorizing of initiands. The suffering is a necessary part of the ritual and may be seen as a means of transforming the individuals or as a test of their fortitude or both" (La Fontaine, *Initiation*, p. 100). Alingi Luba Akombea, an initiated member of the Wagenia people of Zaire, states flatly, "initiation is intended to make the boys suffer" (Droogers, *Dangerous Journey*, p. 236).

180. See Uzoigwe, "Warrior," esp. pp 34–37.

181. DeVries, "Trauma," p. 410. Stamm and Friedman agree that "all humans have the

capacity to experience and express fear, helplessness, or horror, when exposed to traumatic stress" ("Cultural Diversity," p. 70).

182. Hassrick, *Sioux*, p. 92.

183. Alcuin Letter 229 (Duemmler, *Epistolae Karolini*, p. 373).

184. Frank, "*Battle*"; Morgan, "*Spectamur agendo*."

185. *Battle of Maldon*, line 89 (*ASPR* 6, p. 9).

186. *Beowulf*, lines 2596–99 (*ASPR* 4, p. 80).

187. Bately, "Vocabulary," p. 294.

188. E.g., *Maxims I*: "Helm sceal cenum, / ond a þæs heanan hyge hord unginnost" (The helmet goes to the brave man, and the lowly in spirit always gets the slightest treasure; *ASPR* 3, p. 163); see also *Beowulf*, lines 2651–52, 2890–91 (*ASPR* 4, pp. 82, 89).

189. Cavill, *Maxims*, pp. 112–13.

190. *Battle of Maldon*, lines 258–59 (*ASPR* 6, p. 14).

191. *Battle of Maldon*, lines 315–16 (*ASPR* 6, p. 15).

192. *Beowulf*, lines 1534–36 (*ASPR* 4, p. 47).

193. Cavill, *Maxims*, p. 126.

194. Cleary, *Code*, p. 3.

195. Hassrick, *Sioux*, pp. 91–92. Other tribes employed different variations on this complicated code. For instance: "The Comanches recognized two coups struck on the same victim by different persons. Subsequent coups received no credit. The Cheyennes counted coup on an enemy three times, while the Arapahos touched four times" (Wallace and Adamson Hoebel, *Comanches*, p. 248). The authors explain the coup system as a socialization rite: "The game aspect and the survival elements are both a part of the complex, but more important is the functional adjustment of an institution to a social end. The deeds honored are in good part the kind of deeds that toughen a warrior to stand when he is needed, and the numberless opportunities afforded for coup-counters to boast of their exploits were strong ego-builders and the sort of social device that could not but encourage men to fight and fight recklessly" (249).

196. Hassrick, *Sioux*, p. 92.

197. O'Keeffe, "Heroic Values," p. 122.

198. *Battle of Maldon*, lines 198–201 (*ASPR* 6, p. 12).

199. John M. Hill, *Anglo-Saxon Warrior Ethic*, p. 112. For a rejection of Rosemary Woolf's suggestion that the *Maldon* poet simply draws the foreign ideal of a thane not leaving his slain lord on the battlefield from *Bjarkamál* ("Ideal," pp. 63–81), see Harris, "Love," pp. 96–98. Roberta Frank links this literary topos with a handful of other skaldic verses instead (noting that *Bjarkamál* may be a later composition than once thought anyway) and romance/chanson de geste scenes, concluding, "*Maldon* . . . peers, not backward through the mists to Germania, but just around the corner, to an eleventh century Europe in which the profession of warrior was a way of achieving religious perfection and a martyr's crown" ("Ideal," p. 106).

200. Boehnlein, "Culture," p. 520; Bracken, Giller, and Summerfield, "Psychological Responses," p. 1081. Van der Kolk, Van der Hart, and Marmar tend to agree, but warn that few controlled studies have been conducted ("Dissociation," p. 319).

201. Shay, "Learning," p. 574.

202. Cubbin, *Anglo-Saxon Chronicle*, p. 78.

203. See, for instance, Goldman, "Use," pp. 69–80; and Greenfield, *Hero*.

204. *The Wife's Lament*, line 5 (*ASPR* 3, p. 210).

205. See also *The Seafarer*, lines 33–38, 58–64; *The Wanderer* lines 55–57. In a controversial

book, Stephen Glosecki has linked some of these paeans of displacement with psychic dissociation. For him the "external soul" flights implicit in *The Seafarer* and *The Wanderer* may represent reflexes of the archaic psychic journeys associated with pre-Christian shamans (*Shamanism*, pp. 78–91).

206. Jerome, *Vita Hilarionis* 37 (PL 23: col. 48b); Eugippius, *Saint Séverin* 44, p. 286.

207. Felix, *Vita Guthlaci* 42 (Colgrave, *Felix's Life*, pp. 130–32).

208. Butzel et al. "Relationship," pp. 547–49; Farley and Keaney, "Physical Symptoms"; Lipschitz et al. "Childhood Abuse."

209. Gordon C. N. Hall and Amber Phung explore the profile of sexual aggression in collectivist cultures, especially patriarchal ones, in "Cognitive Enculturation," pp. 107–18.

210. This also appears to be Nicholas Orme's assessment for the medieval period in *Medieval Children*, pp. 100–6.

211. Schetky, "Child Sexual Abuse." Ruth S. Kempe and C. Henry Kempe (*Child Abuse*) paint in broad strokes a dreary picture of child maltreatment in all periods and on through the nineteenth and twentieth centuries (3–5), though they believe that modern prevalence of incest in the US is abnormally high due to changing family life situations (47).

212. Finkelhor, "Child Sexual Abuse," p. 105.

213. For overview and criticism see Mayes et al. *Child Sexual Abuse*, pp. 8–12, 164–65.

214. Rogers, "Social Constructions," p. 25.

215. DeMause, *History*, p. 1.

216. David Nicholas states, "The treatment of children in works of art [in early medieval Europe] suggests affection, sympathy, and adults' horror at the violence often visited on the young" ("Childhood," 32); and Jerome Kroll and Bernard Bachrach add that, "historical evidence does not support either sweeping claims for brutality and indifference to children in early medieval Europe or more simplistic notions which stigmatize the childrearing practices of entire civilizations" ("Child Care," p. 563). See also Eleanora Gordon, "Child Health," p. 520; and Herlihy, "Medieval Children," pp. 109–41. Shulamith Shahar distinguishes "controlled beating" (the socially and biblically sanctioned correction of children through corporeal punishment) from "savage ill-treatment" (outbursts by "impulsive, emotionally immature, and ineffectual people"): the latter was undoubtedly present in the Middle Ages, stemming (according to Shahar) from largely the same reasons it still does today, though the prevalence of the phenomenon is by its very nature unknowable (*Childhood*, pp. 109–11).

217. Eleanora Gordon, "Child Health," p. 517.

218. Eleanora Gordon, "Child Health," p. 520.

219. Nicholas, "Childhood," p. 31.

220. Kuefler, "Wryed Existence," p. 830. However, Kuefler also draws attention to a passage in Ælfric's *Colloquy* in which the master asks the pupil whether or not he has been beaten today, and the boy responds, "ic næs, forþam wærlice ic me heold" (I haven't been, because I kept myself careful; Garmonsway, *Ælfric's Colloquy*, p. 45). Gloating masters make their students beg not to be whipped throughout Ælfric Bata's *Colloquy* (Gwara and Porter, *Anglo-Saxon Conversations*, e.g., pp. 92, 132). The ongoing threat of a whipping forms a running conceit in this school exercise, which (in the context of learning vocabulary) may be little more than scholastic humor to keep young students' attention. Still, if so, it is a dark sort of humor: "Hoc est mihi malum nunc. Karius esset mihi mortuum esse modo quam talia flagella sustinere!" (This is hurting me now—it would be better for me to be dead, than to sustain such a whipping!; p. 166). Kuefler comments, "Years of beatings must have created deep psychological scars on children, if modern cases can be used in evidence" ("Wryed Existence," p. 829). In the eleventh century, Anselm of Canterbury

was opposed to beating children in monasteries "because those who suffered violence and threats in childhood would become hate-filled, suspicious, violent, and bestial adults" (Shahar, *Childhood*, pp. 173–74).

221. G. Rattray Taylor, *Sex*, p. 9.

222. Hawkes and Wells, "Crime," p. 119.

223. Hawkes and Wells, "Crime," p. 121.

224. Hawkes and Wells, "Crime," p. 122.

225. Lucy, *Anglo-Saxon Way*, pp. 70–72; Knüsel, "Pagan Charm," pp. 206 (a review of David Wilson, *Anglo-Saxon Paganism*); Nicholas Reynolds, "Rape," pp. 715–18.

226. Lucy, *Anglo-Saxon Way*, pp. 78–80.

227. For a brief review of textual evidence regarding rape over the course of the Anglo-Saxon period, see Julie Coleman, "Rape in Anglo-Saxon England"; and for a study of rape in legal and narrative sources that focuses on the nuances of the different Old English terms for sexual violation, see Horner, "Language."

228. Saunders, *Rape*, pp. 34–36.

229. For a different perspective, see James Brundage: "primitive Germanic legal systems . . . were not much concerned with the protection of women from violent assault" ("Rape," p. 142). Suzanne Fonay Wemple observes that Germanic laws against rape and harassment on the continent are perhaps not so much about protecting women's physical safety as about protecting their honor: "A sexual assault had such a devastating psychological effect on the victim's self-esteem that normally she preferred to conceal her shame rather than take her case into court. Those unfortunate enough to be raped blamed their assaults on demons, and it was not unusual for women who had been defiled to kill themselves" (*Women*, p. 41).

230. Alfred 18: "Gif hwa nunnan mid hæmedþinge oððe on hire hrægl oððe on hire breost butan hire leafe gefo, sie hit twybete swa we ær be læwdum men fundon" (if anyone grabs lustfully at a nun's clothing or breast without her consent, it will be twice the compensation set for a lay woman; Liebermann, *Die Gesetze*, vol. 1, p. 58); II Cnut 73.2: "⁊ þeah heo nydnumen weorðe, þolige þæra æhta, butan heo fram þam ceorle wylle eft ham ongean ⁊ næfre heo eft his ne weorðe" (and even if she was taken by force, she loses those goods, unless she chooses to leave that man to go back home again, and never afterwards be his again; Liebermann, *Die Gesetze*, vol. 1, p. 360); and see also Alfred 11.4 and II Cnut 74 (Liebermann, *Die Gesetze*, vol. 1, pp. 360). Relevant sections from Tacitus, Salic law, and Burgundian law are translated in Amt, *Women's Lives*, pp. 36-49. For discussion see Fell, *Women*, pp. 62–66; Hough, "Alfred's *Domboc*."

231. Alfred 26 (Liebermann, *Die Gesetze*, vol. 1, pp. 64–66); see also Sally Crawford, *Childhood*, p. 52. The age of consent in this context is not specified (112). Crawford notes, however, that "grave goods evidence indicates that girls were buried with adult female grave goods such as chatelaines and brooch sets from as early as ten or twelve years of age, and it must be assumed that this was a feasible age for marriage" (111). According to Fell, children became legally recognized as adults (for purposes of inheritance) at age ten in early Anglo-Saxon England and age twelve in later law codes (*Women*, p. 80). For an alternate interpretation of Alfred 26, see Hough, "New Reading." Hough argues that *ungewintred* could refer to women past childbearing years as well as to those before. She translates the passage: "If anyone rapes a girl not of age, that is to be the same compensation as for a woman past child-bearing age" (12).

232. Theodore's Penitential 2.12.36 (Finsterwalder, *Die Canones*, p. 330). The subsequent provision continues, "puella vero XVI vel XVII annorum quae ante in potestate parentum

sunt. Post hanc aetatem patri filiam suam contra eius voluntatem non licet in matrimonium dare" (a girl of 16 or 17 years who has been in her parent's custody . . . after that age parents are not permitted to give their daughter away in matrimony against her will). The same provisions are given for the same ages in the *Pseudo-Ecgbert Confessional* (or *Old English Confessional*) 3.15 (Spindler, *Das altenglische Bussbuch*, p. 183).

233. *Poenitentiale Pseudo-Ecgberti* 2.15 (Wasserschleben, *Die Bussordnungen*, p. 326).

234. For references, see Julie Coleman, "Rape," p. 196. Coleman notes of the women referred to in these accounts, "no attention is paid to their fate" (196). Barbara Yorke, however, cautions that some accounts of Viking pillage and depredation of nunneries—especially later ones—may be trading in the sensationalistic rewriting of history rather than in facts (*Nunneries*, pp. 58–59).

235. Cogitosus, *Vita Brigidae* (PL 72: col. 785B). The letter of St. Patrick to Coroticus and his soldiers, requesting the return of captured Christians, is heartrending in its implications: Coroticus is said to "mulierculas baptizatas praemia distribuunt" (distribute young baptized women as prizes; *Epistola ad milites Coroticus* 19 [Patrick, *Confession*, p. 150]). So is his statement in the *Confessio* 42: "Sed ex illis maxime laborant quae seruitio detinentur; usque ad terrores et minas assidue perferunt" (but of all these, those women who are held in slavery toil the with greatest distress; they live in constant fear and endure menacing all the time; p. 116). David Pelteret provides a book-length treatment of slavery in Anglo-Saxon England in *Slavery in Early Mediaeval England, from the Reign of Alfred until the Twelfth Century*.

236. II Cnut 54 (Liebermann, *Die Gesetze*, vol. 1, p. 348). The penalty for this is admittedly rather vague: "þolige þære ⁊ bete for hine sylfne wið God ⁊ wið men" (he should suffer for this and make satisfaction for himself with God and with humankind). Pelteret's appendix 1 (on the OE terminology of slavery) demonstrates the existence of a highly nuanced vocabulary managing various levels and relationships of female slaves: *birele* (female slave or bearer), *ham-byrde* (possible interpretation of a gloss, *hm bir*), *in-þinen* (female domestic slave), *mægen-mann* (unmarried or virginal female slave, as used in the Laws of Æthelberht), *mennen* (female slave), *þeow/þeowa* and *þeowen/þeowene* (female slave), *þeow-mennen* (female slave), *þignen* (female slave), *þir* (female slave), *þyften* (female domestic slave), and *wiln* (female slave). For complete semantic data and discussion of these and related terms, see Pelteret, *Slavery*, pp. 261–330.

237. *Decreta Lanfranci*: "Praeter abbatem, priorem, magistrosque eorum, nulli liberum sit in loco custodiae eorum deputato sedere, nec uerbo nec signo aliquid eis innotescere, nisi accepta licentia ab abbate uel priore. Quae licentia cum conceditur, magister sedere debet inter iuuenem et eum, qui iuueni loquitur. . . . Cum dormitum uadunt tamdiu stent ante ipsos magistri usque dum ipsi iuuenes in lectis suis iaceant cooperti. Si nox est, cum candelis accensis assistant. . . . Custos iuuenem non relinquat nisi commendatum alicui fratri, in quo et de quo bene confidant" (Except for the abbot, the prior, and their teachers, no one can sit in the place allotted to be [the boys'] cells, or make themselves known to the boys either by word or sign unless it is with the consent of the abbot or prior. When such consent is given, the master should sit between the youth and the person who speaks with him. . . . When the boys retire to the dormitory, the masters are to stand over them until they lie completely covered over in their beds. If it is nighttime, they should stand by with candles lit. . . . An overseer should not leave a boy without turning him over to another brother, whom he trusts and who trusts him; Knowles, *Monastic Constitutions*, pp. 117–19). The provisions are intended to prevent contact among the *iuvenes* themselves, as well as among *iuvenes* and monks. For greater context, see Frantzen, "Where the Boys Are," pp. 43–66.

238. The church struggled for centuries to curtail consanguinity practices in northwest Europe in the early Middle Ages, where native Germanic marriage practices apparently remained fluid especially among the aristocracy. The nobility, concerned as it was with alliances and property acquisition, was scandalously recalcitrant to the church's efforts to curb what it considered "incest": even as late as 1215, the church reduced the number of prohibited degrees of relationship for a potential suitor from seven to four in a compromise (Archibald, "Incest," p. 10; and see Archibald, *Incest*, pp. 11–52). Ecclesiastical anxiety over consanguinity, however, does not address the sort of nuclear family, intergenerational incest we have in mind in the modern sense. There is no indication that marriage within close consanguinity in the medieval records—while offensive to the church—implied any less consent than did marriages further removed.

239. Freud, *Totem and Taboo*, pp. 3–25.

240. Theodore's Penitential 1 (Finsterwalder, *Die Canones*, pp. 291–92).

241. For the rarity of father-daughter incest in medieval penitentials, see Manselli, "Vie familiale," p. 370; and Payer, *Sex*, pp. 30–32. Of the analogues Payer treats, none seems to discuss father-daughter incest.

242. See *Canones Gregorii*, items 89–101 (Finsterwalder, *Die Canones*, pp. 262–63); *Poenitentiale Bedae* 3.18–32 (Wasserschleben, *Die Bussordnungen*, pp. 222–23).

243. *Poenitentiale Egberti* 4.4 (Wasserschleben, *Die Bussordnungen*, p. 234). The penance is not as great as for fornicating with one's mother (fifteen years, chap. 4.3).

244. Elizabeth Archibald, writing on incest in the Middle Ages, believes that "there seems every reason to believe that the incidence of incest does not change much over the centuries; what does change is the level of public acknowledgment" (*Incest*, p. 7; see also pp. 230–31).

245. Incest is sometimes imputed to others as a slur, though this is scarcely reliable evidence. Vortigern is said to have taken his daughter for a wife in the *Historia Britonum*, for instance (ch. 39; Faral, *La légende Arthurienne*, p. 30). Incest was always a common accusation in medieval polemic, from early apologists (Archibald, *Incest*, p. 242) to Early Modern heresy trials throughout Western Europe (Cohn, *Europe's Inner Demons*, p. 20).

246. Goolden, *Old English Apollonius*, p. 2, lines 8–19.

247. There is some confusion in the manuscript tradition over whether it is the king or the daughter who wishes to conceal the crime in this passage (Goolden, *Old English Apollonius*, p. 45).

248. Goolden, *Old English Apollonius*, p. 44. Note that the Latin text Goolden prints opposite his Old English edition is not from a single, preferred manuscript, but is a reconstructed "conflation" of various manuscripts, each of which seems closest to the Old English readings at various points.

249. Goolden, *Old English Apollonius*, pp. 2–4.

250. Archibald, *Apollonius of Tyre*, p. 112. For further discussion and analogues, see Saunders, *Rape*, pp. 202ff.

251. On this problematic phrase (*nodum virginitatis*), see St. Panayotakis [*sic*], "The Knot and the Hymen."

252. Oedipal patterns resurface in the Middle Ages with the legend of Gregorius, and in Jacobus de Voragine's account of Judas Iscariot in the *Legenda Aurea*, for instance; while father-daughter incest appears in such classical stories as those of Myrrha and Cinyras and of Hippodamia and Oenomaus, as well as in numerous medieval versions of *Apollonius* and the *Clementine Recognitions* cycle. For these references and a basic genealogical relationship among them, see Archibald, "Flight," esp. pp. 267–68. She notes that

the earliest instance of the "flight from incest" motif within the Constance group hails from England, in the twelfth-century *Vita Offae Primi* ("Flight," p. 261). Archibald elsewhere argues that incest suddenly became a popular literary topic in the twelfth century, though there is no reason to think that patterns of incest themselves suddenly changed ("Incest," esp. pp. 1, 5).

253. Archibald, "Flight," p. 267.

254. Geoffrey Chaucer, Man of Law's Prologue, lines 82–85 (Benson, *Riverside Chaucer*, p. 88).

255. Chaucer, Man of Law's Prologue, line 86 (Benson, *Riverside Chaucer*, p. 88). John Fisher discusses this passage, concluding that Chaucer seems to be recalling the drops of blood which fall on the *pauimentum* in the Latin versions (*John Gower*, pp. 289 and 370n18).

256. Chaucer, Man of Law's Prologue, line 88 (Benson, *Riverside Chaucer*, p. 88).

257. Riddle, "Introduction," p. 46: "Wer sæt at wine . . ." (*ASPR* 3, p. 205).

258. Ælfric, "Preface to Genesis" (Sally Crawford, *Childhood*, p. 76).

259. Ælfric, "Preface to Genesis" (Sally Crawford, *Childhood*, p. 76).

260. Thus Fulk and Cain, *History*, p. 85.

261. Bethurum, *Homilies*, p. 270.

262. Bethurum, *Homilies*, p. 271. It is not always clear what Wulfstan means by the term *hæðen* in different contexts: see Meaney, "And we forbeodað," and Meaney, "Old English Legal."

263. On these passages, see Cowen, "*Byrstas* and *bysmeras*," pp. 397–411, esp. pp. 407–10.

264. Finkelhor, "Child Sexual Abuse," p. 102. Stamm and Friedman conclude that race/ethnicity is a "very weak" predictor of PTSD compared to such factors as childhood physical abuse ("Cultural Diversity," p. 76).

265. Yüksel, "Collusion," p. 157.

266. Yüksel, "Collusion," p. 157.

267. Yüksel, "Collusion," p. 157.

268. Yüksel, "Collusion," p. 159.

269. Finkelhor, "Child Sexual Abuse," p. 112.

270. *Vita Caesarii ab eius familiaribus scripta* 2.18 (Morin, *Sancti Caesarii Episcopi Arelatensis*, p. 332).

271. *Vita Caesarii ab eius familiaribus scripta* 2.18 (Morin, *Sancti Caesarii Episcopi Arelatensis*, p. 332).

272. *Vita Caesarii ab eius familiaribus scripta* 2.18 (Morin, *Sancti Caesarii Episcopi Arelatensis*, p. 332).

273. Monahon, *Children*, p. 59.

274. Kocijan-Hercigonja, "Children," p. 170.

275. Interestingly, an institutionalized historical connection between rape and mental illness appears to have arisen in northwest Europe shortly after the close of the Anglo-Saxon period. According to legend, the father of the seventh-century Irish martyr St. Dympna, finding that Dympna resembled her deceased mother, attempted to marry his pubescent daughter. She fled to Gheel, near Antwerp, but he chased her and had her killed. After the thirteenth century, cures of insanity and demonic possession especially were associated with the saint's bones, such that she came to be patron saint of the mentally ill. A mental hospital (which is still today a highly regarded sanitarium) was founded in Gheel at the end of the thirteenth century. A clinical professor of psychiatry at Harvard Medical School writes, "It is appropriate that the patron saint of the mentally afflicted should be an incest victim" (Herman, *Father-Daughter Incest*, p. 3; see also Graham, *Medieval Minds*, p. 35).

Conclusions and Further Questions

A person with Tourette's Syndrome once wrote: "Dignity. How does one live with dignity when you spit constantly, swear involuntarily, and cannot control your movements?"[1] Judging from the occasional portrayals of medieval daily life doled out in popular movies and books, a nonspecialist might think that the only thing worse than to have been born in the Middle Ages is to have been born in the Middle Ages with a serious disease. Serious neurological conditions no doubt impeded the development of normal relations with friends and peers and placed great stress on the family. Without wishing to sentimentalize the desperate responses of medieval society to neurological conditions that are even today only poorly understood, I am struck by the fact that early medieval hagiographers take demoniacs and their unglamorous symptoms seriously, and grant them a right to be seen, heard, and included. Peter Brown and Valerie Flint have argued that the possession and exorcism paradigm allowed for a humane, controlled, and predictable response to public tension for liminal groups in late antiquity. The invisible demons increasingly deflected attention and blame away from "witches," for instance, in late Rome and the early Middle Ages. Similarly, demonization of mental illness deflected potential blame or humiliation away from the individual.[2] Late medieval literature and drama had their share of fools and clowns, including demons and Satan himself, and these embodiments of anxiety are often exorcized, as it were, through mockery and laughter—but the ill themselves are seldom mocked. If there is dignity in granting a public presence and voice, then medieval sources grant this dignity to individuals who, in twenty-first-century America, are kept largely out of sight.

Through many generations, the demon possessed in medieval Europe developed their behavior patterns in the shadow of those few possessions described in the New Testament, which were themselves modeled on hardwired, biological conditions. This is why those functionally possessed foam at the mouth, gnash their teeth, tremble, roll on the ground, and/or thrash (or curl into a fetal position and remain comatose, or "channel" a saint, or speak only in numbers while turning in circles, or any of a range of other possibilities). It is these neurological and motor control disorders that serve at once as a visualization of those conditions which probably did occur from time to time, and as a control group against which more time- and culture-specific behaviors can be assessed. I have attempted to provide a fresh reflection on the sources and an update, of sorts, on the current state of knowledge regarding a few of the most obvious disorders that resemble possession and that have strong cross-cultural profiles. It is my hope that this can serve to help us conceptualize what demon possession may have looked like (etically, or to an outside observer), so far as the available evidence permits.

The English population at the time of the Domesday Book was perhaps somewhere from one-and-a-half to two million people.[3] Despite the growth of some population centers over the eighth through eleventh centuries, Anglo-Saxon England was never much more than a rural agrarian society, with a few towns and thousands of tiny villages, and other large spaces left virtually deserted.[4] Villages varied in size, many based around one or maybe two dozen teams of oxen. Within this sparsely populated island, only a small fraction of people might present with those neurological conditions for which cross-cultural prevalence rates can be ascertained.[5] In mid-tenth-century Raunds, Northamptonshire, for instance, a new church was built—accommodating some twenty adults, half of the population of the eight to ten households of the village—in a space small enough where the priest and congregation were within touching distance.[6] Even taking the most generous of estimated prevalence rates for epilepsy and Tourette's Syndrome, two of the more well-documented conditions with a consistent cross-cultural profile, a village like Raunds might expect something like 1.6 epileptics and 4.8 people with TS every hundred years, or over the course of four generations. Of these, however, only a small fraction of people with either condition would present with such severity that the behavior would lead eventually to an exorcism. The vast majority of people with TS, for instance, would simply tic a little. On the other hand, the rare cases of more severe behavior disorders would likely have formed part of the village lore and family oral history for a long time, and perhaps would have grown disproportionately in the popular imagination. Similarly, accounts of the occasionally striking case in one small community might spread over quite a sizeable geographic area.

Unstable, war-torn nations are known to have a greater number of people suffering from psychoses and trauma-related psychiatric disorders. Nonetheless, the neurological conditions most strongly associated with demon possession behaviors were rare in the extreme, and many generations of Anglo-Saxons within a rural community could live and die without ever seeing an instance of one. Over time saints' tombs could begin to attract the ill and the possessed from increasingly wider geographic ranges, and this could give miracle registers a skewed perception of a disorder's prevalence in the actual population.

Early Anglo-Saxon saints' lives portray demoniacs as common; liturgical books contain dozens of exorcisms. Given the interdependency of literary patterns in the Latin writings of the early Middle Ages as a whole, however, we must be careful not to assume that the literary tropes employed by a certain author necessarily reflect that author's society. Throughout the period of Anglo-Saxon literary culture, authors—in their attempt to emulate continental authors—portrayed many facets of Anglo-Saxon society as congruent with Latin Christendom as a whole. The vast majority of references to demon possession in Anglo-Saxon literature are to events that happened in other times and places: in Judea (the New Testament miracles), Gaul (the numerous materials relating to St. Martin), Italy (Gregory's *Dialogues* and Ælfric's *Passion of Apollonaris*), and India (Ælfric's *Passion of Thomas*), to name but a few. It is probable that many of the references to demon possession in Anglo-Saxon literature represent literary patterning. Old English vernacular poetry, though drawn especially to demonology and to saint-demon conflicts, does not present any episode of possession or exorcism.[7] We have no manuscript illustration or visual depiction of a demoniac from Anglo-Saxon England.[8] That Anglo-Saxons occasionally suffered from severe cases of seizure disorders, TS, and psychosis is certain. If they had a sizeable number of other "demoniacs" beyond that, though, they have left little impression in the documentary record outside of seventh- and eighth-century hagiography. Also, one will learn next to nothing about it from Anglo-Saxon charters, laws, chronicles, or letters.

Historians tacitly assume the widespread presence of possession behavior in Anglo-Saxon England, since that is how we envision the early Middle Ages in general. The healing miracles recorded in saints' lives, references to "the devil" in the medical books, and the presence of exorcisms in liturgical texts seem consistent with that premise. Since there are many ways in which possession behavior can manifest among various societies, I began this project hoping to compile an account of how possession manifested itself particularly in Anglo-Saxon England. I was at first surprised to find how few accounts there were. Eventually I amended my thesis to the current one: that functional demon possession (the unconscious adoption of deliberative behaviors, such as assuming an alternate persona) was quite rare, if not virtually absent, in Anglo-Saxon England. Of course there were on occasion cases of neurological or muscle control disorders, and Anglo-Saxons themselves perceived a wide range of behavioral and physiological compromises as "demon"-induced—not just the trance state involving an alternate persona which forms the core of so many fascinating narrative scenes in hagiography. Possession may have played a role in the social dynamics and tensions of conversion during the seventh and eighth centuries, especially in Northumbria and Anglia, but is not well established as an ongoing dimension of Anglo-Saxon spirituality following the early eighth century. There are no doubt more passages and texts which have not yet come to my attention that can shed further light on the topic. Mine is certainly not the final word on the subject: I see it rather as a starting point. At the very least, I hope to raise a question that has never been sufficiently considered, and to stimulate a fresh examination of sources whose interpretations have long been taken for granted. My hypothesis must necessarily be provisional: I am not married to it, but I believe it is one that currently fits the available evidence most economically.[9]

The usual explanation for why possession is rife in certain times and places as opposed to others is that widespread possession is a sign of cultural crisis.[10] This sort of answer requires further nuance, however, since every people in every century wrestles with its own social anxieties: no century has been without a "cultural crisis" of some sort. There was little or no possession in fifth-century Athens or Victorian England, while in the late twentieth century, Pentecostal and deliverance ministries practicing regular exorcisms have been increasing in heartland and suburban America: a social milieu hardly torn by war, famine, forced exile, or oppression. If possession is better attested in eighth-century Northumbria and Anglia than elsewhere in preconquest England, it may be, as I suggested in chapter 3, because of the particular nexus of competing religious and cultural worlds that came together in that time and place. The widespread appeal to local holy men for healing signifies, perhaps, a population especially receptive to this social dynamic, which easily allows mutual recrimination among peers within the community as well as the expression of resentment against authorities. This sort of speculation remains highly tentative, though. Even in those seventh- and eighth-century texts that have drawn our attention, the problems are largely neurological and muscular, and not behavioral. This weakens the premise that functional demon possession was widespread, even then.

If demon possession did reemerge in postconquest England, it did so as part of an emerging eleventh- and twelfth-century spirituality, which had profound implications for all aspects of personal and public devotion. From the twelfth through the fifteenth centuries, possession and related trance states began to manifest in a great diversity of forms, some of which bear directly on our understanding of demon possession. Communal or epidemic possessions in which entire villages of people jump, dance, and convulse begin to appear in the sources as a new behavioral manifestation, for instance. "Dancing manias" (sometimes called St. Vitus's Dance) are probably better interpreted as spontaneous communal revelries than a widespread neurological disorder. One widely cited cause of such "possessed villages" is the contamination of rye or barley bread with ergot (*Claviceps purpurea*), a fungus containing lysergic acid (the hallucinogenic agent in LSD, *lysergic acid diethylamide*).[11] The hypothesis is often overstated and largely unnecessary to explain possession and trance activity in either an individual or community. In any event, this phenomenon was quite rare in the early Middle Ages as a whole, and virtually undocumented in England (Clarke notes that the first recorded case of ergot poisoning in England is from the nineteenth century).[12] The early Middle

Ages, between the time of Hellenistic oracles and that of late medieval mystics, is a notable period of abatement in ecstatic possession.[13] In contrast, the late Middle Ages evidenced a resurgence in written accounts of ecstatic possession, especially among women. Perhaps these were newly emerging phenomena, or perhaps we are witnessing instead new trends in what was being committed to writing and how it was being presented.[14] At the very least, the accounts left in writing do allow us to trace the validation of a phenomenon—its relative importance—to the literate class and to the intended audience. The growth of lay literacy as a whole may have influenced the selection of what was considered interesting to write about.

In a provocative article André Goddu traces the rising and falling trends of exorcism cases from the fourth through the eighteenth centuries. He finds that possession in Latin Christendom flourished in the sixth and seventh centuries, went into recession from the eighth through the tenth century, and then started again in the eleventh and steadily rose to a culmination in the thirteenth.[15] Regarding our period (roughly), he writes, "In the period from the eighth through the tenth centuries, liturgical sources provide evidence that ritual exorcisms were performed, but there seems to have been a dramatic decline."[16] Goddu's analysis—methodologically problematic at a number of levels—is perhaps most valuable as a case study in how deceptive written sources can be in reconstructing the actual state of affairs. Taking the thirteen volumes of the *Acta Sanctorum* devoted to October (the month containing the greatest amount of material in that collection), Goddu finds 152 exorcism cases related in various saints' lives; in order to assess the relative length and difficulty of exorcisms for the century in which that saint lived, he then counts the number of lines of printed text they occupy. His methodology implicitly presupposes that an equal number of documents from each century from the fourth to the eighteenth were available to the compilers of the *Acta Sanctorum*, and that all writers linger on scenes of exorcism for the same reasons and with predictable consistency. As a result of this approach, Goddu's data passes almost entirely over the otherwise well-documented rise in possession cases in the Early Modern era: the fifteenth and sixteenth centuries appear on his graph as virtually devoid of exorcisms.[17] The article is interesting, then, not because it necessarily has something to tell us about exorcism during the centuries in question, but because it has something to tell us about how exorcisms were written about in certain periods, in a certain genre (hagiography). Goddu's findings do raise important questions, however, such as why more lines of the *Acta Sanctorum* are not devoted to exorcisms for the fifteenth and sixteenth centuries. This would then take us into how hagiography was written and disseminated in that period (with the role of print culture and increased literacy), who the intended audience was (Catholics vs. Protestants, educated vs. popular), how the Catholic Church filtered and controlled hagiographic material differently in different periods, and how the Bollandists (the compilers of the *Acta Sanctorum*) viewed their editorial role over time.[18]

In light of this cautionary tale, the current study must confront the limits of negative evidence. If functional demon possession was in fact an important and vibrant facet of Anglo-Saxon society, would we know? Is possession the sort of thing that should show up in the highly specialized genres of ecclesiastical literary production, such that it is conspicuous by its absence? These are questions that await further discussion, and I hope to learn from the perspectives of others in response to my analysis. I believe this sort of questioning can potentially have a much wider significance. For instance, looking across to Carolingian France and Germany and ahead to Anglo-Norman England, if we subtract the many posthumous miracles at saints' tombs from the equation (since these are not technically exorcisms—they do not imply the dyadic interplay of demoniac and exorcist), historians may find that exorcism proper, as we usually imagine it, did not occur in the Middle Ages quite as frequently as a rough count of the possession references might imply. It could be that we are reading an entirely different phenomenon back into the Middle Ages—or exaggerating its relative proportions or its profile—when we extrapolate (as we inevitably do) from the data derived from the well-documented Early Modern period and from our own contemporary societies that regularly practice possession as religious rite (such as Haiti and Sri Lanka).

Finally, this study can help us rethink the role of diverse genres and textual traditions in Anglo-Saxon England in certain ways. The pharmacologically ineffective recipes in the Anglo-Saxon medical compilations for the treatment of mental disorders point to a society largely incapable of treating those patients who occasionally presented with serious neurological conditions, though that same community was not incapable of integrating their "story" into a communal narrative implying support and validation for their plight. The elemental disease agents of the charms (elves, poisons, worms, and dwarves) bear little resemblance to the articulate and cunning demons (*awyrgedan gastas* or *unclænan gastas*) so prevalent in the saints' lives. The recipes do not seem to imply use for the alleviation of a fragmentation of personality, or for speaking with another voice, blaspheming, exhibiting uncommon strength, seeing hidden or future things, etc. They are more interested in listing plants than describing symptoms, and we are at a loss in many cases even to decide whether or not a recipe referring to elves or to the devil's "temptation" (or "affliction?") is even meant for a mental/behavioral condition in the first place. The charms and recipes with apparent connections to demons or the demonic do not actually paint a scene of a patient "possessed" in any recognizable sense.

For such a scene, we must turn to hagiography, a genre largely modeled on continental exemplars. Early medieval saints' lives portray a lively landscape thronging with the ill, the mad, and the possessed, all of whom find succor immediately and spontaneously through the charismatic powers of the subject saint (either while alive or posthumously). References to exorcism sometimes appear in the lives of native Anglo-Saxon saints and martyrs. This textual tradition, however, conflicts dramatically with the ceremonious exorcisms encoded in liturgical books such as pontificals and benedictionals. There the orderly procedures of church officials imply a carefully controlled monopoly on the ability to correctly perform the rites of exorcism. In these books the possessed are the (passive, from all we can tell) recipients of a series of prayers and gestures designed in part to provide relief to the patient, in part to publicly reinforce the efficacy of ecclesiastical intervention.

In all likelihood none of these three traditions—the medical, the narrative, or the liturgical—presents us with anything like an accurate portrait of what was happening at Anglo-Saxon healing shrines or in Anglo-Saxon churches. They are each mostly closed textual worlds, responding to other texts within the tradition but showing little awareness of the perspectives of competing genres. Perhaps the truth lies somewhere between them all. At the very least, since the texts that constitute our only insight into the possibility of demon possession in Anglo-Saxon England are ultimately derived from the historical traditions of other times and places, it seems best to reserve judgment on whether or not the references to exorcism—for instance, in Felix's *Vita Guthlaci* or the scenes presumed in the Leofric Missal exorcisms—permit us to visualize dramatic scenes of possession and exorcism as any significant or representative part of the Anglo-Saxon everyday experience.

NOTES

1. Seligman and Hilkevich, *Don't Think about Monkeys*, pp. 187–88.

2. On late antique demons as scapegoats that deflect communal blame away from sorcerers, see Peter Brown, "Sorcery, Demons, and the Rise," pp. 28–29. He writes, "if there is misfortune, it is divorced from a human reference and the blame is pinned firmly on the 'spiritual powers of evil'" (33). Flint agrees: "the exorcising of a demon (provided it is done well and without offense) may seem to some to be a far better way of countering human evil than the possibly harsher means taken by the secular powers" ("Demonisation," p. 291, but see also p. 292). Elsewhere she comments, "[Demons] are used to take the panic, much of the blame, and the extreme penalties from the accused maleficus upon themselves. This humane use of a belief in the magical powers of demons by the early medieval church is one deserving of some emphasis, for, in the light especially of later abuses, sight of it can easily be lost" (*Rise*, p. 154).

3. Josiah C. Russell provides a low-end population estimate for late Anglo-Saxon England of 1.1 million people (*British Medieval Population*, p. 54). John Hatcher allows for a range of 1.75 to 2.25 million (*Plague, Population*, p. 68); Stafford accepts a similar range of 1.5 to 2.5 million (*Unification*, p. 202). More recently, John S. Moore calculates around 1.88 million, arguing against any estimate over 2 million ("*Quot homines?*" pp. 333–34).

4. Sally Crawford summarizes: "In the earlier phases of settlement, the Anglo-Saxons lived in small, sprawling hamlets typified by Mucking. There appears to be increasing stratification of settlement into the middle Anglo-Saxon period, as typified by the enclosures and fences at Catholme, Staffordshire, and in the middle Saxon period more concentrated

populations occur, notably at the *wic* sites such as Ipswich and Hamwic. By the later Saxon period, there were small towns or *burhs* scattered throughout the area of Anglo-Saxon settlement" (*Childhood*, p. 107).

5. Prevalence rates for epilepsy are commonly cited as 0.5%–1% of the general population. Prevalence studies for TS yield widely different figures, from 0.05% to 3% (Freeman et al., "An International Perspective," p. 436). A methodic review of the literature indicates a wide range of prevalence rates (in large part because of differing diagnostic mechanisms), concluding that 5–20 cases per 10,000 people is a judicious estimate for the population at large (and not just for clinically reported cases); see Zohar et al., "Epidemiological Studies," pp. 178–79. However, Staley, Wand, and Shandy discuss the factors making prevalence determinations highly problematic ("Tourette Syndrome," pp. 12–13).

6. Blair, *Church*, pp. 391 ("small and rather crowded"), 456; Boddington, *Raunds Furnells*, p. 31.

7. Dendle, *Satan Unbound*, pp. 45–46.

8. See Jordan, "Demonic Elements."

9. I am aware that my conclusions may be mistaken for a polemical attempt to "save" Anglo-Saxon society from charges of superstition such as the post-Enlightenment educated community has commonly understood it; many Victorian scholars, for instance, would certainly have relished the idea that the continent was rife with possession and exorcism while Anglo-Saxon England remained distanced from that unseemly way of behaving. I hope my own analysis will not be taken to endorse any such ideological commitment: if we begin leveling the (usually unhelpful) charge of "superstition" in any meaningful sense, no society of the early Middle Ages would escape it, as indeed, no society of the twentieth or twenty-first century would either.

10. Thus Bourguignon, *Possession*, p. 53 (especially as possession outbreaks are linked with sorcery and periods of high persecution of witches); Hollenbach, "Jesus, Demoniacs," p. 577; Jacobs, "Possession," p. 180; and Rampolla, "Mirror." Pattison observes that "the eruption of demonology is coincident with social situations where there is an oppressive social structure, a loss of trust in the efficacy of social institutions, and a seeming inability to cope with the evils of the social structure" ("Psychosocial Interpretations," p. 7). Swantz observed that possession and exorcism can be a sign of increasing mistrust within a community, correlated for instance with increasing accusations of witchcraft (*Ritual and Symbol*, p. 141).

11. For an ingenious, if ultimately forced, application of this theory to Anglo-Saxon England, see Cameron, "Visions." One hardly needs to appeal to psychogenic poisoning under very particular dietary circumstances in order to account for literary descriptions of demonic temptation in the Antonine tradition. There is one early medieval reference to what may be gangrenous ergotism in the *Annales Xantenses* for the year 857 (Barger, *Ergot and Ergotism*, p. 43); a "plague of fire" is recorded in Paris in 945 (43–44); and an epidemic of similar nature in southern France in 994 reportedly claimed the lives of forty thousand people (44). More recently, see van Dongen and de Groot, "History of Ergot." Robert Bartholomew argues that contemporary constructs of medieval "dancing manias" are rife with reductionism and sexism (*Exotic Deviance*, pp. 127–52).

12. Clarke, *Mental Disorder*, p. 68.

13. Garrett, *Spirit Possession*, p. 10; Waegeman, "Medieval Sybil," p. 103. Some vestiges of oracular possession apparently survived into late antiquity, during which they were being reenvisioned as "demoniacs" by Christian apologists. There are echoes of this phenomenon as late as the time of Gregory of Tours, and perhaps even Walafrid Strabo (*Vita Galli* 1.15–18; Krusch, *Passiones* [MGH, SRM 4], pp. 295–98). See Wiśniewski, "La consultation."

14. For the latter view, see Waegeman, "Medieval Sybil," pp. 103–6.

15. Goddu, "Failure," pp. 548–49.

16. Goddu, "Failure," p. 549.

17. Graph 3 in Goddu, "Failure," p. 547. For further comment on Goddu's argument, see Kieckhefer, *Forbidden Rites*, p. 149.

18. Though the *Acta Sanctorum* began with January in 1643, the Bollandists were only halfway through October at the time of the French Revolution (and it took another hundred years to finish that month). Editorial principles changed over the course of compiling the work; see, for instance, Delehaye, *Work*, p. 209ff.

Works Cited

Abbetmeyer, C. *Old English Poetical Motives Derived from the Doctrine of Sin*. Minneapolis: H. Wilson; New York: Lemcke & Buechner, 1903.

Abusch, Tzvi. "The Demonic Image of the Witch in Standard Babylonian Literature: The Reworking of Popular Conceptions by Learned Exorcists." In *Religion, Science and Magic, in Concert and Conflict*, edited by Jacob Neusner, Ernest Frerichs, and Paul V. M. Flesher, 27–58. New York: Oxford University Press, 1989.

Akanmu, Moses, Kazuki Honda, and Shojiro Inoue. "Hypnotic Effects of Total Aqueous Extracts of Vervain hastata (Verbenaceae) in Rats." *Psychiatry and Clinical Neurosciences* 56 (2002): 309–10.

Akhtar, Salman. *Broken Structures: Severe Personality Disorders and Their Treatment*. Northvale, NJ: Jason Aronson, 1992.

Alarcón, Renato D. "Cross-Cultural Issues." In *Textbook of Personality Disorders*, edited by John M. Oldham, Andrew E. Skodol, and Donna S. Bender, 561–78. Washington, DC: American Psychiatric Publishing, 2005.

Alarcón, Renato D., Edward Foulks, and Mark Vakkur. *Personality Disorders and Culture: Clinical and Conceptual Interactions*. New York: John Wiley & Sons, 1998.

Alcuin. *The Bishops, Kings, and Saints of York*. Edited and translated by Peter Godman. Oxford: Clarendon Press, 1982.

Amt, Emilie. *Women's Lives in Medieval Europe: A Sourcebook*. New York: Routledge, 1993.

Anderson, Alan Orr, and Marjorie Ogilvie Anderson, eds. *Adomnan's Life of Columba*. London: Thomas Nelson and Sons, 1961.

Anderson, Graham. *Philostratus: Biography and Belles Lettres in the Third Century A.D.* London: Croom Helm, 1986.

Andreatini, Roberto, Vânia Sartori, Maria Seabra, and José Leite. "Effect of Valepotriates (Valerian Extract) in Generalized Anxiety Disorder: A Randomized Placebo-Controlled Study." *Phytotherapy Research* 16 (2002): 650–54.

Ankarloo, Bengt, and Stuart Clark, eds. *Witchcraft and Magic in Europe: Ancient Greece and Rome*. Philadelphia: University of Pennsylvania Press, 1999.

Archibald, Elizabeth, ed. and trans. *Apollonius of Tyre: Medieval and Renaissance Themes and Variations*. Cambridge: D. S. Brewer, 1991.

———. "The Flight from Incest: Two Late Classical Precursors of the Constance Theme." *Chaucer Review* 20 (1986): 259–72.

———. *Incest and the Medieval Imagination*. Oxford: Clarendon Press, 2001.

———. "Incest in Medieval Literature and Society." *Forum for Modern Language Studies* 25 (1989): 1–15.

Argenti-Pillen, Alexandra. "The Discourse on Trauma in Non-Western Cultural Contexts." In Shalev, Yehuda, and McFarlane, *International Handbook of Human Response*, 87–102.

Asch, Stuart. "Depression and Demonic Possession: The Analyst as an Exorcist." *Hillside Journal of Psychiatry* 7, no. 2 (1985): 149–64.

Assmann, Bruno, ed. *Angelsächsische Homilien und Heiligenleben*. Kassel: Georg H. Wigand, 1899.

Avalos, Hector. *Health Care and the Rise of Christianity*. Peabody, MA: Hendrickson Publishers, 1999.

———. *Illness and Health Care in the Ancient Near East: The Role of the Temple in Greece, Mesopotamia, and Israel*. Atlanta: Scholars Press, 1995.

Aydin, Süleyman, Rana Beis, Yusuf Öztürk, K. Hüsnü, and C. Baser. "Nepetalactone: A New Opioid Analgesic from *Nepeta caesarea* Boiss." *Journal of Pharmacy and Pharmacology* 50 (1998): 813–17.

Bacher, W. "La légende de l'exorcisme d'un demon." *Revue des âetudes Juives* 35 (1897): 285–87.

Baker, Peter, and Michael Lapidge, eds. *Byrhtferth's Enchiridion*. EETS s.s. 15. Oxford: Oxford University Press, 1995.

Bamberger, Bernard. *Fallen Angels*. Philadelphia: Jewish Publications Society of America, 1952.

Bamberger, John. *Evagrius Ponticus: The Praktikos & Chapters on Prayer*. Kalamazoo, MI: Cistercian Publications, 1981.

Banham, Debbie. "A Millennium in Medicine? New Medical Texts and Ideas in England in the Eleventh Century." In *Anglo-Saxons: Studies Presented to Cyril Roy Hart*, edited by Simon Keynes and Alfred P. Smyth, 230–42. Dublin: Four Courts Press, 2006.

Banting, H. M. J., ed. *Two Anglo-Saxon Pontificals*. HBS 104. Woodbridge, UK: Boydell Press, 1989.

Barger, George. *Ergot and Ergotism: A Monograph*. London: Gurney and Jackson, 1931.

Barrett-Lennard, R. J. S. *Christian Healing after the New Testament: Some Approaches to Illness in the Second, Third, and Fourth Centuries*. Lanham, MD: University Press of America, 1994.

Bartholomew, Robert. *Exotic Deviance: Medicalizing Cultural Idioms; From Strangeness to Illness*. Boulder: University Press of Colorado, 2000.

Bartlett, Robert. *Trial by Fire and Water: The Medieval Judicial Ordeal*. Oxford: Clarendon Press, 1986.

Bately, Janet. "The Vocabulary of Bravery in *Beowulf* and the *Battle of Maldon*." In *Unlocking the Wordhord: Anglo-Saxon Studies in Memory of Edward B. Irving, Jr.*, edited by Mark Amodio and Katherine O'Brien O'Keeffe, 274–301. Toronto: University of Toronto Press, 2003.

Bedingfield, M. Bradford. *The Dramatic Liturgy of Anglo-Saxon England*. Woodbridge, UK: Boydell Press, 2002.

Bennett, Max. *The Idea of Consciousness: Synapses and the Mind*. Amsterdam: Harwood Academic Publishers, 1997.

Ben-Noun, Liubov (Louba). "What Was the Mental Disease That Afflicted King Saul?" *Clinical Case Studies* 2 (2003): 270–82.

Benson, Larry, ed. *The Riverside Chaucer*. 3rd ed. Boston: Houghton Mifflin, 1987.

Benson, Stanley. "The Conquering Sacrament: Baptism and Demon Possession among the Maasai of Tanzania." *Africa Theological Journal* 9 (1980): 52–61.

Berecz, John. *Understanding Tourette Syndrome, Obsessive Compulsive Disorder, and Related Problems*. New York: Springer Publishing, 1992.

Berschin, Walter. "*Opus deliberatum ac perfectum*: Why Did the Venerable Bede Write a Second Prose Life of St Cuthbert?" In *St Cuthbert, His Cult and His Community to AD 1200*, edited by Gerald Bonner, David Rollason, and Clare Stancliffe, 95–102. Woodbridge, UK: Boydell, 1989.

Bethurum, Dorothy, ed. *The Homilies of Wulfstan*. Oxford: Clarendon Press, 1952.

Betz, Hans Dieter. *The Greek Magical Papyri in Translation*. 2nd ed. Chicago: University of Chicago Press, 1992.

Bieler, Ludwig, ed. *The Patrician Texts in the Book of Armagh*. Dublin: Dublin Institute for Advanced Studies, 1979.

Bierbaumer, Peter. *Der botanische Wortschatz des Altenglischen*. 3 vols. Bern: Herbert Lang and Frankfurt: Peter Lang, 1975–79.

Bildhauer, Bettina, and Robert Mills. "Introduction: Conceptualizing the Monstrous." In *The Monstrous Middle Ages*, edited by Bettina Bildhauer and Robert Mills, 1–27. Toronto: University of Toronto Press, 2003.

Bilu, Yoram. "The Taming of the Deviants and Beyond: An Analysis of *Dybbuk* Possession and Exorcism in Judaism." In *Spirit Possession in Judaism: Cases and Contexts from the Middle Ages to the Present*, edited by Matt Goldish, 41–72. Detroit: Wayne State University Press, 2003.

Birch, Walter de Gray. *Cartularium Saxonicum: A Collection of Charters Relating to Anglo-Saxon History*. 3 vols. London: Whiting & Co., 1885–93. Reprint, New York: Johnson Reprint Co., 1964.

Blair, John. *The Church in Anglo-Saxon Society*. Oxford: Oxford University Press, 2005.

Blake, E. O., ed. *Liber Eliensis*. London: Offices of the Royal Historical Society, 1962.

Blanke, Olaf, and Gregor Thut. "Inducing Out of Body Experiences." In *Tall Tales about the Mind and Brain: Separating Fact from Fiction*, edited by Sergio Della Sala, 425–39. Oxford: Oxford University Press, 2007.

Blanke, Olaf, Stéphanie Ortigue, Theodor Landis, and Margitta Seeck. "Stimulating Illusory Out-of-Body Perceptions." *Nature* 419 (2002): 269–70.

Blanke, Olaf, Theodor Landis, Laurent Spinelli, and Margitta Seeck. "Out-of-Body Experience and Autoscopy of Neurological Origin." *Brain* 127 (2004): 243–58.

Bleuler, Eugen. "Dementia Praecox oder Gruppe der Schizophrenien." In *Handbuch der Psychiatrie*, edited by G. Aschaffenburg. Spezieller Teil 4, Abteilung 1, Hälfte. Leipzig: Franz Deuticke, 1911.

———. "Die Prognose der Dementia Praecox-Schizophreniegruppe." *Allgemeine Zeitschrift für Psychiatrie* 65 (1908): 436–64.

Bleuler, Manfred. "The Concept of Schizophrenia in Europe during the Past One Hundred Years." In Flack, Miller, and Wiener, *What Is Schizophrenia?*, 1–15.

Bloomfield, Morton. *The Seven Deadly Sins*. East Lansing: Michigan State College Press, 1952.

Boddington, Andy. *Raunds Furnells: The Anglo-Saxon Church and Churchyard*. London: English Heritage, 1996.

Boddy, Janice. *Wombs and Alien Spirits: Women, Men, and the Zār Cult in Northern Sudan*. Madison: University of Wisconsin Press, 1989.

Boehnlein, James. "Culture and Society in Posttraumatic Stress Disorder: Implications for Psychotherapy." *American Journal of Psychotherapy* 41 (1987): 519–30.

Bonner, Campbell. "Demons of the Bath." In *Studies Presented to F. Ll. Griffith*, edited by S. R. K. Glanville, pp. 203–8. London: Egypt Exploration Society, 1932.

Bonner, Gerald, David Rollason, and Clare Stancliffe, eds. *St. Cuthbert, His Cult and His Community to AD 1200*. Woodbridge, UK: Boydell, 1989.

Bonser, Wilfrid. "Magical Practices against Elves." *Folklore* 37 (1926): 350–63.

———. *The Medical Background of Anglo-Saxon England: A Study in History, Psychology, and Folklore*. London: Wellcome Historical Medical Library, 1963.

Bottéro, Jean. *Myths et Rites de Babylone*. Paris: Éditions Champion, 1985.

Boureau, Alain. *Satan the Heretic: The Birth of Demonology in the Medieval West*. Translated by Teresa Lavender Fagan. Chicago: University of Chicago Press, 2006.

Bourguignon, Erika. Foreword to *Spirit Possession in Judaism: Cases and Contexts from the Middle Ages to the Present*, edited by Matt Goldish, 9–10. Detroit: Wayne State University Press, 2003.

———. *Possession*. San Francisco: Chandler & Sharp, 1976.

———, ed. *Religion, Altered States of Consciousness, and Social Change*. Columbus: Ohio State University Press, 1973.

Bowman, Jeffrey A. "Do Neo-Romans Curse? Law, Land, and Ritual in the Midi (900–1100)." *Viator* 28 (1997): 1–32.

Bowra, C. M. *Pindar*. Oxford: Clarendon Press, 1964.

Boyd, W. J. P. *Aldred's Marginalia: Explanatory Comments in the Lindisfarne Gospels*. Exeter: University of Exeter, 1975.

Bracken, Patrick, Joan Giller, and Derek Summerfield. "Psychological Responses to War and Atrocity: The Limitations of Current Concepts." *Social Science and Medicine* 40 (1995): 1073–82.

Brakke, David. *Demons and the Making of a Monk: Spiritual Combat in Early Christianity*. Cambridge, MA: Harvard University Press, 2006.

Braude, William G., and Israel Kapstein, trans. *Pĕsikta dĕ-Rab Kahăna*. Philadelphia: Jewish Publication Society of America, 1975.

Braune, Wilhelm. *Althochdeutsches Lesebuch*. Tübingen: Max Niemeyer, 1952.

Breasted, James. *Ancient Records of Egypt: Historical Documents from the Earliest Times to the Persian Conquest*. Vol. 3. Chicago: University of Chicago Press, 1906.

Bremner, J. Douglas, Penny Randall, Tammy M. Scott et al. "Does Stress Damage the Brain?" *Biological Psychiatry* 45 (1999): 797–805.

———. "MRI-Based Measurement of Hippocampal Volume in Patients with Combat-Related Posttraumatic Stress Disorder." *American Journal of Psychiatry* 152 (1995): 973–81.

Brennessel, Barbara, Michael D. C. Drout, and Robyn Gravel. "A Reassessment of the Efficacy of Anglo-Saxon Medicine." *ASE* 34 (2005): 183–95.

Brett, Elizabeth. "Classifications of Posttraumatic Stress Disorder in DSM-IV: Anxiety Disorder, Dissociative Disorder, or Stress Disorder?" In *Posttraumatic Stress Disorder: DSM-IV and Beyond*, edited by Jonathan Davidson and Edna Foa, 191–204. Washington, DC: American Psychiatric Press, 1993.

Brock, Sebastian, and Susan Ashbrook Harvey. *Holy Women of the Syrian Orient*. Berkeley: University of California Press, 1987.

Brown, Peter. *The Cult of the Saints: Its Rise and Function in Late Antiquity*. Chicago: University of Chicago Press, 1981.

———. "The Rise and Function of the Holy Man in Late Antiquity." *Journal of Roman Studies* 61 (1971): 80–101.

———. "The Saint as Exemplar in Late Antiquity." In *Persons in Groups: Social Behavior as Identity Formation in Medieval and Renaissance Europe*, edited by Richard C. Trexler, 183–94. Binghamton, NY: Medieval & Renaissance Texts and Studies, 1985.

———. "Sorcery, Demons, and the Rise of Christianity from Late Antiquity into the Middle Ages." In *Witchcraft, Confessions, and Accusations*, edited by Mary Douglas, 17–45. London: Tavistock Publications, 1970.

Brundage, James. "Rape and Seduction in Medieval Canon Law." In *Sexual Practices and the Medieval Church*, edited by Vern Bullough and James Brundage, 141–48. Buffalo, NY: Prometheus Books, 1982.

Bruun, Ruth Dowling, and Cathy Budman. "The Natural History of Gilles de la Tourette Syndrome." In *Handbook of Tourette's Syndrome and Related Tic and Behavioral Disorders*, edited by Roger Kurlan, 27–42. New York: Marcel Dekker, 1993.

Bünning, Silvia, and Olaf Blanke. "The Out-of-Body Experience: Precipitating Factors and Neural Correlates." In *The Boundaries of Consciousness: Neurobiology and Neuropathology*, edited by Steven Laureys, 331–50. Progress in Brain Research 150. Amsterdam: Elsevier, 2005.

Butzel, Jessica, Nancy Talbot, Paul Duberstein et al. "The Relationship between Traumatic Events and Dissociation among Women with Histories of Childhood Sexual Disorder." *Journal of Nervous and Mental Disease* 188 (2000): 547–49.

Caciola, Nancy. "Breath, Heart, Guts: The Body and Spirits in the Middle Ages." In *Communicating with the Spirits*, edited by Gábor Klaniczay and Éva Pócs, 21–37. Budapest: Central European University Press, 2005.

———. *Discerning Spirits: Divine and Demonic Possession in the Middle Ages*. Ithaca, NY: Cornell University Press, 2003.

Caelius Aurelianus. *On Acute Diseases and On Chronic Diseases*. Edited and translated by I. E. Drabkin. Chicago: University of Chicago Press, 1950.

Cameron, M. L. *Anglo-Saxon Medicine*. Cambridge: Cambridge University Press, 1993.

———. "Anglo-Saxon Medicine and Magic." *ASE* 17 (1988): 191–215.

———. "The Visions of Saints Anthony and Guthlac." In Campbell, Hall, and Klausner, *Health, Disease, and Healing*, 152–58.

Campbell, Sheila, Bert Hall, and David Klausner, eds. *Health, Disease, and Healing in Medieval Culture*. New York: St. Martin's Press, 1992.

Carlsson, A. "The Dopamine Theory Revisited." In Hirsch and Weinberger, *Schizophrenia*, 379–400.

Carmody, Francis. "Le diable des bestiaries." *Cahiers de l'association internationale des études françaises* 3, 4, 5 (1953): 79–85.

Cavill, Paul. *Maxims in Old English Poetry*. Cambridge: D. S. Brewer, 1999.

———. "Some Dynamics of Story-Telling: Animals in the Early Lives of St. Cuthbert." *Nottingham Medieval Studies* 43 (1999): 1–20.

Chajes, Jeffrey H. *Between Worlds: Dybbuks, Exorcists, and Early Modern Judaism*. Philadelphia: University of Pennsylvania Press, 2003.

———. "Jewish Exorcism: Early Modern Traditions and Transformations." In *Judaism in Practice, from the Middle Ages through the Early Modern Period*, edited by Lawrence Fine, 386–98. Princeton, NJ: Princeton University Press, 2001.

Chamberlin, John, ed. *The Rule of St. Benedict: The Abingdon Copy*. Toronto: Pontifical Institute of Mediaeval Studies, 1982.

Charcot, Jean-Martin, and Paul Richer. *Les démoniaques dans l'art*. Paris: Delahaye and Lecrosnier, 1887. Reprint, Amsterdam: B. M. Israël, 1972.

Chardonnens, László Sándor. *Anglo-Saxon Prognostics, 900–1100*. Leiden: Brill, 2007.

Charles, R. H. *The Apocrypha and Pseudepigrapha of the Old Testament in English*. 2 vols. 1913. Reprint, Oxford: Clarendon Press, 1963.

Charles-Edwards, Thomas. "The Penitential of Theodore and the *Iudicia Theodori*." In *Archbishop Theodore: Commemorative Studies on His Life and Influence*, edited by Michael Lapidge, 141–74. Cambridge: Cambridge University Press, 1995.

Charlesworth, James H., ed. *The Old Testament Pseudepigrapha*. 2 vols. Garden City, NY: Doubleday & Co., 1983.

Charney, Dennis, Eric Nestler, and Benjamin Bunney, eds. *Neurobiology of Mental Illness*. New York: Oxford University Press, 1999.

Chase, Thomas, Arnold Friedhoff, and Donald Cohen. *Tourette Syndrome: Genetics, Neurobiology, and Treatment, Advances in Neurology*. Vol. 58 of *Advances in Neurology*. New York: Raven Press, 1992.

Chitty, Derwas J. *The Desert a City: An Introduction to the Study of Egyptian and Palestinian Monasticism under the Christian Empire*. Oxford: Basil Blackwell, 1966.

Clarke, Basil. *Mental Disorder in Earlier Britain: Exploratory Studies*. Cardiff: University of Wales Press, 1975.

Clarkin, John F., Elsa Marziali, and Heather Munroe-Blum, eds. *Borderline Personality Disorder: Clinical and Empirical Perspectives*. New York: Guilford Press, 1992.

Clayton, Mary, and Hugh Magennis. *The Old English Lives of St. Margaret*. Cambridge: Cambridge University Press, 1994.

Cleary, Thomas, trans. *Code of the Samurai: A Modern Translation of the Bushido Shoshinsu*. Boston: Tuttle, 1999.

Clemoes, Peter. *Ælfric's Catholic Homilies: The First Series Text*. EETS s.s. 17. Oxford: Oxford University Press, 1997.

———. *The Chronology of Ælfric's Works*. Old English Newsletter Subsidia 5. Binghamton: CEMERS, SUNY-Binghampton, 1980.

Cockayne, Oswald, ed. *Leechdoms, Wortcunning, and Starcraft of Early England*. 3 vols. London: Longman, Green, Longman, Roberts, and Green, 1864–66.

Cohen, Lewis, Joan Berzoff, and Mark Elin, eds. *Dissociative Identity Disorder: Theoretical and Treatment Controversies*. Northvale, NJ: Jason Aronson, 1995.

Cohn, Norman. *Europe's Inner Demons: An Enquiry Inspired by the Great Witch Hunt*. New York: Basic Books, 1975.

Coleman, Julie. "Rape in Anglo-Saxon England." In *Violence and Society in the Early Medieval West*, edited by Guy Halsall, 193–204. Woodbridge, UK: Boydell, 1998.

Coleman, Mary, and Christopher Gillberg. *The Schizophrenias: A Biological Approach to the Schizophrenia Spectrum Disorders*. New York: Springer Publishing Co., 1996.

Colgrave, Bertram, ed. *The Earliest Life of Gregory the Great*. Lawrence: University of Kansas Press, 1968.

———. *Felix's Life of Saint Guthlac*. Cambridge: Cambridge University Press, 1956.

———. *The Life of Bishop Wilfrid, by Eddius Stephanus*. Cambridge: Cambridge University Press, 1927.

———. *Two Lives of Saint Cuthbert*. New York: Greenwood Press, 1969.

Colgrave, Bertram, and R. A. B. Mynors, eds. *Bede's Ecclesiastical History of the English People*. Oxford: Clarendon Press, 1969.

Comings, David. *Tourette Syndrome and Human Behavior*. Duarte, CA: Hope Press, 1990.

Conn, Rex B., William Borer, and Jack Snyder, eds. *Current Diagnosis*. 9th ed. Philadelphia: W. B. Saunders Co., 1997.

Constantius of Lyons. *Vie de Saint Germain d'Auxerre*. Edited by René Borius. Paris: Éditions du Cerf, 1965.

Corrêa, Alicia, ed. *The Durham Collectar*. HBS 107. Woodbridge, UK: Boydell Press, 1992.

Cotter, Wendy. *Miracles in Greco-Roman Antiquity: A Sourcebook*. London: Routledge, 1999.

Coulange, Louis [Joseph Turmel]. *The Life of the Devil*. Translated by Stephen Haden Guest. London: Alfred Knopf, 1929.

Courlander, Harold. *The Tiger's Whisker, and Other Tales from Asia and the Pacific*. New York: Henry Holt & Co., 1987.

Cowen, Alice. "*Byrstas* and *bysmeras*: The Wounds of Sin in the *Sermo Lupi ad Anglos*." In *Wulfstan, Archbishop of York: The Proceedings of the Second Alcuin Conference*, edited by Matthew Townend, 397–411. Turnhout: Brepols, 2004.

Cramer, Peter. *Baptism and Change in the Early Middle Ages, c.200–c.1150*. Cambridge: Cambridge University Press, 1993.

Crapanzano, Vincent, and Vivian Garrison, eds. *Case Studies in Spirit Possession*. New York: John Wiley & Sons, 1977.

Crawford, S. J., ed. *The Old English Version of the Heptateuch, Ælfric's Treatise on the Old and New Testament, and His Preface to Genesis*. EETS o.s. 160. 1922. London: Oxford University Press, 1969.

Crawford, Sally. *Childhood in Anglo-Saxon England*. Stroud: Sutton Publishing, 1999.

Crislip, Andrew. *From Monastery to Hospital: Christian Monasticism and the Transformation of Health Care in Late Antiquity*. Ann Arbor: University of Michigan Press, 2005.

———. "The Sin of Sloth or the Illness of the Demons? The Demon of Acedia in Early Christian Monasticism." *Harvard Theological Review* 98 (2005): 143–69.

Cross-National Collaborative Group. "The Changing Rate of Major Depression: Cross-National Comparisons." *Journal of the American Medical Association* 268 (1992): 3098–105.

Cryer, Frederick H., and Marie-Louise Thomsen. *Witchcraft and Magic in Europe: Biblical and Pagan Societies*. Philadelphia: University of Pennsylvania Press, 2001.

Cubbin, G. P., ed. *The Anglo-Saxon Chronicle: A Collaborative Edition*. Vol. 6, *MS D*. Cambridge: D. S. Brewer, 1996.

Cuneo, Michael W. *American Exorcism: Expelling Demons in the Land of Plenty*. New York: Doubleday, 2001.

Cunningham, Graham. *"Deliver Me from Evil": Mesopotamian Incantations 2500–1500 BC*. Rome: Pontifico Instituto Biblico, 1997.

Cutting, J. "Descriptive Psychopathology." In Hirsch and Weinberger, *Schizophrenia*, 15–27.

Cyprian. *De Lapsis and De Ecclesiae Catholicae Unitate*. Edited by Maurice Bénevot. Oxford: Clarendon Press, 1971.

Dancu, Constance, David Riggs, Diana Hearst-Ikeda et al. "Dissociative Experiences and Posttraumatic Stress Disorder among Female Victims of Criminal Assault and Rape." *Journal of Traumatic Stress* 9 (1996): 253–67.

Danet, Brenda and Bryna Bogoch. "'Whoever Alters This, May God Turn His Face from Him on the Day of Judgment': Curses in Anglo-Saxon Legal Documents." *Journal of American Folklore* 105 (1992): 132–65.

Darlington, Reginald, ed. *The Vita Wulfstani of William of Malmesbury*. London: Offices of the Royal Historical Society, 1928.

D'Aronco, Maria A. "The Benedictine Rule and the Care of the Sick: The Plan of St. Gall and Anglo-Saxon England." In *The Medieval Hospital and Medical Practice*, edited by Barbara S. Bowers, 235–51. Aldershot: Ashgate, 2007.

———. "The Botanical Lexicon of the Old English *Herbarium*." *ASE* 17 (1988): 15–33.

Davis, Edward L. *Society and the Supernatural in Song China*. Honolulu: University of Hawai'i Press, 2001.

Dawes, Elizabeth, and Norman Baynes, trans. *Three Byzantine Saints*. Crestwood, NY: St. Vladimir's Seminary Press, 1996.

De Bellis, Michael D., Stephen R. Hooper, and Jennifer L. Sapia. "Early Trauma Exposure and the Brain." In *Neuropsychology of PTSD: Biological, Cognitive, and Clinical Perspectives*, edited by Jennifer J. Vasterling and Chris R. Brewin, 153–77. New York: Guilford Press, 2005.

Deegan, Marilyn. "A Critical Edition of MS B.L. Royal 12 D.xvii: Bald's Leechbook." Ph.D. diss., University of Manchester, 1991.

Deegan, Marilyn, and Donald G. Scragg. *Medicine in Early Medieval England: Four Papers*. Manchester: Centre for Anglo-Saxon Studies, 1987.

De exorcismis et supplicationibus quibusdam. Vatican City: Libreria Editrice Vaticana, 1999.

Delehaye, Hippolyte. *The Work of the Bollandists through Three Centuries, 1615–1915*. Princeton, NJ: Princeton University Press, 1922.

DeMause, Lloyd, ed. *The History of Childhood*. New York: Psychohistory Press, 1974.

Dendle, Peter. "Cryptozoology in the Medieval and Modern Worlds." *Folklore* 117 (2006): 190–206.

———. "Lupines, Manganese and Devil-Sickness: An Anglo-Saxon Medical Response to Epilepsy." *Bulletin of the History of Medicine* 75 (2001): 91–101.

———. "The Old English *Life of Malchus* and Two Vernacular Tales from the *Vitas Patrum* in MS Cotton Otho C.i: A Translation." Pts. 1 and 2. *English Studies* 90.5 (2009): 505–17; 90.6 (2009): 631–52.

———. "Plants in the Early Medieval Cosmos: Herbs, Divine Potency, and the *Scala natura*." In *Health and Healing from the Medieval Garden*, edited by Peter Dendle and Alain Touwaide, 47–59. Woodbridge, UK: Boydell, 2008.

———. *Satan Unbound: The Devil in Old English Narrative Literature*. Toronto: University of Toronto Press, 2001.

———. "Schizophrenia in the Early Middle Ages: Some Negative Evidence." *Australian and New Zealand Journal of Psychiatry* 39 (2005): 522.

———. "*Solomon and Saturn* 44a: *Đæs deofles dream*." *NM* 98 (1997): 391–96.

des Places, Édouard, ed. *Contre Hiéroclès*. *SC* 333. Paris: Éditions du Cerf, 1986.

De SS. Anatholia Virg. et Audace. *Acta Sanctorum*, July 9. Antwerp: Jacob of Moulin, 1721.

De Vriend, Hubert Jan, ed. *The Old English Herbarium and Medicina de Quadrupedibus*. EETS o.s. 286. Oxford: Oxford University Press, 1984.

DeVries, Marten, ed. *Diagnostic and Statistical Manual of Mental Disorders*. 4th edition. Washington, DC: American Psychiatric Association, 1994. (DSM-IV)

———. "Trauma in Cultural Perspective." In Van der Kolk, McFarlane, and Weisaeth, *Traumatic Stress*, 398–413.

Doble, G. H., ed. *Pontificale Lanaletense*. HBS 74. London: Harrison and Sons, 1937.

Dodds, E. R. "Supernormal Phenomena in Classical Antiquity." In *The Ancient Concept of Progress, and Other Essays on Greek Literature and Belief*, 156–210. Oxford: Clarendon Press, 1973.

Dols, Michael W. *Majnūn: The Madman in Medieval Islamic Society*. Oxford: Clarendon Press, 1992.

Dombart, Bernardus, and Alfonsus Kalb, eds. *Sancti Aurelii Augustini episcopi De civitate*

Dei libri XXII. 2 vols. Leipzig: Teubner, 1928. Reprint, Darmstadt: Wissenschaftliche Buchgesellschaft, 1981.

Doob, Penelope. *Nebuchadnezzar's Children: Conventions of Madness in Medieval English Literature*. New Haven: Yale University Press, 1974.

Dreifuss, Fritz. "Classification of Seizures." In *Comprehensive Epileptology*, edited by Mogens Dam and Lennart Gram, 77–86. New York: Raven Press, 1991.

Droogers, André. *The Dangerous Journey: Symbolic Aspects of Boys' Initiation among the Wagenia of Kisangani, Zaire*. The Hague: Mouton, 1980.

Duchesne, Louis. *Christian Worship: Its Origin and Evolution*. Translated by M. L. McClure. New York: Macmillan, 1949.

Duemmler, E., ed. *Epistolae Karolini aevi* 2. MGH, Epistolarum 4. Berlin: Weidmann, 1895.

Duling, Dennis. "The Eleazar Miracle and Solomon's Magical Wisdom in Flavius Josephus' *Antiquitates Judaicae* 8.42–49." *Harvard Theological Review* 78 (1985): 1–25.

———. "Solomon, Exorcism, and the Son of David." *Harvard Theological Review* 68 (1975): 235–52.

Dupont-Sommer, A. *The Essene Writings from Qumran*. Oxford: Basil Blackwell, 1962.

Dzielska, Maria. *Apollonius of Tyana in Legend and History*. Translated by Piotr Pieńkowski. Rome: L'ERMA di Bretschneider, 1986.

Eadie, Mervyn J. *A Disease Once Sacred: A History of the Medical Understanding of Epilepsy*. Eastleigh, UK: John Libbey & Co., 2001.

———. "The Understanding of Epilepsy across Three Millennia." *Clinical and Experimental Neurology* 31 (1994): 1–12.

Earls, Felton. "Psychosocial Factors in Tourette Syndrome." In Chase, Friedhoff, and Cohen, *Tourette Syndrome*, 55–59.

Eisenman, Robert, and Michael Wise, trans. *The Dead Sea Scrolls Uncovered*. New York: Penguin, 1993.

Ellard, John. "Did Schizophrenia Exist before the Eighteenth Century?" *Australian and New Zealand Journal of Psychiatry* 21 (1987): 306–14.

Ellason, Joan, and Colin Ross. "Positive and Negative Symptoms in Dissociative Identity Disorder and Schizophrenia: A Comparative Analysis." *Journal of Nervous and Mental Disease* 183 (1995): 236–41.

Elliott, Dyan. *Fallen Bodies: Pollution, Sexuality, and Demonology in the Middle Ages*. Philadelphia: University of Pennsylvania Press, 1999.

Erenberg, Gerald. "Treatment of Tourette Syndrome with Neuroleptic Drugs." In Chase, Friedhoff, and Cohen, *Tourette Syndrome*, 241–43.

Eugippius. *Vie de Saint Séverin*. Edited by Philippe Régerat. *SC* 374. Paris: Éditions du Cerf, 1991.

Eusebius. *The History of the Church*. Translated by G. A. Williamson. London: Penguin, 1965.

Evans, K., J. McGrath, and R. Milns. "Searching for Schizophrenia in Ancient Greek and Roman Literature: A Systematic Review." *Acta Psychiatrica Scandinavica* 107 (2003): 323–30.

Evelyn-White, Hugh. *Hesiod: The Homeric Hymns and Homerica*. Cambridge, MA: Harvard University Press; London: William Heinemann, 1914.

Fabrega, Horacia, Jr. "On the Significance of an Anthropological Approach to Schizophrenia." *Psychiatry* 52 (1989): 45–65.

Fairweather, Janet, trans. *Liber Eliensis*. Woodbridge, UK: Boydell, 2005.

Falls, Thomas. *Dialogue with Typho*. Washington, DC: Catholic University of America Press, 2003.

———. *Saint Justin Martyr*. New York: Christian Heritage, 1948.

Faral, Edmond, ed. *La légende Arthurienne*. Vol. 3. Paris: Librairie Ancienne Honoré Champion, 1929.

Farley, Melissa, and Joanne Keaney. "Physical Symptoms, Somatization, and Dissociation in Women Survivors of Childhood Sexual Assault." *Women & Health* 25 (1997): 33–45.

Fehr, Bernhard, ed. *Die Hirtenbriefe Ælfrics in Altenglischer und Lateinischer Fassung*. Bibliothek der angelsächsischen Prosa 9. Hamburg, 1914. Revised and edited by Peter Clemoes. Darmstadt: Wissenschaftliche Buchgesellschaft, 1966.

Fell, Christine. *Women in Anglo-Saxon England*. London: Colonnade Books, 1984.

Ferguson, Everett. *Demonology of the Early Christian World*. New York: Edwin Mellen, 1984.

Férotin, D. Marius, ed. *Le Liber Ordinum*. Paris: Firmin-Didot, 1904.

Ferracuti, Stefano, Roberto Sacco, and Renato Lazzari. "Dissociative Trance Disorder: Clinical and Rorschach Findings in Ten Persons Reporting Demon Possession and Treated by Exorcism." *Journal of Personality Assessment* 66 (1996): 525–39.

Finberg, B. Herbert. *The Early Charters of the West Midlands*. Leicester: Leicester University Press, 1961.

Finkelhor, David. "Child Sexual Abuse: Challenges Facing Child Protection and Mental Health Professionals." In *Childhood and Trauma: Separation, Abuse, War*, edited by Elisabeth Ullmann and Werner Hilweg, 101–15. Aldershot: Ashgate, 1999.

Finsterwalder, Paul Willem. *Die Canones Theodori Cantuariensis und ihre Überlieferungsformen*. Weimar: Hermann Böhlaus Nachfolger, 1929.

Finucane, Ronald. *Appearances of the Dead: A Cultural History of Ghosts*. Buffalo, NY: Prometheus Books, 1984.

———. *Miracles and Pilgrims: Popular Beliefs in Medieval England*. London: Macmillan, 1995.

First, Michael B., and Allan Tasman. *DSM-IV-TR Mental Disorders: Diagnosis, Etiology, and Treatment*. Chichester: John Wiley & Sons, 2004.

Fisher, J. D. C. *Christian Initiation: Baptism in the Medieval West*. London: S.P.C.K., 1965.

Fisher, John. *John Gower: Moral Philosopher and Friend of Chaucer*. New York: New York University Press, 1964.

Flack, William, Jr., Daniel Miller, and Morton Wiener, eds. *What Is Schizophrenia?* New York: Springer-Verlag, 1991.

Flint, Valerie. "The Demonisation of Magic and Sorcery in Late Antiquity: Christian Redefinitions of Pagan Religions." In *Witchcraft and Magic in Europe: Ancient Greece and Rome*, edited by Bengt Ankarloo and Stuart Clark, 277–348. Philadelphia: University of Pennsylvania Press, 1999.

———. *The Rise of Magic in Early Medieval Europe*. Princeton, NJ: Princeton University Press, 1991.

Flobert, Pierre. *La Vie Ancienne de Saint Samson de Dol*. Paris: CNRS Editions, 1997.

Foot, Sarah. "'By Water in the Spirit': The Administration of Baptism in Early Anglo-Saxon Society." In *Pastoral Care before the Parish*, edited by John Blair and Richard Sharpe, 171–92. Leicester: Leicester University Press, 1992.

Forbes, Alexander P., ed. *The Historians of Scotland*. Vol. 5, *Lives of S. Ninian and S. Kentigern*. Edinburgh: Edmonston and Douglas, 1874.

Ford, Gordon B., Jr., trans. *The Letters of St. Isidore of Seville*. Amsterdam: Adolf Hakkert, 1970.

Forster, H. B., H. Niklas, and S. Lutz. "Antispasmodic Effects of Some Medicinal Plants." *Journal of Medicinal Research* 40 (1980): 311–19.
Foster, Benjamin. *Before the Muses: An Anthology of Akkadian Literature*. Vol. 1. Bethesda, MD: CDL Press, 1993.
Foucault, Michel. *Madness and Civilization: A History of Insanity in the Age of Reason*. Translated by Richard Howard. New York: Vintage, 1965.
Frank, Roberta. "*The Battle of Maldon* and Heroic Literature." In *The Battle of Maldon A.D. 991*, edited by Donald Scragg, 196–207. Oxford: Basil Blackwell, 1991.
———. "The Ideal of Men Dying with Their Lord in *The Battle of Maldon*: Anachronism or *Nouvelle Vague*." In *People and Places in Northern Europe, 500–1600: Essays in Honour of Peter Hayes Sawyer*, edited by Ian Wood and Niels Lund, 95–106. Woodbridge, UK: Boydell Press, 1991.
Frantzen, Allen. "Where the Boys Are: Children and Sex in the Anglo-Saxon Penitentials." In *Becoming Male in the Middle Ages*, edited by Jeffrey Jerome Cohen and Bonnie Wheeler, 43–66. New York: Garland, 1997.
Freedy, John, and Stevan Hobfoll, eds. *Traumatic Stress: From Theory to Practice*. New York: Plenum Press, 1995.
Freeman, Roger, Diane Fast, Larry Burd, Jacob Kerbeshian, Mary Robertson, and Paul Sandor. "An International Perspective on Tourette Syndrome: Selected Findings from 3500 Individuals in 22 Countries." *Developmental Medicine and Child Neurology* 42 (2000): 436–47.
Freud, Sigmund. "Eine Teufelsneurose im Siebzehnten Jahrhundert." In *Gessamelte Werke*, vol. 13. London: Imago, 1940.
———. *Totem and Taboo*. Translated by A. A. Brill. New York: Vintage Books, 1918.
Fridrichsen, Anton. "The Conflict of Jesus with the Unclean Spirits." *Theology* 22 (1931): 122–35.
Fry, Timothy, ed. *The Rule of St. Benedict, in Latin and English with Notes*. Collegeville, MN: Liturgical Press, 1981.
Fulk, R. D., and Christopher M. Cain. *A History of Old English Literature*. Malden, MA: Blackwell, 2003.
Gager, John. *Curse Tablets and Binding Spells from the Ancient World*. New York: Oxford University Press, 1992.
Gameson, Richard, ed. *St Augustine and the Conversion of England*. Phoenix Mill, Gloucestershire, UK: Sutton Publishing, 1999.
Gardner, Rex. "Miracles of Healing in Anglo-Celtic Northumbria as Recorded by the Venerable Bede and His Contemporaries: A Reappraisal in the Light of Twentieth Century Experiences." *British Medical Journal* 287 (1983): 1927–33.
Garmonsway, G. N., ed. *Ælfric's Colloquy*. 2nd ed. London: Methuen & Co., 1947.
Garrett, Clarke. *Spirit Possession and Popular Religion: From the Camisards to the Shakers*. Baltimore: The Johns Hopkins University Press, 1987.
Gatch, Milton McC. *Loyalties and Traditions: Man and His World in Old English Literature*. New York: Pegasus, 1971.
Gaudemet, Jean, ed. *Conciles Gaulois du IVe siècle*. Paris: Éditions du Cerf, 1977, 58–62.
Geffcken, Johannes. *The Last Days of Greco-Roman Paganism*. Translated by Sabine MacCormack. Amsterdam: North-Holland Publishing, 1978.
Geller, Markham. *Forerunners to Udug-Hul: Sumerian Exorcistic Incantations*. Stuttgart: Franz Steiner, 1985.
Gerbert, Martin. *Monumenta veteris liturgiae alemannicae*. 2 vols. St. Blasien, 1777–79. Reprint, Hildesheim: Georg Olms, 1967.

Getz, Faye. *Medicine in the English Middle Ages*. Princeton, NJ: Princeton University Press, 1998.

Gildersleeve, Basil. *Pindar: The Olympian and Pythian Odes*. New York: American Book Co., 1885.

Giles, J. A. Vita quorundum Anglo-Saxonum: *Original Lives of Anglo-Saxons and Others Who Lived before the Conquest*. 1854. Reprint, New York: Burt Franklin, 1967.

Giller, Earl, Jr., ed. *Biological Assessment and Treatment of Posttraumatic Stress Disorder*. Washington, DC: American Psychiatric Press, 1990.

Gilmore, David. *Monsters: Evil Beings, Mythical Beasts, and All Manner of Imaginary Terrors*. Philadelphia: University of Pennsylvania Press, 2003.

Gleaves, David H., Mary C. May, and Etzel Cardeña. "An Examination of the Diagnostic Validity of Dissociative Identity Disorder." *Clinical Psychology Review* 21 (2001): 577–608.

Glosecki, Stephen O. *Shamanism and Old English Poetry*. New York: Garland, 1989.

Gneuss, Helmut. "Liturgical Books in Anglo-Saxon England." In *Learning and Literature in Anglo-Saxon England*, edited by Michael Lapidge and Helmut Gneuss, 91–141. Cambridge: Cambridge University Press, 1985.

Godden, Malcolm, ed. *Ælfric's Catholic Homilies: Introduction, Commentary, and Glossary*. EETS s.s. 18. Oxford: Oxford University Press, 2000.

———. *Ælfric's Catholic Homilies: The Second Series Text*. EETS s.s. 5. London: Oxford University Press, 1979.

———. "Ælfric's Saints' Lives and the Problem of Miracles." *Leeds Studies in English* 16 (1985): 83–100.

Goddu, André. "The Failure of Exorcism in the Middle Ages." In *Soziale Ordnungen im Selbstverständnis des Mittelalters*, edited by Albert Zimmermann and Gudrun Vuillemin-Diem. Berlin: De Gruyter, 1980. Reprinted in *Possession and Exorcism*, edited by Brian P. Levack, 540–57. New York: Garland, 1992.

Goff, Donald, Andrew Brotman, Daniel Kindlon et al. "The Delusion of Possession in Chronically Psychotic Patients." *Journal of Nervous and Mental Disease* 179 (1991): 567–71.

Goldish, Matt, ed. *Spirit Possession in Judaism: Cases and Contexts from the Middle Ages to the Present*. Detroit: Wayne State University Press, 2003.

Goldman, Stephen. "The Use of Christian Belief in Old English Poems of Exile." *Res Publica Litterarum* 2 (1979): 69–80.

Golub, Deborah. "Cultural Variations in Multiple Personality Disorder." In *Dissociative Identity Disorder: Theoretical and Treatment Controversies*, edited by Lewis Cohen, Joan Berzoff, and Mark Elin, 285–326. Northvale, NJ: Jason Aronson, 1995.

Gonser, Paul, ed. *Das angelsächsische Prosa-Leben des hl. Guthlac*. Heidelberg: Carl Winter's Universitätsbuchhandlung, 1909. Reprint, Amsterdam: Swets & Zeitlinger, 1966.

Goodman, Felicitas. *How about Demons? Possession and Exorcism in the Modern World*. Bloomington: Indiana University Press, 1988.

Goodwin, Frederick K., and Kay Redfield Jamison. *Manic-Depressive Illness*. New York: Oxford University Press, 1990.

Goolden, Peter, ed. *The Old English Apollonius of Tyre*. London: Oxford University Press, 1958.

Goossens, Louis, ed. *The Old English Glosses of MS. Brussels, Royal Library, 1650 (Aldhelm's De Laudibus Virginitatis)*. Brussels: Paleis der Academiën, 1974.

Gordon, Cyrus. "An Aramaic Exorcism." *Archiv orientalni* 6 (1934): 466–74.

Gordon, Eleanora. "Child Health in the Middle Ages as Seen in the Miracles of Five English Saints, A.D. 1150–1220." *Bulletin of the History of Medicine* 60 (1986): 502–22.

Gordon, Richard. "Imagining Greek and Roman Magic." In *Witchcraft and Magic in Europe: Ancient Greece and Rome*, edited by Bengt Ankarloo and Stuart Clark, 159–275. Philadelphia: University of Pennsylvania Press, 1999.

Goscelin of Saint-Bertin. *The Hagiography of the Female Saints of Ely*. Edited by Rosalind C. Love. Oxford: Clarendon Press, 2004.

Gougaud, L. "Étude sur les *loricae* Celtiques et sur les prières qui s'en rapprochent." *Bulletin d'ancienne littérature et d'archéologie chrétiennes* 1 (1911): 265–81.

Graham, Thomas. *Medieval Minds: Mental Health in the Middle Ages*. London: George Allen & Unwin, 1967.

Grattan, J. H. G., and Charles Singer. *Anglo-Saxon Magic and Medicine*. London: Oxford University Press, 1952.

Greenfield, Stanley. *Hero and Exile: The Art of Old English Poetry*. London: Hambledon Press, 1989.

Gregory of Nyssa. *On the Life and Wonders of Our Father Among the Saints, Gregory the Wonderworker*. In Gregory Thaumaturgus, *Life and Works*.

Gregory the Great. *Dialogues*. Edited by Adalbert de Vogüé. 3 vols. Paris: Éditions du Cerf, 1978–80.

Gregory Thaumaturgus. *Life and Works*. Translated by Michael Slusser. Washington, DC: Catholic University of America Press, 1998.

Grendon, Felix. "The Anglo-Saxon Charms." *Journal of American Folklore* 22 (1909): 105–237.

Griffiths, Bill. *Aspects of Anglo-Saxon Magic*. Frithgarth, UK: Anglo-Saxon Books, 1996.

Grimes, W. F. *Excavations on Defence Sites, 1939–1945*. London: Her Majesty's Stationery Office, 1960.

Grmek, Mirko D., ed. "The Concept of Disease." In *Western Medical Thought from Antiquity to the Middle Ages*, translated by Antony Shugaar, 241–58. Cambridge, MA: Harvard University Press, 1998.

Gruenwald, Ithamar. *Apocalyptic and Merkavah Mysticism*. Leiden: Brill, 1980.

Guo, Qitao. *Exorcism and Money: The Symbolic World of the Five-Fury Spirits in Late Imperial China*. Berkeley: Institute of East Asian Studies, 2003.

Gurvitz, T. V., M. E. Shenton, and R. K. Pitman. "Reduced Hippocampal Volume on Magnetic Resonance Imaging in Chronic Post-Traumatic Stress Disorder." Paper presented at Annual Meeting of International Society for Traumatic Stress Studies, Miami, 1995.

Guthrie, George, and David Szanton. "Folk Diagnosis and Treatment of Schizophrenia: Bargaining with the Spirits in the Philippines." In *Culture-Bound Syndromes, Ethnopsychiatry, and Alternate Therapies*, edited by William Lebra, 147–63. Honolulu: University of Hawaii Press, 1976.

Gwara, Scott, ed. *Aldhelmi Malmesbiriensis Prosa De Virginitate*. 2 vols. CCSL 124 and 124A. Turnhout: Brepols, 2001.

Gwara, Scott, ed., and David Porter, trans. *Anglo-Saxon Conversations: The Colloquies of Ælfric Bata*. Woodbridge, UK: Boydell Press, 1997.

Haddan, Arthur West, and William Stubbs. *Councils and Ecclesiastical Documents Relating to Great Britain and Ireland*. Vol. 3. Oxford: Clarendon Press, 1871.

Haldipur, C. V. "Madness in Ancient India: Concept of Insanity in Charaka Samhita (1st Century A.D.)." *Comprehensive Psychiatry* 25 (1984): 335–44.

Hale, Anthony, and Narsimha Pinninti. "Exorcism-Resistant Ghost Possession Treated with Clopenthixol." *British Journal of Psychiatry* 165 (1994): 386–88.

Hall, Alaric T. P. "Calling the Shots: The Old English Remedy *Gif Hors Ofscoten Sie* and Anglo-Saxon 'Elf-Shot.'" *NM* 106 (2005): 195–209.

———. *Elves in Anglo-Saxon England: Matters of Belief, Health, Gender, and Identity.* Woodbridge, UK: Boydell, 2007.

———. "The Meanings of Elf and Elves in Medieval England." Ph.D. diss., University of Glasgow, 2004.

Hall, Gordon C. N., and Amber Phung. "Cognitive Enculturation and Sexual Abuse." In *Cultural Cognition and Psychopathology*, edited by John Schumaker and Tony Ward, 107–18. Westport, CT: Praeger, 2001.

Halm, Charles, ed. *Sulpicii Severi libri qui supersunt.* CSEL 1. Vienna: Geroldus, 1866.

Hamilton, Sarah. "Remedies for 'Great Transgressions': Penance and Excommunication in Late Anglo-Saxon England." In *Pastoral Care in Late Anglo-Saxon England*, edited by Francesca Tinti, 83–105. Woodbridge, UK: Boydell, 2005.

Hare, Edward. "Commentary One" (addendum to John Ellard's "Did Schizophrenia Exist before the Eighteenth Century?"). *Australian and New Zealand Journal of Psychiatry* 21 (1987): 315–16.

Harkness, Kate L., and Scott M. Monroe. "Childhood Adversity and the Endogenous Versus Nonendogenous Distinction in Women with Major Depression." *American Journal of Psychiatry* 159 (2002): 387–93.

Harmon, Austin Morris, ed. and trans. *Lucian.* Vol. 3. Cambridge, MA: Harvard University Press, 1921.

Harris, Joseph. "Love and Death in the *Männerbund.*" In *Heroic Poetry in the Anglo-Saxon Period*, edited by Helen Damico and John Leyerle, 77–114. Kalamazoo, MI: Medieval Institute Publications, 1993.

Hart, Cyril. *Learning and Culture in Late Anglo-Saxon England and the Influence of Ramsey Abbey on the Major English Monastic Schools.* 2 vols. Lewiston, NY: Edwin Mellen, 2003.

Hartranft, Chester, ed. *Ecclesiastical History of Sozomen.* In *NPNF*, vol. 2, edited by Philip Schaff and Henry Wace, 179–427. New York: Christian Literature Co.; Oxford: Parker & Co., 1890.

Harvey, Allison G., Michael D. Kopelman, and Chris R. Brewin. "PTSD and Traumatic Brain Injury." In *Neuropsychology of PTSD: Biological, Cognitive, and Clinical Perspectives*, edited by Jennifer J. Vasterling and Chris R. Brewin, 230–46. New York: Guilford Press, 2005.

Hassrick, Royal. *The Sioux: Life and Customs of a Warrior Society.* Norman: University of Oklahoma Press, 1964.

Hatcher, John. *Plague, Population, and the English Economy, 1348–1530.* London: Macmillan, 1977.

Hauser, Allen, and Dale Hesdorffer. *Epilepsy: Frequency, Causes and Consequences.* New York: Epilepsy Foundation of America/Demos Publications, 1990.

Hawkes, Sonia, and Calvin Wells. "Crime and Punishment in an Anglo-Saxon Cemetery?" *Antiquity* 49 (1975): 118–22.

Headland, Thomas N., Kenneth L. Pike, and Marvin Harris, eds. *Emics and Etics: The Insider/Outsider Debate.* Newbury Park, CA: Sage Publications, 1990.

Healey, Antonette diPaolo. "Old English Glossaries: Creating a Vernacular." *Computing in the Humanities Working Papers* B.36. University of Toronto, November 1997.

———. *The Old English Vision of St. Paul.* Cambridge, MA: Mediaeval Academy of America, 1978.

Hecht, Hans, ed. *Dialoge Gregors des Grossen.* Bibliothek der angelsächsischen Prosa 5, part 1. Leipzig: Georg H. Wigand's Verlag, 1900.

Henderson, James. "Exorcism and Possession in Psychotherapy and Practice." *Canadian Journal of Psychiatry* 27 (1982): 129–34.

Herlihy, David. "Medieval Children." In *The Walter Prescott Webb Memorial Lectures: Essays on Medieval Civilization*, edited by Bede Karl Lackner and Kenneth Roy Philip, 109–41. Austin: University of Texas Press, 1978.

Herman, Judith L. *Father-Daughter Incest.* Cambridge, MA: Harvard University Press, 2000.

Herrmann, Léon. "Les premiers exorcismes juifs et judéo-chrétiens." *Revue de l'Université de Bruxelles*, n.s., 7 (1954–55): 305–8.

Hessels, John H., ed. *A Late Eighth-Century Latin-Anglo Saxon Glossary.* Cambridge: Cambridge University Press, 1906.

Higham, Nicholas. *Rome, Britain, and the Anglo-Saxons.* London: Seaby, 1992.

Hilgard, Ernest. *Divided Consciousness: Multiple Controls in Human Thought and Action.* New York: John Wiley, 1977.

Hill, John M. *The Anglo-Saxon Warrior Ethic: Reconstructing Lordship in Early English Literature.* Gainesville: University Press of Florida, 2000.

Hill, Joyce. "Monastic Reform and the Secular Church: Ælfric's Pastoral Letters in Context." In *England in the Eleventh Century*, edited by Carola Hicks, 103–17. Stamford: Paul Watkins, 1992.

Hill, Peter. *Whithorn and St. Ninian: The Excavation of a Monastic Town, 1984–91.* Stroud: Sutton Publishing, 1997.

Hill, Thomas D. "The Devil's Forms and the Pater Noster's Powers: 'The Prose Solomon and Saturn *Pater Noster* Dialogue' and the Motif of the Transformation Combat." *Studies in Philology* 85 (1985): 164–76.

———. "Tormenting the Devil with Boiling Drops: An Apotropaic Motif in the Old English Solomon and Saturn I and Old Norse–Icelandic Literature." *JEGP* 92 (1993): 157–66.

———. "When God Blew Satan Out of Heaven: The Motif of Exsufflation in Vercelli Homily XIX and Later English Literature." *Leeds Studies in English* 16 (1985): 132–41.

Hippocrates. "On the Sacred Disease." In vol. 2 of *Hippocrates*, edited and translated by W. H. S. Jones, 127–83. Cambridge: Harvard University Press; London: William Heinemann, 1967.

Hirsch, Steven, and Daniel Weinberger. *Schizophrenia.* Oxford: Blackwell Science, 1995.

Hollenbach, Paul. "Jesus, Demoniacs, and Public Authorities: A Socio-Historical Study." *Journal of the American Academy of Religion* 49 (1981): 567–88.

Hollis, Stephanie, and Michael Wright. *Old English Prose of Secular Learning.* Woodbridge, UK: D. S. Brewer, 1992.

Homer. *The Iliad.* Edited and translated by A. T. Murray. Cambridge, MA: Harvard University Press; London: William Heinemann, 1960.

———. *The Odyssey.* Edited and translated by A. T. Murray. Cambridge, MA: Harvard University Press; London: William Heinemann, 1966.

Horner, Shari. "The Language of Rape in Old English Literature and Law: Views from the Anglo-Saxon(ist)s." In *Sex and Sexuality in Anglo-Saxon England: Essays in Memory of Daniel Gillmore Calder*, edited by Carol Braun Pasternack and Lisa M. C. Weston, 149–81. Tempe: Arizona Center for Medieval and Renaissance Studies, 2004.

Hough, Carole. "Alfred's *Domboc* and the Language of Rape: A Reconsideration of Alfred Ch. 11." *Medium Ævum* 66 (1997): 1–27.

———. "A New Reading of Alfred, Ch. 26." *Nottingham Medieval Studies* 41 (1997): 1–12.

Houghton, P. J. "The Scientific Basis for the Reputed Activity of Valerian." *Journal of Pharmacy and Pharmacology* 51 (1999): 505–12.

Hucbald of St. Amand. *Vita Rictrudis. Acta Sanctorum*, May, vol. 3. Paris and Rome: Victor Palm, 1866.

Hultkrantz, Åke. "Aspects of Saami (Lapp) Shamanism." In *Northern Religions and Shamanism*, edited by Mihály Hoppál and Juha Pentikäinen, 138–45. Helsinki: Finnish Literature Society, 1992.

Hunter, Erica. "Aramaic-Speaking Communities of Sasanid Mesopotamia." *Aram* 7 (1995): 319–35.

Hunter, Richard, and Ida Macalpine, eds. *Three Hundred Years of Psychiatry, 1535–1860: A History Presented in Selected English Texts*. London: Oxford University Press, 1963.

Hyams, Paul R. "Trial by Ordeal: The Key to Proof in the Early Common Law." In *On the Laws and Customs of England*, edited by Morris Arnold et al., 90–126. Chapel Hill: University of North Carolina Press, 1981.

Isaacs, Haskell D. *Medical and Para-Medical Manuscripts in the Cambridge Genizah Collections*. Cambridge: Cambridge University Press, 1994.

Jablensky, A., N. Sartorius, G. Ernberg et al. *Schizophrenia: Manifestations, Incidence and Course in Different Cultures*. Cambridge: Cambridge University Press, 1992.

Jackson, Peter. "The *Vitas Patrum* in Eleventh-Century Worcester." In *England in the Eleventh Century*, edited by Carola Hicks, 119–34. Stamford: Paul Watkins, 1992.

Jackson, Stanley. *Melancholia and Depression: From Hippocratic Times to Modern Times*. New Haven: Yale University Press, 1986.

———. "Unusual Mental States in Medieval Europe, I. Medical Syndromes of Mental Disorder: 400–1100 A.D." *Journal of the History of Medicine and Allied Sciences* 27 (1972): 262–97.

Jacobs, Donald. "Possession, Trance State, and Exorcism in Two East African Communities." In *Demon Possession: A Medical, Historical, Anthropological, and Theological Symposium*, edited by John W. Montgomery, 175–87. Minneapolis: Bethany Fellowship, 1976.

Jadhav, Sushrut. "The Cultural Origins of Western Depression." *International Journal of Social Psychiatry* 42 (1996): 269–86.

Jagiello-Wojtowicz, Ewa, Leon Jusiak, Jaroslaw Szponar, and Zdzislaw Kleinrok. "Preliminary Pharmacological Evaluation of Chelidonine in Rodents." *Polish Journal of Pharmacology and Pharmacy* 41 (1989): 125–31.

Janet, Pierre. "Un cas de possession et l'exorcisme moderne." *Bulletin de l'Université de Lyon* 8 (1894): 41–57.

Janowitz, Naomi. *Icons of Power: Ritual Practice in Late Antiquity*. University Park: Pennsylvania State University Press, 2002.

———. *Magic in the Roman World: Pagans, Jews, and Christians*. London: Routledge, 2001.

Jessopp, Augustus, and Montague R. James, eds. *The Life and Miracles of St. William of Norwich*. Cambridge: Cambridge University Press, 1896.

Jeste, Dilip, Rebecca del Carmen, James Lohr, and Richard Jed Wyatt. "Did Schizophrenia Exist before the Eighteenth Century?" *Comprehensive Psychiatry* 26 (1985): 493–503.

John, Eric. *Land Tenure in Early England*. Leicester: Leicester University Press, 1960.

Johnson, David. "The *Crux Usualis* as Apotropaic Weapon in Anglo-Saxon England." In

The Place of the Cross in Anglo-Saxon England, edited by Catherine E. Karkov, Sarah Larratt Keefer, and Karen L. Jolly, 80–95. Woodbridge, UK: Boydell, 2006.

———. "Euhemerisation versus Demonisation: The Pagan Gods and Ælfric's *De falsis diis*." In *Pagans and Christians: The Interplay between Christian Latin and Traditional Germanic Cultures in Early Modern Europe*, edited by T. Hofstra, L. A. J. R. Houwen, and A. A. MacDonald, 35–69. Groningen: Egbert Forsten, 1995.

Johnson, Felix Y. Attah. "Gilles de la Tourette Syndrome in Papua New Guinea." *Papua and New Guinea Medical Journal* 38 (1995): 127–32.

Johnson, Richard F. *Saint Michael the Archangel in Medieval English Legend*. Woodbridge, UK: Boydell, 2005.

Jolly, Karen. "Elves in the Psalms? The Experience of Evil from a Cosmic Perspective." In *The Devil, Heresy, and Witchcraft in the Middle Ages: Essays in Honor of Jeffrey B. Russell*, edited by Alberto Ferreiro, 19–44. Leiden: Brill, 1998.

———. "Magic, Miracle, and Popular Practice in the Early Medieval West: Anglo-Saxon England." In *Religion, Science and Magic, in Concert and Conflict*, edited by Jacob Neusner, Ernest Frerichs, and Paul V. M. Flesher, 166–82. New York: Oxford University Press, 1989.

———. "On the Margins of Orthodoxy: Devotional Formulas and Protective Prayers in Cambridge, Corpus Christi College MS 41." In *Signs on the Edge: Space, Text, and Margin in Medieval Manuscripts*, edited by Sarah Larratt Keefer and Rolf H. Bremmer, 135–83. Paris: Peeters, 2007.

———. *Popular Religion in Late Saxon England: Elf Charms in Context*. Chapel Hill: University of North Carolina Press, 1996.

———. "Prayers from the Field: Practical Protection and Demonic Defense in Anglo-Saxon England." *Traditio* 61 (2006): 95–147.

———. "Tapping the Power of the Cross: Who and for Whom?" In *The Place of the Cross in Anglo-Saxon England*, edited by Catherine E. Karkov, Sarah Larratt Keefer, and Karen L. Jolly, 58–79. Woodbridge, UK: Boydell, 2006.

Joly, Robert, ed. and trans. *Hermas le Pasteur*. *SC* 53 Paris: Éditions du Cerf, 1958.

Jones, Charles. *Saints' Lives and Chronicles in Early England*. Ithaca, NY: Cornell University Press, 1947.

Jones, Timothy S., and David A. Sprunger, eds. *Marvels, Monsters, and Miracles: Studies in the Medieval and Early Modern Imagination*. Kalamazoo, MI: Medieval Institute Publications, 2002.

Jordan, Louis. "Demonic Elements in Anglo-Saxon Iconography." In *Sources of Anglo-Saxon Culture*, edited by Paul Szarmach, 283–317. Studies in Medieval Culture 20. Kalamazoo, MI: Medieval Institute Publications, 1986.

Jost, Karl, ed. *Die "Institutes of Polity, Civil and Ecclesiastical."* Bern: Francke, 1959.

Joynes, Andrew. *Medieval Ghost Stories: An Anthology of Miracles, Marvels and Prodigies*. Woodbridge, UK: Boydell Press, 2001.

Kales, Anthony, Costas Stefanis, and John Talbott, eds. *Recent Advances in Schizophrenia*. New York: Springer-Verlag, 1990.

Kantor, Martin. *Diagnosis and Treatment of the Personality Disorders*. St. Louis: Ishiyaku EuroAmerica, 1992.

Karkov, Catherine E., Sarah Larratt Keefer, and Karen L. Jolly, eds. *The Place of the Cross in Anglo-Saxon England*. Woodbridge, UK: Boydell, 2006.

Karlsen, Carol. *The Devil in the Shape of a Woman: Witchcraft in Colonial New England*. New York: W. W. Norton, 1987.

Kaviratna, Avinash Chandra, trans. *Charaka-Samhita*. Fascicle 7. Calcutta: D. C. Dass & Co., n.d.

Kealey, Edward. *Medieval Medicus: A Social History of Anglo-Norman Medicine*. Baltimore: Johns Hopkins University Press, 1981.

Kee, Howard Clark. *Miracle in the Early Christian World*. New Haven: Yale University Press, 1983.

Keefer, Sarah Larratt. "Manuals." In Pfaff, *Liturgical Books*, 99–109.

———. "*Ut in omnibus honorificetur Deus*: The *Corsnæd* Ordeal in Anglo-Saxon England." In *The Community and the Saint: Patterns of Power in Early Medieval Europe*, edited by Joyce Hill and Mary Swan, 237–64. Turnhout: Brepols, 1998.

Keller, Edmund. "Glimpses of Exorcism in Religion." In Nauman, *Exorcism through the Ages*, 259–311. New York: Philosophical Library, 1974.

Keller, Mary. *The Hammer and the Flute: Women, Power, and Spirit Possession*. Baltimore: The Johns Hopkins University Press, 2002.

Kelly, Henry A. *The Devil, Demonology, and Witchcraft: The Development of Christian Beliefs in Evil Spirits*. Garden City, NY: Doubleday, 1968.

———. *The Devil at Baptism: Ritual, Theology, and Drama*. Ithaca: Cornell University Press, 1985.

———. "The Devil in the Desert." *Catholic Biblical Quarterly* 26 (1964): 190–220.

———. "The Struggle against Satan in the Liturgies of Baptism and Easter." *Chronica* 24 (1979): 9–10.

Kemp, Simon. "'Ravished of a Fiend': Demonology and Medieval Madness." In Colleen Ward, *Altered States*, 67–78.

Kempe, Ruth S., and C. Henry Kempe. *Child Abuse*. Cambridge, MA: Harvard University Press, 1978.

Kendell, Robert. "Schizophrenia: A Medical View of a Medical Concept." In Flack, Miller, and Wiener, *What Is Schizophrenia?*, 59–72.

Ker, Neil R. *Catalogue of Manuscripts Containing Anglo-Saxon*. Oxford: Clarendon Press, 1957.

Kershaw, Paul. "Illness, Power and Prayer in Asser's *Life of King Alfred*." *Early Medieval Europe* 10 (2001): 201–24.

Kerwin, Robert. "The Neuropharmacology of Schizophrenia: Past, Present, and Future." In *The Psychopharmacology of Schizophrenia*, edited by Michael Reveley and J. F. William Deakin, 41–55. London: Arnold, 2000.

Khouzam, Hani Raoul, Bita Ghafoori, and Robert Hierholzer. "Progress in the Identification, Diagnosis, and Treatment of Posttraumatic Stress Disorder." In *Trends in Posttraumatic Stress Disorder Research*, edited by Thomas A. Corales, 1–28. New York: Nova Science Publishers, 2005.

Kieckhefer, Richard. *Forbidden Rites: A Necromancer's Manual of the Fifteenth Century*. University Park: Pennsylvania State University Press, 1998.

———. *Magic in the Middle Ages*. Cambridge: Cambridge University Press, 1989.

Kiev, Ari, ed. *Magic, Faith, and Healing: Studies in Primitive Psychiatry Today*. New York: Free Press, 1964.

Kilger, Dom Laurent. "The Devil and the Conversion of the Pagan." In *Satan*, edited by Bruno de Jesus-Marie, 213–22. London: Sheed and Ward, 1951.

Kindschi, Lowell. "The Latin-Old English Glossaries in Plantin-Moretus MS 32 and British Museum MS Additional 32246." Ph.D. diss., Stanford University, 1955.

King, Robert A., Lawrence Scahill, Diane Findley, and Donald Cohen. "Psychosocial and Behavioral Treatments." In Leckman and Cohen, *Tourette's Syndrome*, 338–59.

Kirmayer, Laurence J. "Pacing the Void: Social and Cultural Dimensions of Dissociation." In Spiegel, *Dissociation*, 91–122.

Kitchen, John. "Saints, Doctors, and Soothsayers: The Dynamics of Healing in Gregory of Tours's *De virtutibus Sancti Martini*." *Florilegium* 12 (1993): 15–32.

Kitson, Peter. "From Eastern Learning to Western Folklore: The Transmission of Some Medico-Magical Ideas." In Scragg, *Superstition and Popular Medicine*, 57–71.

Klaniczay, Gábor, and Éva Pócs, eds. *Communicating with the Spirits*. Budapest: Central European University Press, 2005.

Klerman, Gerald L., and Myrna M. Weissman. "Increasing Rates of Depression." *Journal of the American Medical Association* 261 (1989): 2229–35.

Klingshirn, William. *Caesarius of Arles: The Making of a Community in Late Antique Gaul*. Cambridge: Cambridge University Press, 1994.

Klutz, Todd. *The Exorcism Stories in Luke-Acts: A Sociostylistic Reading*. Cambridge: Cambridge University Press, 2004.

———. *Rewriting the Testament of Solomon: Tradition, Conflict and Identity in a Late Antique Pseudepigraphon*. London: T & T Clark, 2005.

Knowles, David, ed. *The Monastic Constitutions of Lanfranc*. New York: Oxford University Press, 1951.

Knox, Wilfred Lawrence. "Jewish Liturgical Exorcism." *Harvard Theological Review* 31 (1938): 191–203.

Knüsel, Christopher. "Pagan Charm and the Place of Anthropological Theory." Review of *Anglo-Saxon Paganism*, by David Wilson. *Journal of European Archaeology* 1 (1993): 205–8.

Kocijan-Hercigonja, Dubravka. "Children in War: Experiences from Croatia." In *Childhood and Trauma: Separation, Abuse, War*, edited by Elisabeth Ullmann and Werner Hilweg, 157–72. Aldershot: Ashgate, 1999.

Kofsky, Aryeh. *Eusebius of Caesarea against Pagansim*. Leiden: Brill, 2000.

Kotzor, Günter, ed. *Das altenglische Martyrologium*. 2 vols. Munich: Bayerische Akademie der Wissenschaften, 1981.

Krippner, Stanley. "Cross-Cultural Treatment Perspectives on Dissociative Disorders." In *Dissociation: Clinical and Theoretical Perspectives*, edited by Steven Jay Lynn and Judith Rhue, 338–61. New York: Guilford Press, 1994.

Kroll, Jerome. "A Reappraisal of Psychiatry in the Middle Ages." *Archives of General Psychiatry* 29 (1973): 276–83.

Kroll, Jerome, and Bernard Bachrach. "Child Care and Child Abuse in Early Medieval Europe." *Journal of the American Academy of Child Psychiatry* 25, no. 4 (1986): 562–68.

———. "Medieval Visions and Contemporary Hallucinations." *Psychological Medicine* 12 (1982): 709–21.

———. "Sin and Mental Illness in the Middle Ages." *Psychological Medicine* 14 (1984): 507–14.

———. "Sin and the Etiology of Disease in Pre-Crusade Europe." *Journal of the History of Medicine and Allied Sciences* 41 (1986): 395–414.

Krusch, Bruno, ed. *Fredegarii et aliorum chronica*. MGH, SRM 2. Hanover: Hahn, 1888.

———. *Gregorii episcopi Turonensis historiarum libri X*. MGH, SRM 1, part 1, fascicle 2. Hanover: Hahn, 1942.

———. *Gregorii episcopi Turonensis miracula et opera minora*. MGH, SRM 1, part 2. Hanover: Hahn, 1885.

———. *Passiones vitaeque sanctorum aevi Merovingici*. MGH, SRM 4. Hanover: Hahn, 1902.

———. *Passiones vitaeque sanctorum aevi Merovingici et antiquiorum aliquot*. MGH, SRM 3. Hanover: Hahn, 1896.

———. *Venanti Honori Clementiani Fortunati presbyteri Italici Opera pedestrian*. MGH, AA 4, part 2. Berlin: Weidmann, 1885.

Krusch, Bruno, and Wilhelm Levison, eds. *Passiones vitaeque sanctorum aevi Merovingici (V)*. MGH, SRM 7. Hanover: Hahn, 1920.

Kuefler, Mathew S. "'A Wryed Existence': Attitudes toward Children in Anglo-Saxon England." *Journal of Social History* 24 (1991): 823–34.

Kurlan, Roger, ed. *Handbook of Tourette's Syndrome and Related Tic and Behavioral Disorders*. New York: Marcel Dekker, 1993.

Kurtz, Benjamin. "From St. Anthony to St. Guthlac: A Study in Biography." *University of California Publications in Modern Philology* 12 (1926): 103–46.

Kushner, Howard. *A Cursing Brain? The Histories of Tourette Syndrome*. Cambridge, MA: Harvard University Press, 1999.

Kuypers, Dom A. B., ed. *The Prayer Book of Aedeluald the Bishop, Commonly Called the Book of Cerne*. London: Cambridge University Press, 1902.

Kytzler, Bernhard, ed. *M. Minuci Felicis Octavius*. Leipzig: B. G. Teubner, 1982.

Labat, René, ed. and trans. *Traité Akkadien de diagnostics et pronostics médicaux*. Paris: Academie Internationale d'Histoires des Sciences; Leiden: Brill, 1951.

Lacroix, Paul. *Military and Religious Life in the Middle Ages*. 1874. Reprint, New York: Frederick Ungar, 1964.

La Fontaine, J. S. *Initiation*. Manchester: Manchester University Press, 1985.

Lake, Stephen. "Knowledge of the Writings of John Cassian in Early Anglo-Saxon England." *ASE* 32 (2004): 27–41.

Lambek, Michael. "From Disease to Discourse: Remarks on the Conceptualization of Trance and Spirit Possession." In Colleen Ward, *Altered States*, 36–61.

Lambert, Catherine. "The Old English Medical Vocabulary." *Proceedings of the Royal Society of Medicine* 33 (1939–40): 137–45.

Langslow, D. R. *The Latin Alexander Trallianus: The Text and Transmission of a Late Latin Medical Book*. Journal of Roman Studies Monograph 10. London: Society for the Promotion of Roman Studies, 2006.

Langton, Edward. *Satan, A Portrait: A Study of the Character of Satan through All the Ages*. London: Skeffington & Son, 1946.

Lapidge, Michael. *The Cult of St. Swithun*. Oxford: Clarendon Press, 2003.

———. "A Metrical *Vita S. Iudoci* from Tenth-Century Winchester." *Journal of Medieval Latin* 10 (2000): 255–306.

Lapidge, Michael, and Rosalind C. Love. "The Latin Hagiography of England and Wales (600–1550)." In vol. 3 of *Hagiographies: Histoire Internationale de la Littérature Hagiographique Latine et Vernaculaire en Occident des Origines à 1550*, edited by Guy Philippart, 203–325. Turnhout: Brepols, 2001.

Laungani, Pittu. "Culture, Cognition, and Trauma: Crosscultural Evaluations." In *Cultural Cognition and Psychopathology*, edited by John Schumaker and Tony Ward, 119–43. Westport, CT: Praeger, 2001.

Lea, Henry Charles. *A History of Auricular Confession and Indulgences in the Latin Church*. Vol. 1. New York: Greenwood Press, 1968.

Leavitt, John. "Are Trance and Possession Disorders?" *Transcultural Psychiatric Research Review* 30 (1993): 51–57.

Le Bourdellès, Hubert. "Vie de St Josse avec commentaire historique et spiritual." *Studi Medievali*, 3rd series, 34, fascicle 2 (1993): 861–958.

Lebra, William. *Culture-Bound Syndromes, Ethnopsychiatry, and Alternate Therapies*. Honolulu: University of Hawaii Press, 1976.

Leckman, James, and Donald Cohen, eds. *Tourette's Syndrome—Tics, Obsessions, Compulsions: Developmental Psychopathology and Clinical Care*. New York: John Wiley and Sons, 1999.

LeDoux, Joseph. "Emotion as Memory: Anatomical Systems Underlying Indelible Neural Traces." In *The Handbook of Emotion and Memory*, edited by Sven-Åke Christianson, 269–88. Hillsdale, NJ: Lawrence Erlbaum Associates, 1992.

Leeper, Elizabeth Ann. "Exorcism in Early Christianity." Ph.D. diss., Duke University, 1991.

Lennox, William G. *Epilepsy and Related Disorders*. Vol. 2. Boston: Little, Brown, and Co., 1960.

Lesses, Rebecca. "Exe(o)rcising Power: Women as Sorceresses, Exorcists, and Demonesses in Babylonian Jewish Society of Late Antiquity." *Journal of the American Academy of Religion* 69, no. 2 (2001): 343–75.

Levison, Wilhelm, ed. *Vitae Sancti Bonifatii Archiepiscopi Moguntini*. MGH, Scriptores 52. Hanover: Hahn, 1905.

Lewine, Richard. "Epilogue: Comments on the Origins and Development of Schizophrenia." In *Origins and Development of Schizophrenia*, edited by Mark Lenzenweger and Robert Dworkin, 493–503. Washington, DC: American Psychological Association, 1998.

Lewis, I. M. "Spirit Possession and Deprivation Cults." *Man*, n.s., 1 (1966): 307–29.

Lieberman, Leo. "The Concept of the 'Dybbuk' (Demon) in Hebrew Literature and Thought." In Nauman, *Exorcism through the Ages*, 99–104. New York: Philosophical Library, 1974.

Liebermann, F., ed. *Die Gesetze der Angelsachsen*. 3 vols. Halle: Max Niemeyer. 1903–16.

Lindelöf, U., ed. *Rituale Ecclesiae Dunelmensis: The Durham Collectar*. Publications of the Surtees Society 140. London: Andrews & Co., 1927.

Lindsay, W. M., ed. *The Corpus Glossary*. Cambridge: Cambridge University Press, 1921.

Ling, Trevor. *The Significance of Satan: New Testament Demonology and Its Contemporary Relevance*. London: S.P.C.K., 1961.

Lipschitz, Deborah, Margaret Kaplan, Jodie Sorkenn et al. "Childhood Abuse, Adult Assault, and Dissociation." *Comprehensive Psychiatry* 37 (1996): 261–66.

Lisowski, F. P. "Prehistoric and Early Historic Trepanation." In *Diseases in Antiquity: A Survey of the Diseases, Injuries and Surgery of Early Populations*, edited by Don Brothwell and A. T. Sandison, 651–72. Springfield, IL: Charles C. Thomas, 1967.

Little, Lester. *Benedictine Maledictions: Liturgical Cursing in Romanesque France*. Ithaca, NY: Cornell University Press, 1993.

Liuzza, Roy M. "Anglo-Saxon Prognostics in Context: A Survey and Handlist of Manuscripts." *ASE* 30 (2001): 181–230.

———, ed. *The Old English Version of the Gospels*. EETS o.s. 304. Oxford: Oxford University Press, 1994.

Lloyd, Paul M. "On the Names of Languages (and Other Things)." In *Latin and the Romance Languages in the Early Middle Ages*, edited by Roger Wright. University Park: Pennsylvania State University Press, 1996.

Locherbie-Cameron, M. A. L. "Ælfric's Devils." *Notes & Queries* 238 (1993): 286–87.

Logan, F. Donald. "Excommunication." In vol. 4 of *Dictionary of the Middle Ages*, edited by Joseph Strayer, 536–48. New York: Charles Scribner's Sons, 1984.

Logeman, H. "New Aldhelm Glosses." *Anglia* 13 (1891): 26–41.

Lohr, Evelyn. "Patristic Demonology in Old English Literature." Ph.D. diss., New York University, 1947.

Lubac, Henri de. *Exégèse médiévale: Les quatre sens de l'écriture.* 2 vols. Paris: Aubier, 1959–64.

———. *Medieval Exegesis: The Four Senses of Scripture.* Vol. 1, translated by Mark Sebanc; vol. 2, translated by E. M. Macierowski. Grand Rapids, MI: W. B. Eerdmans; Edinburgh: T&T Clark, 1998–2000.

Lucy, Sam. *The Anglo-Saxon Way of Death: Burial Rites in Early England.* Stroud, UK: Sutton Publishing, 2000.

Lukken, G. M. *Original Sin in the Roman Liturgy.* Leiden: Brill, 1973.

Lynn, Steven Jay, and Judith Rhue, eds. *Dissociation: Clinical and Theoretical Perspectives.* New York: Guilford Press, 1994.

Lysaght, Gary A. "Fleury and S. Benedict: Monastery and Patron Saint (640–877)." Ph.D. diss., Magdalen College, Oxford, 1984.

Maddicott, J. R. "Plague in Seventh-Century England." *Past and Present* 156 (1997): 7–54.

Maldonado, José R., and David Spiegel. "Dissociative States." In *Textbook of Personality Disorders,* edited by John M. Oldham, Andrew E. Skodol, and Donna S. Bender, 493–521. Washington, DC: American Psychiatric Publishing, 2005.

Manfield, Philip. *Split Self/Split Object: Understanding and Treating Borderline, Narcissistic, and Schizoid Disorders.* Northvale, NJ: Jason Aronson, 1992.

Manselli, Raoul. "Vie familiale et éthique sexuelle dans les pénitentiels." In *Famille et Parenté dans l'Occident Médiéval,* edited by Georges Duby and Jacques Le Goff, 363–83. Rome: École française de Rome, 1977.

Marcus, Eric. *Psychosis and Near Psychosis: Ego Function, Symbol Structure, Treatment.* New York: Springer-Verlag, 1992.

Marsden, C. David, and Edward H. Reynolds. "Seizures in Adults." In *A Textbook of Epilepsy,* edited by John Laidlaw, Alan Richens, and Jolyon Oxley, 144–82. 3rd ed. Edinburgh: Churchill Livingstone, 1988.

Marsella, Anthony. "Culture and Mental Health: An Overview." In *Cultural Conceptions of Mental Health and Therapy,* edited by Anthony Marsella and Geoffrey White, 359–88. Dordrecht: D. Reidel, 1982.

Martin, Malachi. *Hostage to the Devil: The Possession and Exorcism of Five Living Americans.* New York: Reader's Digest Press, 1976.

Martine, François, ed. *Vie des Pères du Jura. SC* 142. Paris: Éditions du Cerf, 1968.

Mayes, G. M., et al. *Child Sexual Abuse: A Review of Literature and Educational Materials.* Edinburgh: Scottish Academic Press, 1992.

McCasland, S. Vernon. *By the Finger of God: Demon Possession and Exorcism in Early Christianity in the Light of Modern Views of Mental Illness.* New York: Macmillan, 1951.

McCready, William. *Signs of Sanctity: Miracles in the Thought of Gregory the Great.* Toronto: Pontifical Institute of Mediaeval Studies, 1989.

McHugh, Paul, and Frank Putnam. "Resolved: Multiple Personality Disorder Is an Individually and Socially Created Artifact." *Journal of the American Academy of Child and Adolescent Psychiatry* 34 (1995): 957–63.

McKenna, P. J. *Schizophrenia and Related Syndromes.* New York: Oxford University Press, 1994.

McKillop, Alan. "Illustrative Notes on Genesis B." *JEGP* 20 (1921): 28–38.

McNeill, John, and Helena Gamer, trans. *Medieval Handbooks of Penance: A Translation of the Principal Libri Poenitentiales and Selections from Related Documents.* New York: Columbia University Press, 1938.

Meaney, Audrey L. "'And we forbeodað eornostlice ælcne hæðenscipe': Wulfstan and Late Anglo-Saxon and Norse 'Heathenism.'" In *Wulfstan, Archbishop of York: The Proceedings of the Second Alcuin Conference*, edited by Matthew Townend, 461–500. Turnhout: Brepols, 2004.

———. *Anglo-Saxon Amulets and Curing Stones*. Oxford: B.A.R., 1981.

———. "The Anglo-Saxon View of the Causes of Illness." In Campbell, Hall, and Klausner, *Health, Disease, and Healing*, 12–33.

———. "Felix's Life of St. Guthlac: Hagiography and/or Truth." *Proceedings of the Cambridge Antiquarian Society* 90 (2001): 29–48.

———. "Old English Legal and Penitential Penalties for 'Heathenism.'" In *Anglo-Saxons: Studies Presented to Cyril Roy Hart*, edited by Simon Keynes and Alfred P. Smyth, 127–58. Dublin: Four Courts Press, 2006.

———. "Women, Witchcraft, and Magic." In Scragg, *Superstition and Popular Medicine*, 9–40.

Menner, Robert, ed. *The Poetical Dialogues of Solomon and Saturn*. New York: Modern Language Association of America; London: Oxford University Press, 1941.

Meritt, Herbert D. *Old English Glosses*. New York: Modern Language Association of America; London: Oxford University Press, 1945.

Merrifield, Ralph. *The Archaeology of Ritual and Magic*. London: B. T. Batsford, 1987.

Metzger, Bruce, and Roland Murphy. *The New Oxford Annotated Bible*. New York: Oxford University Press, 1991.

Meyer, Marvin, and Richard Smith, eds. *Ancient Christian Magic: Coptic Texts of Ritual Power*. Princeton, NJ: Princeton University Press, 1999.

Middle English Dictionary. Ann Arbor: University of Michigan Press, 1959–2001. http://quod.lib.umich.edu/m/med/.

Midelfort, H. C. Erik. "Madness and Civilization in Early Modern Europe: A Reappraisal of Michel Foucault." In *After the Reformation: Essays in Honor of J. H. Hexter*, edited by Barbara C. Malament, 247–65. Philadelphia: University of Pennsylvania Press, 1980.

Miller, Carol Lynn. "The Old High German and Old Saxon Charms: Text, Commentary, and Critical Bibliography." Ph.D. diss., Washington University, 1963.

Miller, Thomas, ed. *The Old English Version of Bede's Ecclesiastical History of the English People*. EETS o.s. 95, 96. London: Trübner and Co., 1890–91.

Millon, Theodore. "The Borderline Personality: A Psychosocial Epidemic." In *Borderline Personality Disorder: Etiology and Treatment*, edited by Joel Paris, 197–210. Washington, DC: American Psychiatric Press, 1993.

Minucius Felix, Marcus. *The Octavius of Marcus Minucius Felix*. Translated by G. W. Clarke. *ACW* 39. New York: Newman Press, 1974.

Miracula S. Austrebertæ. *Acta Sanctorum*, February, vol. 2. Antwerp: J. Mersius, 1658.

Mittman, Asa Simon. *Maps and Monsters in Medieval England*. New York: Routledge, 2006.

Mittman, Asa Simon, and Peter Dendle, eds. *The Ashgate Research Companion to Monsters and the Monstrous*. Farnham, UK, and Burlington, VT: Ashgate, 2012.

Moltke, Erik. *Runes and Their Origin: Denmark and Elsewhere*. Translated by Peter Foote. Copenhagen: Nationalmuseets, 1985.

Monahon, Cynthia. *Children and Trauma*. New York: Lexington Books, 1993.

Montgomery, John W., ed. *Demon Possession: A Medical, Historical, Anthropological, and Theological Symposium*. Minneapolis: Bethany Fellowship, 1976.

Mooneyham, W. Stanley. "Demonism on the Mission Field: Problems of Communicating a Difficult Phenomenon." In *Demon Possession: A Medical, Historical, Anthropological, and Theological Symposium*, edited by John W. Montgomery, 209–19. Minneapolis: Bethany Fellowship, 1976.

Moore, John S. "*Quot homines?* The Population of Domesday England." *Anglo-Norman Studies* 19 (1997): 307–34.

Moore, Norman, ed. *The Book of the Foundation of St. Bartholomew's Church in London*, EETS o.s. 163. London: Oxford University Press, 1923.

Morgan, Gerald. "*Spectamur agendo*: The Universality of the Battle of Maldon." In *Text and Gloss: Studies in Insular Learning and Literature Presented to Joseph Donovan Pheifer*, edited by Helen Conrad O'Briain, Anne Marie D'Arcy, and John Scattergood, 182–205. Dublin: Four Courts Press, 1999.

Morgan, Michael, trans. *Sepher Ha-Razim: The Book of the Mysteries*. Chico, CA: Scholars Press, 1983.

Morin, Dom Germain, ed. *Sancti Caesarii Arelatensis Sermones*. Vol. 1. CCSL 103. Turnhout: Brepols, 1953.

———. *Sancti Caesarii Episcopi Arelatensis, Opera Omnia*. Vol. 2, *Opera Varia*. Denée: Maredsous, 1942.

Morris, Brian. *Anthropology of the Self: The Individual in Cultural Perspective*. London: Pluto Press, 1994.

Morris, Colin. "*Judicium Dei*: The Social and Political Significance of the Ordeal in the Eleventh Century." In *Church, Society and Politics*, edited by Derek Baker, 95–111. Oxford: Basil Blackwell, 1975.

Morris, R., ed. *The Blickling Homilies*. Oxford: Oxford University Press, 1967.

Motz, Lotte. "Of Elves and Dwarfs." *Arv. Tidskrift för Nordisk Folkminnesforskning* 29–30 (1973–74): 93–127.

Munier, Charles, ed. *Concilia Africae, A.345–A.525*. Turnhout: Brepols, 1974.

———. *Les Statuta ecclesiae antiqua*. Paris: Presses Universitaires de France, 1960.

Murdoch, Brian. "But Did They Work? Interpreting the Old High German *Merseburg Charms* in Their Medieval Context." *NM* 89 (1988): 358–69.

———. "Charms, Recipes, and Prayers." In *German Literature of the Early Middle Ages*, edited by Brian Murdoch, 57–72. Rochester, NY: Camden House, 2004.

———. "*Peri Hieres Nousou*: Approaches to the Old High German Medical Charms." In *"Mit regulu bithuungan": Neue Arbeiten zur Althochdeutschen Poesie und Sprache*, edited by John Flood and David Yeandle, 142–60. Göppingen: Kümmerle Verlag, 1989.

Napier, Arthur, ed. *Old English Glosses*. Oxford: Clarendon Press, 1900. Reprint, Hildesheim: Georg Olms, 1969.

———, ed. *The Old English Version of the Enlarged Rule of Chrodegang together with the Latin Original*. London: Kegan Paul, Trench, Trübner & Co., 1916.

Nash, Victor. "The Other Satan: A Study of the Watcher Devil in Patristics, Folklore, and English Literature." Ph.D. diss., University of Oregon, 1977.

Nauman, St. Elmo, ed. *Exorcism through the Ages*. New York: Philosophical Library, 1974.

Naveh, Joseph, and Shaul Shaked. *Magic Spells and Formulae: Aramaic Incantations of Late Antiquity*. Jerusalem: Magnes Press/Hebrew University, 1993.

Nelson, Janet L., and Richard W. Pfaff. "Pontificals and Benedictionals." In Pfaff, *Liturgical Books*, 87–98.

Neusner, Jacob, Ernest Frerichs, and Paul V. M. Flesher, eds. *Religion, Science and Magic, in Concert and Conflict*. New York: Oxford University Press, 1989.

Nevius, John L. *Demon Possession and Allied Themes*. 3rd ed. Chicago: Fleming H. Revell, 1896.

New Catholic Encyclopedia. New York: McGraw Hill, 1967.

Newman, Barbara. "Possessed by the Spirit: Devout Women, Demoniacs, and the Apostolic Life in the Thirteenth Century." *Speculum* 73 (1998): 733–70.

Nicholas, David. "Childhood in Medieval Europe." In *Children in Historical and Comparative Perspective*, edited by Joseph M. Hawes and N. Ray Hiner, 31–52. New York: Greenwood Press, 1991.

Nie, Giselle de. *Views from a Many-Windowed Tower: Studies of Imagination in the Works of Gregory of Tours*. Amsterdam: Rodopi, 1987.

Niedermeyer, Ernst. *The Epilepsies: Diagnosis and Management*. Baltimore: Urban & Schwarzenberg, 1990.

North, Richard. *Heathen Gods in Old English Literature*. Cambridge: Cambridge University Press, 1997.

Nualláin, Tomás P. Ua. "A Prayer to the Archangels for Each Day of the Week." *Ériu* 2 (1905): 92–94.

Nucifora, T. L., and M. H. Malone. "Comparative Psychopharmacologic Investigation of Cryogenine, Certain Non-Steroid Anti-Inflammatory Compounds, Lupine Alkaloids and Cyproheptadine." *Archives Internationales de Pharmacodynamie et de Thérapie* 191 (1971): 345–56.

Obeyesekere, Gananath. "The Idiom of Demonic Possession: A Case Study." *Social Science and Medicine* 4 (1970): 97–111.

O'Donovan, John. *Annals of the Kingdom of Ireland*. Vol. 1. Dublin: Hodges, Smith, and Co., 1856.

Oesterreich, Traugott K. *Possession and Exorcism among Primitive Races, in Antiquity, the Middle Ages, and Modern Times*. Translated by D. Ibberson. New York: Causeway Books, 1974.

Ogden, Daniel. "Binding Spells: Curse Tablets and Voodoo Dolls in the Greek and Roman Worlds." In *Witchcraft and Magic in Europe: Ancient Greece and Rome*, edited by Bengt Ankarloo and Stuart Clark, 3–90. Philadelphia: University of Pennsylvania Press, 1999.

O'Keeffe, Katherine O'Brien. "Body and Law in Late Anglo-Saxon England." *ASE* 27 (1998): 209–32.

———. "Heroic Values and Christian Ethics." In *The Cambridge Companion to Old English Literature*, edited by Malcolm Godden and Michael Lapidge, 107–25. Cambridge: Cambridge University Press, 1991.

O'Laughlin, Michael. "The Bible, the Demons and the Desert: Evaluating the *Antirrheticus* of Evagrius Ponticus." *Studia Monastica* 34 (1992): 201–5.

———. "Evagrius Ponticus: *Antirrheticus* (Selections)." In *Ascetic Behavior in Greco-Roman Antiquity: A Sourcebook*, edited by Vincent Wimbush, 243–62. Minneapolis: Fortress Press, 1990.

Oldham, John M., Andrew E. Skodol, and Donna S. Bender, eds. *Textbook of Personality Disorders*. Washington, DC: American Psychiatric Publishing, 2005.

Olds, Barbara M. "The Anglo-Saxon Leechbook III: A Critical Edition and Translation." Ph.D. diss., University of Denver, 1984.

O'Leary, Aideen M. "Apostolic *Passiones* in Early Anglo-Saxon England." In Powell and Scragg, *Apocryphal Texts and Traditions*, 103–19.

Oliphant, Robert, ed. *The Harley Latin-Old English Glossary*. The Hague: Mouton & Co., 1966.

Olsen, K. E., and L. A. J. R. Houwen, eds. *Monsters and the Monstrous in Medieval Northwest Europe*. Leuven: Peeters, 2001.

Orchard, Andy. *Pride and Prodigies: Studies in the Monsters of the Beowulf-Manuscript*. Cambridge: D. S. Brewer, 1995.

Orchard, Nicholas, ed. *The Leofric Missal*. 2 vols. HBS 113–14. Woodbridge, UK: Boydell Press, 2002.

Origen. *Contra Celsum*. Edited by Henry Chadwick. Cambridge: Cambridge University Press, 1953.

Orme, Nicholas. *Medieval Children*. New Haven: Yale University Press, 2001.

Orme, Nicholas, and Margaret Webster. *The English Hospital, 1070–1570*. New Haven: Yale University Press, 1995.

Orr, Scott, and Danny Kaloupek. "Psychophysiological Assessment of Posttraumatic Stress Disorder." In *Assessing Psychological Trauma and PTSD*, edited by John Wilson and Terence Keane, 69–97. New York: Guilford Press, 1997.

Paciaudi, Paulli M. *De sacris Christianorum balneis*. Rome: Palearini Brothers, 1758.

Palladius. *The Lausiac History*. Translated by Robert Meyer. *ACW* 34. Westminster, MD: Newman Press; London: Longmans, Green, and Co., 1965.

Panayotakis, St. [*sic*]. "The Knot and the Hymen: A Reconsideration of *Nodus Virginitatis* (*Hist. Apoll.* 1)." *Mnemosyne* 53 (2000): 599–608.

Paris, Joel. "Personality Disorders, Parasuicide, and Culture." *Transcultural Psychiatric Research Review* 28 (1991): 25–39.

Parker, S. J. "Skulls, Symbols and Surgery: A Review of the Evidence for Trepanation in Anglo-Saxon England and a Consideration of the Motives behind the Practice." In Scragg, *Superstition and Popular Medicine*, 73–84.

Parpola, Simo, ed. *Letters from Assyrian and Babylonian Scholars*. State Archives of Assyria 10. Helsinki: Helsinki University Press, 1993. Pp. 149–250.

Patrick. *Confession et Lettre à Coroticus*. Edited by Richard P. C. Hanson. *SC* 249. Paris: Éditions du Cerf, 1978.

Pattison, E. Mansell. "Psychosocial Interpretations of Exorcism." *Journal of Operational Psychiatry* 8, no. 2 (1977): 5–21.

Pausanias. *Description of Greece*. Edited and translated by W. H. S. Jones. Vol. 3. Cambridge, MA: Harvard University Press; London: William Heinemann: 1966.

Payer, Pierre. *Sex and the Penitentials: The Development of a Sexual Code, 550–1150*. Toronto: University of Toronto Press, 1984.

Payne, Joseph Frank. *English Medicine in the Anglo-Saxon Times*. Oxford: Clarendon Press, 1904.

Pelteret, David A. E. *Slavery in Early Mediaeval England, from the Reign of Alfred until the Twelfth Century*. Woodbridge, UK: Boydell, 1995.

Penney, Douglas L., and Michael O. Wise. "By the Power of Beelzebub: An Aramaic Incantation Formula from Qumran (4Q560)." *Journal of Biblical Literature* 113 (1994): 627–50.

Percival, Henry. *The Seven Ecumenical Councils of the Undivided Church*. Vol. 14 of *NPNF*, 2nd series, edited by Philip Schaff and Henry Wace. New York: Christian Literature Company, 1900.

Pertz, George, ed. *Eigilis Vita Sturmi*. MGH, Scriptores 2. Hanover: Hahn, 1829. Reprint, New York: Kraus, 1963.

Pertzii, G. H. ed. *Annales Fuldenses*. 1891. Reprint, Hanover: Hahn, 1978.

Petersen, Joan M. *The Dialogues of Gregory the Great in Their Late Antique Cultural Background*. Toronto: Pontifical Institute of Mediaeval Studies, 1984.

Petitpierre, Dom Robert. *Exorcism: The Report of a Commission Convened by the Bishop of Exeter*. London: S.P.C.K., 1971.

Petschenig, Michael, ed. *Cassiani Opera: De Institutis Coenobiorum*. CSEL 17. 1888. Reprint, Vienna: Österreichischen Akademie der Wissenschaften, 2004. Pp. 173–74.

———. *Iohannis Cassiani Conlationes XXIIII*. CSEL 13. Vienna: C. Geroldus Sons, 1886.

Pettit, Edward. *Anglo-Saxon Remedies, Charms, and Prayers from British Library MS Harley 585*. 2 vols. Lewiston, NY: Edwin Mellen, 2001.

Pfaff, Richard, ed. *The Liturgical Books of Anglo-Saxon England*. Old English Newsletter Subsidia 23. Kalamazoo, MI: Medieval Institute Publications, 1995.

Pheifer, J. D., ed. *Old English Glosses in the Épinal-Erfurt Glossary*. Oxford: Clarendon Press, 1974.

Philo of Alexandria. *The Contemplative Life; The Giants; and Selections*. Translated by David Winston. New York: Paulist Press, 1981.

Philostratus. *The Life of Apollonius of Tyana*. Edited and translated by F. C. Conybeare. Vol. 1. 1912. Reprint, Cambridge, MA: Harvard University Press; London: William Heinemann, 1960.

———. *The Life of Apollonius of Tyana*. Translated by Christopher P. Jones. Vol. 1. Cambridge, MA: Harvard University Press, 2005.

Pitman, James Hall, ed. *The Riddles of Aldhelm*. New Haven: Yale University Press, 1925.

Pitman, Roger K. "Hippocampal Diminution in PTSD: More (or Less?) Than Meets the Eye." *Hippocampus* 11 (2001): 73–74.

Plummer, Charles, ed. *Venerabilis Baedae Opera Historica*. 2 vols. Oxford: Clarendon Press, 1896.

———. *Vitae Sanctorum Hiberniae*. 2 vols. 1910. Reprint, Dublin: Four Courts Press, 1997.

Plutarch. "Oracles in Decline." In *Plutarch: Selected Essays*, translated by Donald Russell. Oxford: Oxford University Press, 1993.

Pócs, Éva. "Possession Phenomena, Possession-Systems: Some East-Central European Examples." In *Communicating with the Spirits*, edited by Gábor Klaniczay and Éva Pócs, 84–151. Budapest: Central European University Press, 2005.

Pollington, Stephen. *Leechcraft: Early English Charms, Plant Lore, and Healing*. Frithgarth, UK: Anglo-Saxon Books, 2000.

Pope, John C., ed. *Homilies of Ælfric: A Supplementary Collection*, 2 vols. EETS o.s. 259, 260. London: Oxford University Press, 1967–68.

Porterfield, Amanda. *Healing in the History of Christianity*. Oxford: Oxford University Press, 2005.

Pothier, J., S.-L. Cheav, N. Galand, C. Dormeau, and C. Viel. "A Comparative Study of the Effects of Sparteine, Lupanine, and Lupin Extract on the Central Nervous System of the Mouse." *Journal of Pharmacy and Pharmacology* 50 (1998): 949–54.

Powell, Kathryn, and Donald Scragg, eds. *Apocryphal Texts and Traditions in Anglo-Saxon England*. Cambridge: D. S. Brewer, 2003.

Pratt, David. "The Illnesses of King Alfred the Great." *ASE* 30 (2001): 39–90.

Prince, Raymond, Alexander Leighton, and Rollo May. "The Therapeutic Process in Cross-Cultural Perspective: A Symposium." *American Journal of Psychiatry* 124 (1968): 1171–83.

Puech, Émile. "11QPsAp[a]: Un rituel d'exorcismes. Essai de reconstruction." *Revue de Qumran* 14 (1990): 377–408.

Quammen, David. *Monster of God: The Man-Eating Predator in the Jungles of History and the Mind*. New York: W. W. Norton & Co., 2003.

Raine, James, ed. *The Historians of the Church of York and Its Archbishops*. Vol. 1. London: Longman & Co., 1879.

Raiswell, Richard, and Peter Dendle. "Demon Possession in Anglo-Saxon and Early Modern England: Continuity and Evolution in Social Context." *Journal of British Studies* 47 (2008): 738–67.

———, eds. *The Devil in Premodern Society.* Toronto: Centre for Reformation and Renaissance Studies, 2012.

Rampolla, Mary Lynn. "'A Mirror of Sanctity': Madness as Metaphor in the *Vita Wulfstani.*" In *Saints: Studies in Hagiography*, edited by Sandro Sticca, 95–114. Binghamton, NY: Center for Medieval and Early Renaissance Studies, 1996.

Rauch, Scott L., Paul J. Whalen, Lisa M. Shin et al. "Exaggerated Amygdala Response to Masked Facial Stimuli in Posttraumatic Stress Disorder: A Functional MRI Study." *Biological Psychiatry* 47 (2000): 769–76.

Reichel, Oswald J. *A Complete Manual of Canon Law.* Vol. 1. London: John Hodges, 1896.

Rendall, Thomas. "Bondage and Freeing from Bondage in Old English Religious Poetry." *JEGP* 73 (1974): 497–512.

Reynolds, Nicholas. "The Rape of the Anglo-Saxon Women." *Antiquity* 62 (1988): 715–18.

Reynolds, Roger E. "Christ as Cleric: The Ordinals of Christ." In *Clerics in the Early Middle Ages: Hierarchy and Image*, edited by Roger E. Reynolds, 1–50. Aldershot: Ashgate/Variorum, 1999.

———. *The Ordinals of Christ from Their Origins to the Twelfth Century.* Berlin: Walter de Gruyter, 1978.

Riddle, John. "The Introduction and Use of Eastern Drugs in the Early Middle Ages." *Sudhoffs Archiv für Geschichte der Medizin und der Naturwissenschaften* 49 (1965): 185–98.

———. "Theory and Practice in Medieval Medicine." *Viator* 5 (1974): 157–84.

Roberts, Alexander, and James Donaldson, eds. *The Apostolic Fathers, Justin Martyr, Iranaeus. ANF* 1. 1885. Reprint, Grand Rapids, MI: William Eerdmans, 1993.

———. *Fathers of the Third Century: Hippolytus, Cyprian, Caius, Novation, Appendix. ANF* 5. 1885. Reprint, Grand Rapids, MI: William Eerdmans, 1981.

———. *Fathers of the Third and Fourth Centuries. ANF* 7. 1886. Repr. New York: Charles Scribner's Sons, 1905.

———. *The Writings of Methodius, Etc.* Vol. 14 of *Ante-Nicene Christian Library.* Edinburgh: T. & T. Clark, 1869.

Roberts, C. M. *A Treatise on the History of Confession.* London: C. J. Clay and Sons, 1901.

Robertson, A. J., ed. *Anglo-Saxon Charters.* Cambridge: Cambridge University Press, 1956.

Robertson, James C., ed. *Materials for the History of Thomas Becket.* 2 vols. London: Longman & Co., 1875–76.

Robertson, Mary M. "Self-Injurious Behavior and Tourette Syndrome." In Chase, Friedhoff, and Cohen, *Tourette Syndrome*, 105–14.

Robertson, Mary, and Simon Baron-Cohen. *Tourette Syndrome: The Facts.* Oxford: Oxford University Press, 1998.

Robinson, F. N. "A Note on the Sources of the Old Saxon 'Genesis.'" *Modern Philology* 4 (1906): 389–96.

Robinson, Fred. "The Devil's Account of the Next World: An Anecdote from Old English Homiletic Literature." *NM* 73 (1972): 362–71.

Rodewyk, Adolf. *Possessed by Satan: The Church's Teaching on the Devil, Possession, and Exorcism.* Translated by Martin Ebon. Garden City, NY: Doubleday & Co., 1975.

Rogers, Rex Stainton. "The Social Constructions of Childhood." In *Child Abuse and Neglect: Facing the Challenge*, edited by Wendy Stainton Rogers, Denise Harvey, and Elizabeth Ash, 23–29. London: B. T. Batsford, 1989.

Roper, Lyndal. *Oedipus and the Devil: Witchcraft, Sexuality and Religion in Early Modern Europe*. London: Routledge, 1994.

Rosenthal, Constance. *The Vitae Patrum in Old and Middle English Literature*. Philadelphia, 1936.

Ross, Colin A. *Dissociative Identity Disorder: Diagnosis, Clinical Features, and Treatment of Multiple Personality*. New York: John Wiley & Sons, 1997.

Rothschild, Babette. *The Body Remembers: The Psychophysiology of Trauma and Trauma Treatment*. New York: W. W. Norton, 2000.

Rubin, Stanley. "The Anglo-Saxon Physician." In *Medicine in Early Medieval England: Four Papers*, edited by Marilyn Deegan and Donald G. Scragg, 7–15. Manchester: Centre for Anglo-Saxon Studies, 1987.

———. "The Medical Practitioner in Anglo-Saxon England." *Journal of the Royal College of General Practitioners* 20 (1970): 63–71.

———. *Medieval English Medicine, AD 500–1300*. New York: Barnes & Noble, 1974.

Rufinus of Aquileia. *Historia Monachorum*. Edited by Eva Schultz-Flügel. Berlin: Walter de Gruyter, 1990.

Russell, Jeffrey Burton. *The Devil: Perceptions of Evil from Antiquity to Primitive Christianity*. Ithaca, NY: Cornell University Press, 1977.

———. *Lucifer: The Devil in the Middle Ages*. Ithaca, NY: Cornell University Press, 1984.

———. *Satan: The Early Christian Tradition*. Ithaca, NY: Cornell University Press, 1981.

Russell, Josiah C. *British Medieval Population*. Albuquerque: University of New Mexico Press, 1948.

Russell, Norman. *The Lives of the Desert Fathers*. Kalamazoo, MI: Cistercian Publications, 1981.

Sack, William, John Seeley, and Gregory Clarke. "Does PTSD Transcend Cultural Boundaries? A Study from the Khmer Adolescent Refugee Project." *Journal of the American Academy of Child and Adolescent Psychiatry* 36 (1997): 49–54.

Sarbin, Theodore. "The Social Construction of Schizophrenia." In Flack, Miller, and Wiener, *What Is Schizophrenia?*, 173–97.

Sartorius, N., A. Jablensky, A. Korten, G. Ernberg, M. Anker, J. E. Cooper, and R. Day. "Early Manifestations and First-Contact Incidence of Schizophrenia in Different Cultures." *Psychological Medicine* 16 (1986): 909–28.

Saunders, Corinne. *Rape and Ravishment in the Literature of Medieval England*. Cambridge: D. S. Brewer, 2001.

Sawyer, Peter H. "Fairs and Markets in Early Medieval England." In *Danish Medieval History: New Currents*, edited by Niels Skyum-Nielsen and Niels Lund, 153–68. Copenhagen: Museum Tusculanum Press, 1981.

Scharer, Anton. *Die angelsächsische Königsurkunde im 7. und 8. Jahrhundert*. Vienna: Hermann Böhlaus Nachf, 1982.

Schetky, Diane. "Child Sexual Abuse in Mythology, Religion, and History." In *Child Sexual Abuse: A Handbook for Health Care and Legal Professionals*, edited by Diane Schetky and Arthur Green, 19–29. New York: Brunner/Mazel, 1988.

Schiffman, Lawrence H., and Michael D. Swartz. *Hebrew and Aramaic Incantation Texts from the Cairo Genizah*. Sheffield: Sheffield Academic Press, 1992.

Schmitt, Jean-Claude. *Ghosts in the Middle Ages: The Living and the Dead in Medieval Society*. Translated by Teresa Lavender Fagan. Chicago: University of Chicago Press, 1998.

Schoedel, William. *Athenagoras: Legatio and De resurrectione*. Oxford: Clarendon Press, 1972.

Schreiber, Shaul. "Migration, Traumatic Bereavement and Transcultural Aspects of

Psychological Healing: Loss and Grief of a Refugee Woman from Begameder County in Ethiopia." *British Journal of Medical Psychology* 68 (1995): 135–42.

Schröer, Arnold, ed. *Die Angelsächsischen Prosabearbeitungen der Benediktinerregel.* Darmstadt: Wissenschaftliche Buchgesellschaft, 1964.

Schumaker, John, and Tony Ward, eds. *Cultural Cognition and Psychopathology.* Westport, CT: Praeger, 2001.

Scragg, Donald G. "'The Devil's Account of the Next World' Revisited." *American Notes and Queries* 24 (1986): 107–10.

———, ed. *Superstition and Popular Medicine in Anglo-Saxon England.* Manchester: Manchester Centre for Anglo-Saxon England, 1989.

———, ed. *The Vercelli Homilies and Related Texts.* EETS o.s. 300. Oxford: Oxford University Press, 1992.

Scull, Andrew. *The Most Solitary of Afflictions: Madness and Society in Britain 1700–1900.* New Haven: Yale University Press, 1993.

Seabourne, Alice, and Gwen Seabourne. "Suicide or Accident: Self-Killing in Medieval England." *British Journal of Psychiatry* 178 (2001): 42–47.

Seidel, Jonathan. "Possession and Exorcism in the Magical Texts of the Cairo Geniza." In *Spirit Possession in Judaism: Cases and Contexts from the Middle Ages to the Present,* edited by Matt Goldish, 73–95. Detroit: Wayne State University Press, 2003.

Seligman, Adam W., and John Hilkevich, eds. *Don't Think about Monkeys: Extraordinary Stories Written by People with Tourette Syndrome.* Duarte, CA: Hope Press, 1992.

Sengers, Gerda. *Women and Demons: Cult Healing in Islamic Egypt.* Leiden: Brill, 2003.

Shahar, Shulamith. *Childhood in the Middle Ages.* London: Routledge, 1990.

Shakespeare, William. *The First Part of Henry the Fourth.* In G. Blakemore Evans, gen. ed., *The Riverside Shakespeare.* Boston: Houghton Mifflin, 1974.

Shalev, Arieh, Rachel Yehuda, and Alexander McFarlane, eds. *International Handbook of Human Response to Trauma.* New York: Kluwer, 2000.

Shapiro, Arthur, and Elaine Shapiro. "Neuroleptic Drugs." In *Handbook of Tourette's Syndrome and Related Tic and Behavioral Disorders,* edited by Roger Kurlan, 347–75. New York: Marcel Dekker, 1993.

Shapiro, Arthur, Elaine Shapiro, J. Gerald Young, and Todd Feinberg. *Gilles de la Tourette Syndrome.* 2nd ed. New York: Raven Press, 1988.

Sharpe, Richard. *Medieval Irish Saints' Lives: An Introduction to Vitae Sanctorum Hiberniae.* Oxford: Clarendon Press, 1991.

Shay, Jonathan. *Achilles in Vietnam: Combat Trauma and the Undoing of Character.* New York: Atheneum, 1994.

———. "Learning about Combat Stress from Homer's *Iliad.*" *Journal of Traumatic Stress* 4 (1991): 561–79.

Shweder, Richard, and Edmund Bourne. "Does the Concept of the Person Vary Cross-Culturally?" In *Cultural Conceptions of Mental Health and Therapy,* edited by Anthony Marsella and Geoffrey White, 97–137. Dordrecht: D. Reidel Publishing, 1982.

Siegel, George, Bernard Agranoff, R. Wayne Albers, and Perry Molinoff, eds. *Basic Neurochemistry: Molecular, Cellular, and Medical Aspects.* New York: Raven Press, 1989.

Simons, Ronald, and Charles Hughes, eds. *The Culture-Bound Syndromes: Folk Illnesses of Psychiatric and Anthropological Interest.* Dordrecht: D. Reidel Publishing, 1985.

Simpson, Michael. "Gullible's Travels, or the Importance of Being Multiple." In *Dissociative Identity Disorder: Theoretical and Treatment Controversies,* edited by Lewis Cohen, Joan Berzoff, and Mark Elin, 87–134. Northvale, NJ: Jason Aronson, 1995.

Simpson, William Kelly. *The Literature of Ancient Egypt*. 3rd ed. New Haven: Yale University Press, 2003.

Singer, Charles. *A Short History of Medicine*. Oxford: Clarendon Press, 1928.

Skeat, Walter W., ed. *Ælfric's Lives of Saints*. 2 vols. EETS o.s. 76, 82, 94, 114. London: Trübner & Co., 1881 (vol. 1); London: Oxford University Press, 1890 (vol. 2).

———. *The Holy Gospels, in Anglo-Saxon, Northumbrian, and Old Mercian Versions, Synoptically Arranged*. Cambridge: Cambridge University Press, 1871–87.

Skemer, Don C. *Binding Words: Textual Amulets in the Middle Ages*. University Park: Pennsylvania State University Press, 2006.

Smedt, Charles de, and Joseph de Backer, eds. *Acta Sanctorum Hiberniae ex codice Salmanticensi*. Edinburgh: Blackwood and Sons, 1888.

Smith, Wesley. "So-Called Possession in Pre-Christian Greece." *Transactions and Proceedings of the American Philological Association* 96 (1965): 403–26.

Smith, William, and Samuel Cheetham. *A Dictionary of Christian Antiquities*. Vol. 1. Hartford: J. B. Burr, 1876.

Smyth, Alfred P. *The Medieval Life of King Alfred the Great: A Translation and Commentary on the Text Attributed to Asser*. Houndmills, UK: Palgrave, 2002.

Sonnenberg, Stephen. "A Transcultural Observation of Posttraumatic Stress Disorder." *Hospital & Community Psychiatry* 33 (1982): 58–59.

Sorensen, Erik. *Possession and Exorcism in the New Testament and Early Christianity*. Tübingen: Mohr Siebeck, 2002.

Southwick, Steve, Ann Rasmusson, Jill Barron, and Amy Arnsten. "Neurobiological and Neurocognitive Alterations in PTSD: A Focus on Norepinephrine, Serotonin, and the Hypothalamic-Pituitary-Adrenal Axis." In *Neuropsychology of PTSD: Biological, Cognitive, and Clinical Perspectives*, edited by Jennifer J. Vasterling and Chris R. Brewin, 27–58. New York: Guilford Press, 2005.

Spiegel, David, ed. *Dissociation: Culture, Mind, and Body*. Washington, DC: American Psychiatric Press, 1994.

Spindler, Robert, ed. *Das altenglische Bussbuch*. Leipzig: Bernhard Tauchnitz, 1934.

Stafford, Pauline. *Unification and Conquest: A Political and Social History of England in the Tenth and Eleventh Centuries*. New York: Edward Arnold, 1989.

Staley, Douglas, Roxburgh Wand, and Gary Shady. "Tourette Syndrome: A Cross-Cultural Review." *Comprehensive Psychiatry* 38 (1997): 6–16.

Stamm, B. Hudnall, and Matthew Friedman. "Cultural Diversity in the Appraisal and Expression of Trauma." In Shalev, Yehuda, and McFarlane, *International Handbook of Human Response*, 69–85.

Stancliffe, Clare. "The British Church and the Mission of Augustine." In Gameson, *St. Augustine*, 107–51.

———. "Cuthbert and the Polarity between Pastor and Solitary." In *St Cuthbert, His Cult and His Community to AD 1200*, edited by Gerald Bonner, David Rollason, and Clare Stancliffe, 21–44. Woodbridge, UK: Boydell, 1989.

Stefanis, Costas. "On the Concept of Schizophrenia." In Kales, Stefanis, and Talbott, *Recent Advances in Schizophrenia*, 25–57.

Stein, M. B., C. Hannah, C. Koverola et al. "Neuroanatomical and Neuroendocrine Correlates in Adulthood of Severe Sexual Abuse in Childhood." Paper presented at the Annual Meeting of the American College of Neuropsychopharmacology, San Juan, Puerto Rico, 1994.

Steinberg, Marlene. *Handbook for the Assessment of Dissociation: A Clinical Guide.* Washington, DC: American Psychiatric Press, 1995.

———. "Systematizing Dissociation: Symptomatology and Diagnostic Assessment." In Spiegel, *Dissociation*, 59–88.

Stephens, Walter. *Demon Lovers: Witchcraft, Sex, and the Crisis of Belief.* Chicago: University of Chicago Press, 2002.

Stevenson, William Henry, ed. *Asser's Life of King Alfred.* Oxford: Clarendon Press, 1959.

Stewart, Columbia. *The World of the Desert Fathers.* Kalamazoo, MI: Cistercian Publications, 1986.

Stol, Marten. *Epilepsy in Babylonia.* Groningen: Styx Publications, 1993.

Stone, Michael E., ed. *Jewish Writings of the Second Temple Period: Apocrypha, Pseudepigrapha, Qumran Sectarian Writings, Philo, Josephus.* Assen: Van Gorcum; Philadelphia: Fortress Press, 1984.

Storms, G. *Anglo-Saxon Magic.* The Hague: Martinus Nijhoff, 1948.

Storr, F. *Sophocles.* Vol. 1. Cambridge, MA: Harvard University Press; London: William Heinemann, 1968.

Strack, Hermann, and Paul Billerbeck. *Exkurse zu Einzelnen Stellen des Neuen Testaments.* Vol. 4 of *Kommentar zum Neuen Testament aus Talmud und Midrash.* Munich: C. H. Beck, 1928.

Stracke, J. Richard. *The Laud Herbal Glossary.* Amsterdam: Rodopi, 1974.

Straube, Eckart, and Robert Oades. *Schizophrenia: Empirical Research and Findings.* San Diego: Academic Press, 1992.

Strickland, Debra Higgs. *Saracens, Demons, and Jews: Making Monsters in Medieval Art.* Princeton, NJ: Princeton University Press, 2003.

Strömgren, Erik. "Autism: Core of the Schizophrenic Reaction." In Flack, Miller, and Wiener, *What Is Schizophrenia?*, 33–44.

Stryker, William G. "The Latin-Old English Glossary in MS Cotton Cleopatra A.iii." Ph.D. diss., Stanford University, 1951.

Stuart, Heather. "The Anglo-Saxon Elf." *Studia Neophilologica* 48 (1976): 313–20.

Stubbs, William, ed. *Memorials of Saint Dunstan.* London: Longman, Trübner, & Co., 1874.

Sugaya, E., W. Jin, A. Sugaya, K. Sunaga, and T. Tsuda, "Inhibitory Effects of Peony Root Extract on the Large Conductance Calcium-Activated Potassium Current Essential in Production of Bursting Activity." *Journal of Herbal Pharmacotherapy* 6 (2006): 65–77.

Swantz, Marja-Liisa. *Ritual and Symbol in Transitional Zaramo Society.* Lund: C. W. K. Gleerup, 1970.

Sweeten, Alan. *Christianity in Rural China: Conflict and Accommodation in Jiangxi Province, 1860–1900.* Ann Arbor: University of Michigan, 2001.

Symons, Dom Thomas, ed. and trans. *Regularis Concordia: The Monastic Agreement of the Monks and Nuns of the English Nation.* New York: Oxford University Press, 1953.

Talbot, C. H. *Medicine in Medieval England.* London: Oldbourne, 1967.

Tambornino, Julius. *De Antiquorum Daemonismo.* Giessen: Alfred Töpelmann, 1909.

Tamminga, Carol. "Principles of the Pharmacotherapy of Schizophrenia." In Charney, Nestler, and Bunney, *Neurobiology of Mental Illness*, 272–85.

Tangl, Michael, ed. *Die Briefe des Heiligen Bonifatus und Lullus.* MGH, Epistolae Selectae 1. Berlin: Weidmann, 1955.

Taylor, G. Rattray. *Sex in History.* London: Thames and Hudson, 1953.

Taylor, Graeme. "Demoniacal Possession and Psychoanalytic Theory." *British Journal of Medical Psychology* 51 (1978): 53–60.

Taylor, Kenneth, ed. *Demon Experiences in Many Lands*. Chicago: Moody Bible Institute of Chicago, 1960.

Temkin, Owsei. *The Falling Sickness: A History of Epilepsy from the Greeks to the Beginnings of Modern Neurology*. Baltimore: The Johns Hopkins Press, 1945.

Testaments of the Twelve Patriarchs. Translated by Robert Sinker. In *The Twelve Patriarchs, Excerpts and Epistles, The Clementina, Apocrypha, Decretals, Memoirs of Edessa, and Syriac Documents, Remains of the First Age*, edited by Alexander Roberts and James Donaldson. *ANF* 8. New York: Christian Literature Co., 1886. Repr. Grand Rapids, MI: W. B. Eerdmans, 1989.

Thacker, Alan. "Bede's Ideal of Reform." In *Ideal and Reality in Frankish and Anglo-Saxon Society: Studies Presented to J. M. Wallace-Hadrill*, edited by Patrick Wormald, Donald Bullough, and Roger Collins, 130–53. Oxford: Basil Blackwell, 1983.

Thackeray, H. St. J., trans. *Josephus*. Vol. 3. Cambridge, MA: Harvard University Press; London: William Heinemann, 1968.

Thackeray, H. St. J., and Ralph Marcus, trans. *Josephus*. Vol. 5. Cambridge, MA: Harvard University Press; London: William Heinemann, 1958.

Thigpen, Corbett, and Hervey Cleckley. "On the Incidence of Multiple Personality Disorder: A Brief Communication." *International Journal of Clinical and Experimental Hypnosis* 32 (1984): 63–66.

Thomas, John Christopher. *The Devil, Disease and Deliverance: Origins of Illness in New Testament Thought*. Sheffield: Sheffield Academic Press, 1998.

Thompson, R. Campbell. *The Devils and Evil Spirits of Babylonia*. 2 vols. London: Luzac and Co., 1903–4.

Thorpe, Benjamin, ed. *Ancient Laws and Institutes of England*. Vol. 2. London, 1840.

Thun, Nils. "The Malignant Elves." *Studia Neophilologica* 41 (1969): 378–96.

Tierney, Lawrence, Stephen McPhee, and Maxine Papadakis, eds. *Current Medical Diagnosis & Treatment, 1999*. 38th ed. Stamford, CT: Appleton & Lange, 1999.

Tillman, Jane, Michael Nash, and Paul Lerner. "Does Trauma Cause Dissociative Pathology?" In *Dissociation: Clinical and Theoretical Perspectives*, edited by Steven Jay Lynn and Judith Rhue, 395–414. New York: Guilford Press, 1994.

Tomlin, R. S. O. *Tabellae Sulis: Roman Inscribed Tablets of Tin and Lead from the Sacred Spring at Bath*. Oxford: Oxford University Committee for Archaeology, 1988.

Torrey, E. Fuller. *Schizophrenia and Civilization*. New York: Jason Aronson, 1980.

Toso, Fotini. "'And Then There Was Silence': The Lack of Transmission of Anglo-Saxon Attitudes towards Suicide." *Journal of the Australian Early Medieval Association* 2 (2006): 237–42.

Treharne, Elaine M. "A Unique Old English Formula for Excommunication from Cambridge, Corpus Christi College 303." *ASE* 24 (1995): 185–211.

Tseng, Wen-Shing, and Jon Streltzer, eds. *Culture and Psychopathology: A Guide to Clinical Assessment*. New York: Brunner/Mazel, 1997.

Tsuda, T., A. Sugaya, H. Ohguchi, N. Kishida, and E. Sugaya. "Protective Effects of Peony Root Extract and Its Components on Neuron Damage in the Hippocampus Induced by the Cobalt Focus Epilepsy Model." *Experimental Neurology* 146 (1997): 518–25.

Turkat, Daniel. *The Personality Disorders: A Psychological Approach to Clinical Management*. New York: Pergamon Press, 1990.

Twelftree, Graham. *Jesus the Exorcist*. Peabody, MA: Hendrickson Publishers, 1993.

Ullmann, Elisabeth, and Werner Hilweg, eds. *Childhood and Trauma: Separation, Abuse, War*. Aldershot: Ashgate, 1999.

Ullrich, Helen. "Cultural Shaping of Illness: A Longtitudinal Perspective on Apparent Depression." *Journal of Nervous and Mental Disease* 181, no. 10 (1993): 647–49.

Uzoigwe, G. N. "The Warrior and the State in Precolonial Africa." In *The Warrior Tradition in Modern Africa*, edited by Ali A. Mazrui, 20–47. Leiden: E. J. Brill, 1977.

Van Acker, Lieven, ed. *Agobardi Lugdunensis, Opera Omnia*. CCCM 52. Turnholt: Brepols, 1981.

Van Arsdall, Anne. *Medieval Herbal Remedies: The Old English Herbarium and Anglo-Saxon Medicine*. New York: Routledge, 2002.

Van Dam, Raymond. *Saints and Their Miracles in Late Antique Gaul*. Princeton, NJ: Princeton University Press, 1993.

Van der Kolk, Bessel. "The Body Keeps the Score: Approaches to the Psychobiology of Posttraumatic Stress Disorder." In Van der Kolk, McFarlane, and Weisaeth, *Traumatic Stress*, 214–41.

Van der Kolk, Bessel, and Mark Greenberg. "The Psychobiology of the Trauma Response: Hyperarousal, Constriction, and Addiction to Traumatic Reexposure." In *Psychological Trauma*, edited by Bessel A. Van der Kolk, pp. 63–87. Washington, DC: American Psychiatric Press, 1987.

Van der Kolk, Bessel, Alexander McFarlane, and Lars Weisaeth, eds. *Traumatic Stress: The Effects of Overwhelming Experience on Mind, Body, and Society*. New York: Guilford Press, 1996.

Van der Kolk, Bessel, Onno Van der Hart, and Charles Marmar. "Dissociation and Information Processing in Posttraumatic Stress Disorder." In Van der Kolk, McFarlane, and Weisaeth, *Traumatic Stress*, 303–27.

van Dongen, Pieter W. J., and Akosua N. J. A. de Groot. "History of Ergot Alkaloids from Ergotism to Ergometrine." *European Journal of Obstetrics & Gynecology and Reproductive Biology* 60 (1995): 109–16.

Van Slyke, Daniel G. "The Ancestry and Theology of the Rite of Major Exorcism (1999/2004)." *Antiphon* 10, no. 1 (2006): 70–116.

———. "Augustine and Catechumenal *Exsufflatio*: An Integral Element of Christian Initiation." *Ephemerides Liturgicae* 118 (2004): 175–208.

———. "The Emergence of *Insufflatio* as a Distinct Ritual Gesture in Christian Initiation." Paper presented at 41st International Congress on Medieval Studies, Kalamazoo, MI, May 2006.

Vasterling, Jennifer J., and Chris R. Brewin, eds. *Neuropsychology of PTSD: Biological, Cognitive, and Clinical Perspectives*. New York: Guilford Press, 2005.

Verdun, Paul. *Le diable dans les missions*. 2 vols. Paris, 1893–95.

Vermes, Geza. *The Complete Dead Sea Scrolls in English*. New York: Penguin, 1962.

Verner, Lisa. *The Epistemology of the Monstrous in the Middle Ages*. New York: Routledge, 2005.

Versnel, Henk. "An Essay on Anatomical Curses." In *Ansichten Griechischer Rituale*, edited by Fritz Graf, 217–67. Stuttgart: Teubner, 1998.

Vita Genovefae. *Acta Sanctorum*, January, vol. 1. Antwerp: Johannes Meursius, 1643.

Vita Willehadi. *Acta Sanctorum*, November 8. Brussels: Bollandist Society, 1910.

Voelkle, William M. "Morgan Manuscript M.1001: The Seven Deadly Sins and the Seven Evil Ones." In *Monsters and Demons in the Ancient and Medieval Worlds*, edited by Ann E. Farkas, Prudence O. Harper, and Evelyn B. Harrison, 101–14 and plates XXXVII–LIV. Mainz: Philipp von Zabern, 1987.

Vogel, Cyrille, and Reinhard Elze, eds. *Le Pontifical Romano-Germanique du dixième siècle*.

3 vols. Studi e Testi 226, 227, and 269. Vatican City: Biblioteca Apostolica Vaticana, 1963–72.

Voigts, Linda E. "Anglo-Saxon Plant Remedies and the Anglo-Saxons." *Isis* 70 (1979): 250–68.

Voigts, Linda E., and Robert Hudson. "*A drynke þat men callen dwale to make a man to slepe whyle men kerven him*: A Surgical Anesthetic from Late Medieval England." In Campbell, Hall, and Klausner, *Health, Disease, and Healing*, 34–56.

von Erhardt-Siebold, Erika. "The Hellebore in Anglo-Saxon Pharmacy." *Englische Studien* 71 (1936–37): 161–70.

von Storch, T. C. "An Essay on the History of Epilepsy." *Annals of Medical History* 2 (1930): 614–50.

Waddington, J. L. "The Clinical Psychopharmacology of Antipsychotic Drugs in Schizophrenia." In Hirsch and Weinberger, *Schizophrenia*, 341–57.

Waegeman, Annick. "The Medieval Sibyl." In *The Pagan Middle Ages*, edited by Ludo J. R. Milis and translated by Tanis Guest, 83–107. Woodbridge, UK: Boydell, 1998.

Waitz, G., ed. *Translatio et miracula sanctorum Marcellini et Petri*. MGH, Scriptores 15, part 1. Hanover: Hahn, 1887.

———. *Vita Anskarii*. MGH Scriptores rerum Germanicarum 55. Hanover: Hahn, 1884.

Walker, Nigel. *Crime and Insanity in England*. Vol. 1, *The Historical Perspective*. Edinburgh: Edinburgh University Press, 1968.

Wallace, Ernest, and E. Adamson Hoebel. *The Comanches: Lords of the South Plains*. Norman: University of Oklahoma Press, 1952.

Wallace-Hadrill, J. M. *Bede's Ecclesiastical History of the English People: A Historical Commentary*. Oxford: Clarendon Press, 1988.

Walzel, Diana Lynn. "Sources of Medieval Demonology." *Rice University Studies* 60 (1974): 83–99.

Ward, Benedicta, trans. *The Sayings of the Desert Fathers: The Alphabetical Collection*. Kalamazoo, MI: Cistercian Publications, 1975.

———. *The Wisdom of the Desert Fathers*. Oxford: SLG Press, 1975. Reprint, Kalamazoo, MI: Cistercian Publications, 1997.

Ward, Colleen, ed. *Altered States of Consciousness and Mental Health: A Cross-Cultural Perspective*. New York: Sage Publications, 1989.

———. "Possession and Exorcism: Psychopathology and Psychotherapy in a Magico-Religious Context." In Colleen Ward, *Altered States*, 125–44.

Warner, Richard. "Commentary Two" (addendum to John Ellard's "Did Schizophrenia Exist before the Eighteenth Century?") *Australian and New Zealand Journal of Psychiatry* 21 (1987): 317–18.

Warner, Richard, and Giovanni de Girolamo. *Schizophrenia: Epidemiology of Mental Disorders and Psychological Problems*. Geneva: World Health Organization, 1995.

Warren, F. E. *The Liturgy and Ritual of the Celtic Church*. Oxford: Clarendon Press, 1881.

Wasserschleben, F. W. H., ed. *Die Bussordnungen der abendländischen Kirche*. Halle: Graeger, 1851.

Watkins, Calvert. *How To Kill a Dragon: Aspects of Indo-European Poetics*. New York: Oxford University Press, 1995.

Waxler, Nancy. "Is Mental Illness Cured in Traditional Societies? A Theoretical Analysis." *Culture, Medicine, and Psychiatry* 1 (1977): 233–53.

Way, Arthur. *Euripides*. Vol. 4. Cambridge, MA: Harvard University Press; London: William Heinemann, 1964.

Weathers, Frank, Brett Litz, and Terence Keane. "Military Trauma." In *Traumatic Stress: From Theory to Practice*, edited by John Freedy and Stevan Hobfoll, 103–28. New York: Plenum Press, 1995.

Weber, Robert, ed. *Biblia Sacra*. Stuttgart: Deutsche Bibelgesellschaft, 1969.

Wemple, Suzanne Fonay. *Women in Frankish Society: Marriage and the Cloister, 500 to 900*. Philadelphia: University of Pennsylvania Press, 1981.

Wenzel, Siegfried. *The Sin of Sloth: Acedia in Medieval Thought and Literature*. Chapel Hill: University of North Carolina Press, 1960.

Weston, L. M. C. "Women's Medicine, Women's Magic: The Old English Metrical Childbirth Charms." *Modern Philology* 92 (1995): 279–93.

White, Stephen. "Proposing the Ordeal and Avoiding It: Strategy and Power in Western French Litigation, 1050–1110." In *Cultures of Power: Lordship, Status, and Process in Twelfth-Century Europe*, edited by Thomas N. Bisson, 89–123. Philadelphia: University of Pennsylvania Press, 1995.

Whitehouse, Harvey. "Cultural Cognition and Psychopathology: Anthropological Perspectives." In *Cultural Cognition and Psychopathology*, edited by John Schumaker and Tony Ward, 17–30. Westport, CT: Praeger, 2001.

Whitney, William Dwight, trans. *Atharva-Veda Saṁhitā*. 2 vols. Delhi, Patna, and Varanasi: Motilal Banarsidass, 1962.

Wiener, Morton. "Schizophrenia: A Defective, Deficient, Disrupted, Disorganized Construct." In Flack, Miller, and Wiener, *What Is Schizophrenia?*, 199–222.

Wilcox, Jonathan, ed. *Ælfric's Prefaces*. 1994. Reprint, Durham: Durham Medieval Texts, 1996.

Wildhagen, Karl, ed. *Der Cambridger Psalter*. Darmstadt: Wissenschaftliche Buchgesellschaft, 1964.

Willems, R., ed. *In Iohannis Evangelium Tractatus CXXIV*. CCSL 36. Turnhout: Brepols, 1954.

Williams, Hugh, trans. *Two Lives of Gildas*. Cymmrodon Record Series. 1899. Reprint, Felinfach: Llanerch Enterprises, 1990.

Willis, G. G. *Further Essays in Early Roman Liturgy*. Alcuin Club Collections 50. London: S.P.C.K., 1968.

Wilmer, Harry, and Richard Scammon. "Neuropsychiatric Patients Reported Cured at St. Bartholomew's Hospital in the Twelfth Century." *Journal of Nervous and Mental Disease* 119, no. 1 (1954): 1–22.

Wilson, David. *Anglo-Saxon Paganism*. London: Routledge, 1992.

Wilson, H. A., ed. *The Gelasian Sacramentary*. Oxford: Clarendon Press, 1894.

———. *The Gregorian Sacramentary*. London, 1915.

———. *The Missal of Robert of Jumièges*. 1896. Reprint, Woodbridge, UK: Boydell, 1994.

Wilson, J. V. Kinnier, and E. H. Reynolds. "Translation and Analysis of a Cuneiform Text Forming Part of a Babylonian Treatise on Epilepsy." *Medical History* 34 (1990): 185–98.

Wiśniewski, Robert. "La consultation des possédés dans l'Antiquité tardive: *Pythones*, *engastrimythoi* et *arrepticii*." *Revue d'études augustiniennes et patristiques* 51 (2005): 127–52.

Woolf, Rosemary. "The Ideal of Men Dying with Their Lord in the *Germania* and in *The Battle of Maldon*." *ASE* 5 (1976): 63–81.

———, ed. *Juliana*. New York: Appleton-Century-Crofts, 1966.

Wright, C. E., ed. *Bald's Leechbook: British Museum Royal Manuscript 12 D.xvii*. Early English Manuscripts in Facsimile 5. Copenhagen: Rosenkilde and Bagger, 1955.

Wright, Charles. *The Irish Tradition in Old English Literature*. Cambridge: Cambridge University Press, 1993.

Wright, Thomas. *Anglo-Saxon and Old English Vocabularies*. 2nd ed., edited by R. P. Wülcker. 2 vols. London: Trübner & Co., 1884.

Wulfstan of Winchester. *The Life of St. Æthelwold*. Edited by Michael Lapidge and Michael Winterbottom. Oxford: Clarendon Press, 1991.

Yates, Roy. "Jesus and the Demonic in the Synoptic Gospels." *Irish Theological Quarterly* 44 (1977): 39–57.

Yorke, Barbara. *Nunneries and the Anglo-Saxon Royal Houses*. London: Continuum, 2003.

———. "The Reception of Christianity at the Anglo-Saxon Royal Courts." In Gameson, *St. Augustine*, 152–73.

Yüksel, Sahika. "Collusion and Denial of Childhood Sexual Trauma in Traditional Societies." In Shalev, Yehuda, and McFarlane, *International Handbook of Human Response*, 153–62.

Zika, Charles. *Exorcising Our Demons: Magic, Witchcraft, and Visual Culture in Early Modern Europe*. Leiden: Brill, 2003.

Zinkin, Joseph. *Dementia Praecox or the Group of Schizophrenias*. New York: International Universities Press, 1950.

Zohar, Ada H., Alan Apter, Robert A. King, David L. Pauls, James F. Leckman, and Donald Cohen. "Epidemiological Studies." In Leckman and Cohen, *Tourette's Syndrome*, 177–92.

Zupitza, Julius, trans. *Aelfrics Grammatik und Glossar*. 1880. Reprint, Berlin: Weidmann/Max Niehan, 1966.

Zycha, Joseph, ed. *Sancti Aurelii Augustini, Opera Selecta*. CSEL 28, part 1. Vienna: F. Tempsky, 1894.

Index

Typeset in 10/13 Adobe Caslon Pro
Composed by Tom Krol
Manufactured by McNaughton & Gunn, Inc.

Medieval Institute Publications
College of Arts and Sciences
Western Michigan University
1903 W. Michigan Avenue
Kalamazoo, MI 49008-5432
http:/ /www.wmich.edu/medieval/mip

WESTERN MICHIGAN UNIVERSITY